Dietary and Medicinal Significance of Wild Edible Fruiting Plants

This book explores the roles of wild edible fruit plants in combating malnutrition and diseases through their use in food and medicine. It delves into the chemical composition of these plants, providing both qualitative and quantitative analyses, and explains how these compounds contribute to their healing properties. This book also provides a detailed presentation of evidence-based applications in medicine and food supplements. These chapters include pharmacological research on these plants, offering concrete examples of how interactions between different herbs can lead to synergistic or even pleiotropic effects while ensuring the safety of these herbal products. Furthermore, this book highlights the industrial potential of phytochemicals and standardized extracts from these plants, showing their relevance across various sectors, such as cosmetics, food, health, chemicals, and textiles. It also addresses the efficient use of by-products, emphasizing sustainability. This book presents insights into ethnopharmacology and phytopharmacology and is tailored for researchers, academicians, and professionals in the fields of pharmacology, ethnobotany, and natural product chemistry.

Key Features

- Presents a clear overview of how wild edible fruit plants can be used in medicine and as food supplements
- Provides an in-depth qualitative and quantitative analysis of the chemical profiles of wild edible fruit plants
- Explores the interactions between different herbs, highlighting the synergistic and pleiotropic effects of these combinations
- Details the industrial applications of phytochemicals and plant extracts derived from wild edible fruit plants
- Offers valuable insights into the ethnopharmacology and phytopharmacology properties of wild edible fruit plants

Dietary and Medicinal Significance of Wild Edible Fruiting Plants

Devi Datt Joshi and Harendra Kharkwal

CRC Press
Taylor & Francis Group
Boca Raton London New York

CRC Press is an imprint of the
Taylor & Francis Group, an **informa** business

Designed cover image: Devi Datt Joshi and Harendra Kharkwal

First edition published 2026
by CRC Press
2385 NW Executive Center Drive, Suite 320, Boca Raton FL 33431

and by CRC Press
4 Park Square, Milton Park, Abingdon, Oxon, OX14 4RN

CRC Press is an imprint of Taylor & Francis Group, LLC

ISBN: 9781032844770 (hbk)
ISBN: 9781032844787 (pbk)
ISBN: 9781003512868 (ebk)

DOI: 10.1201/9781003512868

Typeset in Times
by codeMantra

Contents

About the Authors

Devi Datt Joshi is a distinguished scientist with extensive experience in phytochemistry and phytomedicine. He is currently serving as the Director of the Himalayans Herbs Research and Cultural Welfare Society in Ghaziabad. His career includes important positions such as Assistant Director & Head of Institute at the Amity Institute of Phytochemistry & Phytomedicines, and Scientist E at IBSD-Imphal. Dr. Joshi holds a Ph.D. in Chemistry (Natural Product Chemistry) from ITRC Lucknow and KU Nainital. He has filed 56 patents, with 14 granted; published 52 papers; presented at 18 conferences; contributed as an independent author to eight chapters; and authored four books, demonstrating his commitment to advancing knowledge in his field.

Harendra Kharkwal has a Ph.D. in Medicinal and Aromatic Plants from Kumaun University in Nainital. He is currently the Director Scientist at the Ministry of Environment, Forest and Climate Change in New Delhi, India. His main focus is on research and development to improve environmental research in natural resources and clean technologies aimed at minimizing waste. Dr. Kharkwal is also a member of the Working Group on Remediation for Soil and Groundwater Pollution in the Asian and Pacific Region, headquartered in Taiwan. He serves on the editorial boards of several international research publishing groups as well.

Section I

Introduction

1 Ethnobotany, Ethnopharmacology, and Bioprospecting

INTRODUCTION

Ancient herbal knowledge (ethnobotany) has passed through two distinct evolutionary phases with time, namely folk and traditional practices, and has been influenced by global socioeconomic revolutions. All traditional herbal healing practices evolved with folk culture and gradually obtained the tag of traditional healing systems and, subsequently, traditional medicines. The knowledge that evolved and was confined to certain geopolitical regions, yet remains effective with an innovative spirit, has been termed folk practices and folk medicines. Currently, these folk medicines have gained increased scientific attention as sources for modern green medicines via reverse pharmacology. The WHO has launched a fresh initiative to support traditional practices under the 'Traditional Medicine Strategy 2014–2023',[1] and related information is now available with a single click through systematic computerized databases such as the AYUSH Research Portal, ScienceDirect, PubMed, Google Scholar, ResearchGate, WHO ICTRP, etc. However, folk knowledge remains quite intact and needs a fresh global initiative. The term wild edible fruiting plants is a part of these folk practices, which bear edible fruits and are targeted to explore their hidden therapeutic and food potential.

The domestication of fruiting plants since the prehistoric period is based on their numerous health-promoting bioactivities and a few wild fruiting species have been reported richer in bioactive ingredients compared to the domesticated variant. Traditionally, the wild collection from the neat and clean environment of *Aegle marmelos* (L.) Correa (Hindi: Bel) is preferred to treat fever, dysentery, seminal weakness, urinary problems, etc.[2,3] The consumption and utilization of some wild fruits have been increasing, either as such or in value added products. The domestication of a wild plant species may result in decreased biological value due to a reduced quantity of secondary metabolites or their complete absence.[4] Additionally, excessive exploitation of the species from its natural habitat may lead to a depauperation of the natural environment.

CURRENT SCENARIO

The post-Stone Age scenario of human civilization still can be observed from the aboriginal people of the Andaman and Nicobar Islands, India, who still have and practice the ethnomedicinal information of that period, and there is a lot of scientific curiosity to understand their health-healing process and procedure. Additionally, these people use mostly pteridophytes as a source in their healing practices, which chronologically coincides with the dominance of pteridophytes on earth and the settlement of the oldest human population, tribal groups inhabiting the Andaman & Nicobar Islands around 35 to 60 thousand years ago.[5]

Ingestion is a natural thing, an inherently basic instinct of life, and forms a biological web to survive as the instinct of eating, even a few-hours-old baby grabs his palm and takes it to the mouth. This practice continues as a means of survival, even for the feeling of satiety. Most humans have migrated from their native shelters to open areas in search of better life opportunities, settling as communities that gradually developed into societies with previous settlers in and around the new area. The moving population's patterns have been recorded in several parts of the world, while isolated communities have appeared as 'tribes'. The ancestral knowledge of these tribes, which could not be shared among the societies and remained confined to certain zones, is currently a folk knowledge.[5]

Food choice depended on the availability of resources (plants or animals) around the human settlement, compelled by the environmental surroundings. Thousands of plant species of all forms (trees, shrubs, herbs, lichens, and aquatic) in all kinds of ecosystems have been meticulously exploited for medicines, food, and fodder. After several generations, these tribes must have been descendants of the conclusion to be able to identify the good and bad fruiting plants, their other tasteful parts, and their poisonous properties, if any. They uninterruptedly used them as supplements with cereals and grains in the form of decoctions, mixed vegetables, curries, tisanes, fermented brews, etc. This knowledge may take a thousand years to become a part of human society, so it needs to be deciphered, even in the present context of wild edible fruiting plants.[5]

Currently, wild fruiting plants are mostly considered exotic in urban societies and, if available, are underutilized or less known for utility, even though many wild fruiting species are safe to consume and have medicinal value. Due to various environmental factors, fruits from wild sources are rich in phytochemicals such as flavonoids and anthocyanins and are often considered an option for healthy foods. As a result, wild fruiting plants are currently receiving increased attention for investigating their bio-impacts, such as anticancer, anti-inflammatory, antioxidant, and antimicrobial effects.[6] These studies have revealed that wild fruiting plants have an appreciable quality and quantity of secondary metabolites (terpenoids, alkaloids, steroids, polysaccharides, amino acids, flavonoids, antibiotics, fatty acids, etc.) and are suitable as a medicine for many chronic diseases/ailments along with the prevention of cancers.[5]

DOI: 10.1201/9781003512868-2

PHYTOCHEMICAL KNOWLEDGE

Plants develop secondary metabolites for self-protection against abiotic and biotic stress and are used to reduce reactive oxygen species (ROS) in the human body, which are generated during metabolic processes and pathogenic infections in the body. The overproduction of ROS in the body (due to pollution, stress, food habits, etc.) is the main cause of chronic diseases (e.g., cardiovascular, aging, rheumatoid arthritis, cancer, atherosclerosis, etc.). The results of the biomolecular research on these wild fruiting plants have revealed the synergistic effects of their various ingredients.[7] In purified form, they are not as effective as in their whole natural state, highlighting the need to promote the whole consumption of these fruits and different parts of these plants. Tribal communities and local inhabitants residing around forest areas are frequent users of these wild products as food supplements and staple foods globally.[8] Wild edible fruiting plants are an indispensable constituent of the human diet, providing certain hormone precursors in addition to protein, carbohydrates, fat, minerals, vitamins, etc.,[9] and are relevant to household food security in remote and rural areas, especially during famines and natural calamities. Additionally, these plants are an additional and valuable source of income by means of trade, resulting in economic prosperity. As per the Food and Agricultural Organization, at least one billion people are supposed to use wild food in their diet, and other parts, including seeds, fruits, rhizomes, and leaves, are nutritionally rich and have health-oriented properties as well.[10,11]

Pandey et al. have reported that more than 2000 plant species are used by the aborigines inhabiting the Andaman and Nicobar Islands, the most primitive people to treat different health ailments. These tribal groups use fruits, leaves, and roots selectively or in combination orally before or after dietary intake or as per body requirement and have been well versed in the medicine.[12] Wild fruits have been used in folk and traditional medicine, as well as a part of the diet, for centuries. Tribal people have reported that one ripe fruit of *A. marmelos* can fulfill the average hunger of an adult.[5] Its fruit pulp contains sugars and digestive enzymes, and a ripened fruit can be stored for several months as it remains protected by a hard fruit cover, which is stony. *Madhuca longifolia* (L.) J.F. Macbr. (Hindi name: Mahua) is a nutritious species with several ethnomedical properties like anticancer, antibacterial, analgesic, antihyperglycemic, hepatoprotective, etc. Its flowers are widely used in the manufacturing of liquor rather than in the preparation of medicine and food supplements such as jam, jelly, laddu, biscuits, candy, cake, bars, sauces, etc., and are still underutilized.[13] *Syzygium cumini* (Linn) Skeels is distributed in the forests of Australia, Sri Lanka, India, and Malaysia and has edible fruits, which are good for health at the ripened stage, and has been used for controlling blood sugar levels for centuries as a medicinal food for patients with diabetes and hypertension. The fruit pulp extract of Indian origin provokes insulin secretion within half an hour of use; however, the Brazilian product under the same conditions has no metabolic or physiological changes.[2,14] Pepato et al. have reported that the differing results are due to the varied chemical ingredients of fruit pulps, influenced by abiotic and biotic factors of the cultivation sites.[14]

Phoenix dactylifera Linn (common name: date palm), native to North Africa and the Middle East, is extensively cultivated and is naturalized in subtropical and tropical regions globally. The ripened fruits have ample sugar and are liked by inhabitants of both urban and rural areas. These fruits are used as laxatives, in jams, and as expectorants, and are prescribed to patients with high fever and respiratory problems.[5]

MOLECULAR MEDICINE FROM CUMULATIVE AND PROGRESSIVE KNOWLEDGE

During the settlement phases, humans used different plant parts (leaves, flowers, fruits, rhizomes, roots, and their combinations) of selected plants and must have gained folk knowledge, often at the cost of many lives of their co-workers.[15] Time, a great teacher, resulted in developing the cultivation practices for the regular availability of different forms of food.[5] Currently, several pure compounds extracted from different parts of plants (twigs, leaves, flowers, whole aerial parts, and roots) and many in vivo and in vitro trials have been carried out all over the world before being recommended for medicinal use. The modern pharmaceutical industry has a good share of medicines rooted in ethnobotany, and examples can be cited from the cross-continental references below. In ancient times, in almost all parts of the world, isolated human groups (tribes) used locally available plants to treat common body ailments, such as *Andrographis paniculata* (Burm.f.) Wall. ex Nees, *Cinchona* L., *Rauwolfia* L., *Terminalia* L., *Garcinia mangostana* L., etc., and this folk knowledge gradually advanced into modern molecular medicine. The use of *A. paniculata* in India and *Cinchona* bark in South America to treat malarial fever, as well as the pungency of *Capsicum* spp. for self-defense, are a few examples. There are several legends for the historical ethno-phytopharmacological applications of each species, which have academic utility; hence, two cases are described below:

i. **A stagnant water pond with a tree on the bank**: There is a legend that a thirsty Indian with a high fever in an Andean Forest drank from a pond of stagnant water that was surrounded by quina-quina trees. Surprisingly, very soon his fever abated, and he shared the incident with fellow villagers, with his realization that taste like *A. paniculata* used to treat fever in India; thereafter, villagers frequently used the water from the same pond to treat fever. Once, a Spanish countess, 'Chinchon', was in Peru and contracted a fever. She was cured by the stagnant water of the same pond. Returning to Spain, she ordered scientific research on the water of the pond. Researchers have concluded that a few roots and branches of quina-quina trees were submerged in the water, and dissolved ingredients resulted in their febrifuge properties. The plant quina-quina was introduced in Europe (1638 AD), and later (1742 AD), it was called 'Cinchona' (botanical name: *Cinchona officinalis* L.) by the botanist Carl Linnaeus in honor of the countess.[16]

Cinchona (*C. officinalis* L.) (Fam.: Rubiaceae) is indigenous to South America. Its bark, known as 'Peruvian Bark' or 'Jesuit's Bark', is renowned for therapeutic properties and has several alkaloids, namely cinchonidine, cinchonine, quinidine, quinine, quinamine, etc. Since 1638 AD Cinchona bark has been used to treat malaria, and quinine, a drug used to treat malaria, is extracted from its bark. All the cinchona alkaloids, except cinchonine sulfate, are known for their febrifugal action, and quinine has the highest potency among all. Malaria is a distinct fever from at least 128 different types recorded between 1774 and 1794. Sir Ronald Ross discovered the malarial parasite (1897), a protozoan, and established that malaria is transmitted by mosquitoes. The use of quinine, a chemical compound to treat malaria, continued to be challenged by its poor compliance with complex dosing regimens, poor tolerability, and the availability of more efficacious antimalarial drugs.[16]

Before 1820, the bark of the Cinchona tree was used as medicine to cure malaria. After drying, bark was ground to a fine powder and mixed into a liquid (commonly wine) before being drunk to treat malaria.[16] In 1820, quinine was extracted from the bark, and the purified quinine replaced it. Quinine, along with other Cinchona alkaloids such as cinchonine, quinidine, and cinchonidine (Figure 1.1), is an effective treatment for malaria.

The efficacies of these four alkaloids were evaluated (1866–1868) in 3600 patients using sulfate salts of these alkaloids, and all four alkaloids have been reported for comparison, with cure rates of >98%. Quinine was preferred for malaria treatment until the 1920s, as chloroquine was preferred over quinine. However, heavy use of chloroquine gradually led to development of resistance in *Plasmodium falciparum* populations in parts of Southeast Asia and South America. By the late 1950s, the rate of resistance was highest and had become widespread globally, resulting in quinine once again becoming a key medicine to treat severe malaria[16,17] and continuing to play a significant role in the management and treatment.[16,17]

Quinine is an extremely basic compound and, therefore, exists as a salt. Its various derivatives, including dihydrochloride, hydrochloride, bisulfate, sulfate, and gluconate, are used, of which dihydrochloride is widely used. Quinine has rapid schizonticide action against intra-erythrocytic malaria parasites (*Plasmodium vivax* and *Plasmodium malariae*) but not for *Plasmodium falciparum*. Quinine has analgesic properties but is not antipyretic. The antimalarial mechanism of quinine is unknown. It is rapidly absorbed both parenterally and orally, obtaining peak concentrations within 1–3 hours.[16]

The development of resistance against quinine has been slow. Its use started in the 17th century; the first resistance was reported in 1910, compared to chloroquine and proguanil emerged within only 12 and 1 year of their introduction, respectively. The recrudescence rates for quinine over the past 30 years have remained roughly constant. These results suggest the efficacy of quinine and opportunities for its safe use. The therapeutic response of quinine varies with age, immunity, disease severity, and pregnancy.[16] For quality control, there is a wide variation in quinine content in the bark of the species, which also varies depending on the collection sites.[18]

Currently, investigations for improving quinine treatment outcomes by combining it with antibiotics to treat HIV and tuberculosis-infected populations are in strategic planning[18–20]

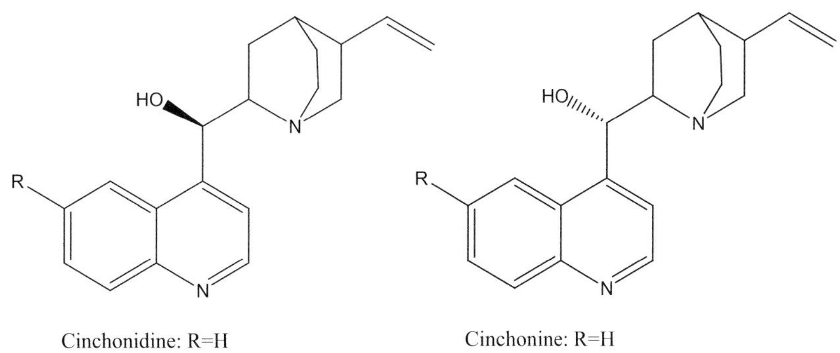

Cinchonidine: R=H
Quinine: R= $-CH_3O$

Cinchonine: R=H
Quinidine: R=$-CH_3O$

FIGURE 1.1 Different cinchona alkaloids.

ii. **Pungency of chili and different value-added products:** Chili fruits cause burning sensation on contact with mucous membranes such as those in the eyes, mouth, and renal system, etc., with feeling of burning ranging from simple to severe based on the concentration of capsaicinoids. In Mexico, chiles are instrumental in countering the effects of 'salting', a ritual to save an individual from a bad soul. In Zambia and Northeast India, farmers and crop fields are protected from elephants that may enter the fields during harvest time by burning chili smoke. These elephants leave behind droppings on the ground, which serve as a natural and organic form of fertilizer (Figure 1.2).[20,21]

Fruits of *Capsicum chinense Jacq.* from Northeast India have a unique aroma. Alcohols, aldehydes, esters, ketones, lactones, terpenoids, etc., are the main chemical classes of aromas. These fruits have a very short lifespan if not protected. These fruits are rich in carotenoids, vitamin C, phenolics, and capsaicinoids. Its name varies as per location; it is commonly known as 'Bhut Jolokia' in Assam, 'Naga Raja Mircha'/Naga King Chili in Nagaland, and 'U-Morok' in Manipur. The aroma of fruits of *C. chinense* has been practiced for therapeutic purposes in the folklore healing art of Northeast India and is used to treat night blindness, headache, rheumatism, gastritis, arthritis, spondylitis, digestive diseases, and to reduce chronic congestion.[20,21] Aromas and flavors occur in the cytoplasm of the cell in liquid form. Various methods of mechanical grinding are used for herbs, but further distillation causes the aroma and its ingredients to lose their originality. As an innovation to trap aroma and flavors, the fruits were ground at a defined range of temperatures. An edible liquid phase was used for pursing and trapping the aroma with other therapeutic ingredients of the fruits at a defined range temperature (Figure 1.3). The edible liquid phase (after 'pursed and trap' treatment) was re-analyzed for major ingredients of *C. chinense* fruits; all were found intact in the carrier. Chromatographic (Figure 1.4) and spectral fingerprints were developed as evidence for claims made for the product.[22]

The natural fragrance captured within the herbal matrix is a superior food ingredient that

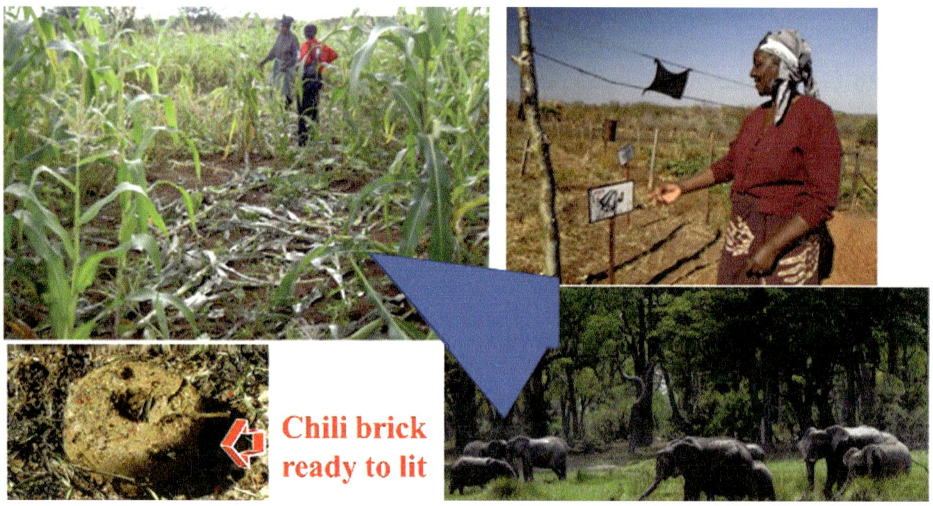

FIGURE 1.2 Folk application of chili smoke.

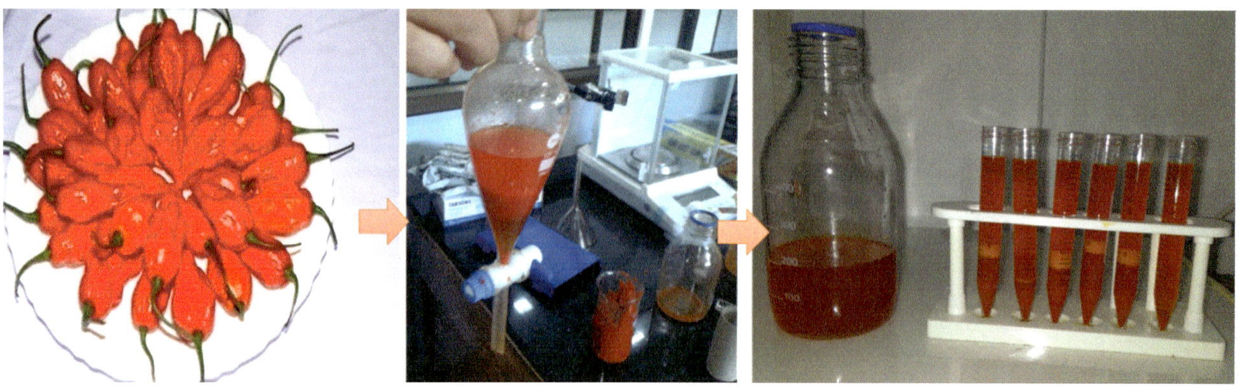

FIGURE 1.3 Tapping of *C. chinense* fruit's aroma in edible herbal matrix.[22]

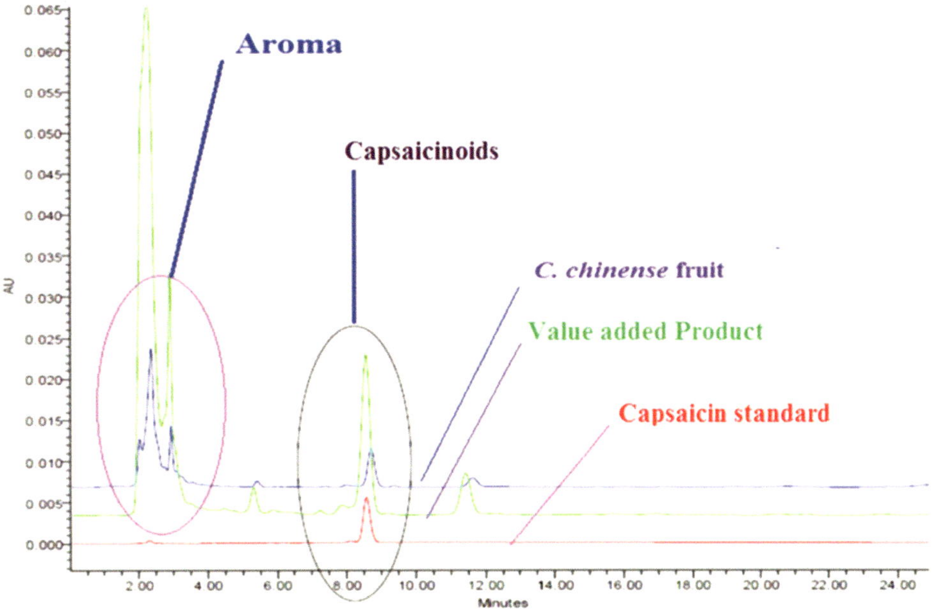

FIGURE 1.4 High Performance Liquid Chromatography (HPLC) fingerprints; Trapped aroma and fruits of *C. chinense*.[22]

requires less effort. It is convenient to transport and has an extended shelf life while providing the flavor of fresh fruits that are typically available locally and seasonally throughout the year. This product retains all of the unique qualities and characteristics of the original fruit cultivar.

The low concentration of aroma and many promising compounds, localized distribution of *C. chinense,* the impact of both biotic and abiotic factors/stresses, and human intervention for better food with fewer efforts all highlight the need for crop improvement and breeding programs, along with improved global distribution.

RELEVANCE OF ETHNO-PHYTO-PHARMACOLOGY FOR A HEALTHY PHYSIQUE

Herbals were a primary health-healing supplement in ancient times to treat different metabolic syndromes and infections. The different extracts of herbals in practice protect the human body against cellular redox stress and pathogens either safely or with a low toxicity. On oral ingestion, herbals interact with about 10^{14} microorganisms in the gut,[23,24] and a few gut microbes can induce immune cells in the gut wall to release proinflammatory cytokines, affecting the permeability of the blood-brain barrier. As per the World Health Organization (WHO), 60% of the population uses herbal medicine and deciphers traditional herbal medicines as complete drugs in the absence of adequate analytical methods, or otherwise uses therapeutic fractions to standardize their ingredients. Molecular research has revealed that herbals promote the development of beneficial *Bifidobacteria* and *Lactobacillus*, along with the reduction in the growth of harmful gut microbes. Different herbals have been described in the form of beverages that are prepared by steeping, infusion, decoction, maceration, and fermentation processes to balance the gut microbiota.[23]

The interaction of gut microbiota with herbal beverages generates a series of metabolites such as vitamins, short-chain fatty acids (SCFAs), indole derivatives, and polyamines, which are used to regulate homeostasis. Furthermore, these ingredients interact with archaeons, bacteria, viruses, and eukaryotes (microorganisms about 10^{14}) in the intestine. The human body does not produce enzymes to catalyze the fermentation of carbohydrates, but gut microbiotas secrete a series of enzymes, called propionaldehyde dehydratase and propionate-CoA transferase, to convert carbohydrates into SCFAs. SCFAs protect colonic epithelium and increase the differentiation and proliferation of cell membrane assembly, colonocytes, and mucosal cell migration.[23] The non-pathogenic bacteria of the gut help in the prevention of the settlement of harmful microbes, digest food and medicine, and protect different intestinal functions. Diet is a deciding factor for the composition, richness, and diversity of gut microbiota at every stage of life. A fruit-rich diet is associated with a healthy gut microbiota, while animal-based diets result in a reduction of the number of Firmicutes.[23] Jandhyala et al. (2015) have reported that a diet rich in herbals promotes gut microbiota health,[25] and obesity has resulted in enhanced numbers of body ailments.[26]

Tuber powder of *Dioscorea deltoidea* Wall. Ex Griseb. fruits is prescribed with honey and milk for its antiaging effects and has the potential to induce the cells and tissues for rejuvenation, improving both the quantity and quality of semen and sperm. Its folk utilization has been validated to use to treat impotency and infertility, as well as a reproductive tonic for both male and female utilization. Traditionally its tubers are used to treat asthma, leprosy, colds, coughs, tuberculosis, constipation, muscular pain, indigestion, abdominal pain, bone fractures, sore throats, dysentery, wounds, cuts, boils, injuries, and tumors and are used to reduce body heat during summer.[27] These properties are due to the richness of various chemical classes in tubers (e.g., diosgenin, saponins, flavonoids, dioscorin, and other important constituents), and include antimicrobial, anticancer, CNS effects, and many more cardiac activities. Diosgenin is a main compound in *Dioscorea* species and serves as a precursor of steroidal drugs such as estrogen and a medicines for different body ailments.[27,28]

MODERN GREEN MEDICINES AND REGULATORY NORMS

The old proverb, 'one's meal is another's poison', deciphers the need for assurance and control of quality along with the prescribed dose. Certain ingredients, though health-friendly, can be extremely harmful if ingested in large quantities, for example, 'accutane', a derivative of vitamin A, which can cause abortions.[13] During pregnancy, the excess consumption of vitamins A and C develops many complications in the developing fetus; hence, expecting mothers are often advised to take only prescribed doses. However, malnutrition and vitamin-deficient diets also have resulted in abortions.[13] Similarly, excess milk consumption can cause many intestinal and digestive problems, even though it is a complete food. Similarly, chemical compounds extracted from plants need specification along with clinical data after rigorous microbiological tests to be used before a medicine.

The advancement of human civilization coincides with enhanced knowledge of plant-based remedies, and even today, the WHO cites that about 80% of the world's population using herbals from traditional and folk practices for their primary healthcare. These systems are free of side effects, more natural, and environmentally friendly to treat various illnesses such as diarrhea, hemorrhage, gallstones, mouthwash, wounds, inflammation, burns, chronic diabetes, etc.[23] However, the scientific reports on the chemical profile and pharmacological evidence supporting the claims made about these species have not been validated, representing a major knowledge gap and an essential requirement for designing future studies for modern green medicines. Evaluation of nutritional ingredients, along with the quantification of antinutritional factors such as tannins and phytic acid, which can diminish the bioavailability of nutritional ingredients, is a matter of concern, as a certain quantity of these compounds may help treat and prevent several fatal diseases.[29] At present, the isolation of endophytic entities from medicinal plants has revolutionized the path of discovering modern green medicines. Endophyte species may produce similar bioactives as the host plant species, along with others that may have utility for a variety of human health ailments. A research approach for the bioprospecting of endophytes from the wild edible fruiting plant species for different food supplements and medicines is needed for hours to combat future human health threats,[30] such as the COVID-19 pandemic, blood cancer, etc.

CONCLUSION

Wild edible fruits are not only a source of food but also contain potent nutrients and medicines. They can be used for fuel, fiber, and other purposes. The plant species discussed in this text have high economic value beyond their use as fodder and wood. They are also capable of colonizing degraded ecosystems and meeting the needs of local people for food and medicine. Marginal lands have limited nutrients and water, which can result in low plant production. However, higher nutrient availability can support the development of new branches and foliage. Therefore, if we want to cultivate these plants commercially, we should select suitable lands. It is essential to screen more wild fruit resources for their bioactivities, identify their therapeutic and food properties, and evaluate their toxicity for safe human consumption. We need to understand the mechanisms of action of these resources to apply them effectively.

REFERENCES

1. World Health Organization. 2013. *WHO: Traditional Medicine Strategy: 2014–2023*. World Health Organization, Geneva.
2. Joshi DD, Deb L, Somkuwar BG, Rana VS. 2023. Relevance of Indian traditional tisanes in the management of type 2 diabetes mellitus: a review. *Saudi Pharmaceutical Journal* 31: 626–638. https://doi.org/10.1016/j.jsps.2023.03.003
3. Singh U, Kocher A, Boora R. 2012. Proximate composition, available carbohydrates, dietary fibres, and anti-nutritional factors in bael (*Aegle marmelos* L.) leaf, pulp and seed powder. *International Journal of Scientific and Research Publications*. 2: 1–4.
4. Dyduch-Sieminska M, Najda A, Dyduch J, Gantner M, Klimek K. 2015. The content of secondary metabolites and antioxidant activity of wild strawberry fruit (*Fragaria vesca* L.). *Journal of Analytical Methods in Chemistry*. 2015: 1–8.
5. Goswami HT, Ram HK. 2017. Ancient food habits dictate that food can be medicine but medicine cannot be food. *Medicines*. 4 (4): 82. https://doi.org/10.3390/medicines4040082
6. Li Y, Zhang JJ, Xu DP, Zhou T, Zhou Y, Li S, Li HB. 2016. Bioactivities and health benefits of wild fruits. *International Journal of Molecular Sciences*. 17 (8): 1258. https://doi.org/10.3390/ijms17081258
7. Tamang JP. 2022. "Ethno-microbiology" of ethnic Indian fermented foods and alcoholic beverages. *Journal of Applied Microbiology*. 133: 145–161. https://doi.org/10.1111/jam.15382

8. Aberoumand A, Deokule SS. 2009. Studies on nutritional values of some wild edible plants from Iran and India. *Pakistan Journal of Nutrition*. 8 (1): 26–31. https://doi.org/10.3923/pjn.2009.26.31
9. Akubugwo IE, Obasi NA, Chinyere GC, Ugbogu A. 2007. Nutritional and chemical value of Amaranthus hybridus L. leaves from Afikpo, Nigeria. *African Journal of Biotechnology*. 6 (24): 2833–2839.
10. FAO. 2003. Food energy methods of analysis and conversion factors. Food and nutrition paper 77. Food and Agriculture Organisation of the United Nations, Rome, Italy, pp: 1–93.
11. FAO, IFAD, UNICEF, WFP and WHO. 2019. The State of Food Security and Nutrition in the World 2019. Safeguarding against economic slowdowns and downturns. Rome, FAO.
12. Pandey RP, Rasingam L, Lakra GS. 2011. Ethnomedicinal plants of the Aborigines in Andaman & Nicobar Islands, India. *Nelumbo*. 51: 5–40.
13. Sinha J, Singh V, Singh J, Rai AK. 2017. Phytochemistry, ethnomedical uses and prospects of Mahua *(Madhuca longifolia*) as a food: A review. *Journal of Nutrition & Food Sciences*. 7: 573.
14. Pepato MT, Mori DM, Baviera AM, Harami JB, Vendramini RC, Brunetti IL. 2005. Fruit of the jambolan tree (*Eugenia jambolana* Lam.) and experimental diabetes. *Journal of Ethnopharmacology*. 96: 43–48. https://doi.org/10.1016/j.jep.2004.07.029
15. Joshi B, Tiwari AP, Sikarwar RLS. 2013. Poisonous plants with medicinal values from Bilaspur District, Chhatisgarh. *Bionature*. 33: 37–45
16. Achan J, Talisuna AO, Erhart A, Yeka A, Tibenderana JK, Baliraine FN, Rosenthal PJ, D'Alessandro U. 2011. Quinine, an old anti-malarial drug in a modern world: role in the treatment of malaria. *Malaria Journal*. 10: 144. https://doi.org/10.1186/1475-2875-10-144
17. Hellgren U, Ericsson O, Ericsson O, Gustafsson LL. 1995. *Handbook of Drugs for Tropical Parasitic Infections*. CRC Press. https://doi.org/10.1201/9781482272536
18. Products of the Empire: Cinchona: A Short Story. https://www.lib.cam.ac.uk/rcs/projects-exhibitions/products-empire-cinchona-short-history, as on 13th April 2024.
19. Gachelin G, Garner P, Ferroni E, Trohler U, Chalmers I. 2017. Evaluating *Cinchona* bark and quinine for treating and preventing malaria. *Journal of the Royal Society of Medicine*. 110 (1): 31–40. https://doi.org/10.1177/0141076816681421
20. Maldonado C, Barnes CJ, Cornett C, Holmfred E, Hansen SH, Persson C, Antonelli A, Rønsted N. 2017. Phylogeny predicts the quantity of antimalarial alkaloids within the iconic yellow *Cinchona* bark (Rubiaceae: *Cinchona calisaya*). *Frontiers in Plant Science*. 8: 391. https://doi.org/10.3389/fpls.2017.00391
21. Joshi DD, Changkija S, Sujata W, Somkuwar B G. 2018. Characterization of pungent red chilies (*Capsicum* spp.); Cultivars of Manipur and Nagaland, part of Indo-Burma mega biodiversity hotspot. *Bulletin of Environment, Pharmacology and Life Sciences*. 7 (11): 116–126.
22. Joshi DD, Changkija S, Sujata W, Somkuwar BG, Rana VS, Talukdar NC. 2017. Nutraceutical from *Capsicum chinense* fruits in shelf-stable herbal matrix. *Innovative Food Science & Emerging Technologies*. 42: 130–137.
23. Joshi DD, Deb L, Kaul K, Somkuwar BG, Rana VS, Singh R. 2024. Relevance of Indian traditional herbal brews for gut microbiota balance. *Indian Journal of Microbiology*. https://doi.org/10.1007/s12088-024-01251-4
24. Sekirov I, Russell SL, Antunes LCM, Finlay BB. 2010. Gut microbiota in health and disease. *Physiological Reviews*. 90: 859–904. doi: 10.1152/physrev.00045.2009.
25. Jandhyala SM, Talukdar R, Subramanyam C, Vuyyuru H, Sasikala M, Reddy ND. 2015. Role of the normal gut microbiota. *World Journal of Gastroenterology* 21:8787–8803. https://doi.org/10.3748/wjg.v21.i29.8787
26. Carbone S, Lavie CJ, Elagizi A, Arena R, Ventura HO. 2022. The impact of obesity in heart failure. *Cardiology Clinics*. 40: 209–218. https://doi.org/10.1016/j.ccl.2021.12.009
27. Mustafa A, Ahmad A, Tantray AH, Parry PA. 2018. Ethnopharmacological potential and medicinal uses of miracle herb *Dioscorea* spp. *Journal of Ayurvedic and Herbal Medicine*. 4 (2): 79–85.
28. Guo Y, Xing E, Liang X, Song H, Dong W. 2016. Effects of total saponins from Rhizome *Dioscoreae nipponicae* on expression of vascular endothelial growth factor and angiopoietin-2 and Tie-2 receptors in the synovium of rats with rheumatoid arthritis. *Journal of the Chinese Medical Association*. 79 (5): 264–271.
29. Alshehri B. 2024. The *Geranium* genus: A comprehensive study on ethnomedicinal uses, phytochemical compounds, and pharmacological importance. *Saudi Journal of Biological Sciences*. 31 (4):103940. https://doi.org/10.1016/j.sjbs.2024.103940
30. Sharma S, Chaitanya MVNL, Sharma S, Kumar S, Rustagi S, Singh S, Shreaz S, Rai AK, Negi R, Yadav AN. 2024. The medicinal plant *Berberis aristata* and its endophytes for pharmacological applications: Current research and future challenges. *Journal of Applied Biology and Biotechnology*. X(XX): 1–10. https://doi.org/10.7324/JABB.2024.167591

2 Nutrient Analysis, Methodologies, and Outcomes

INTRODUCTION

Since ancient times, nutrition has been considered one of the vital ingredients of a healthy life; therefore, the universal medical science concepts have recognized it as one of the integral components of healing and health care since the time of Galen and Aristotle. Galen and Aristotle have described nutrition as a vital part of performance, health, healing, and disease. In short, the energy in each part of the body depends on the blood flow, and blood results from nutrients absorbed from food.[1] The Ayurvedic, Roman, Greek, and Chinese classical healing literature describes that diet should be mainly fruits, grains, honey, legumes, cereal, milk, and fish-based, and wine, meat, and confectionary should be used in moderation. The modern theory of nutrition adds minerals and vitamins to it. Currently, nutrition and lifestyle metabolic disorders (e.g., dyslipidemia and associated complications, obesity, diabetes, etc.) and social patterns of food as an experience for instant gratification and pleasure have resulted in weaknesses in our fundamental biology because the human body has a natural liking for fatty foods and sweetness, and human fatty food preference has been fueled by the easy availability of fast foods globally. These changes in food habits have resulted in different metabolic syndromes and deterioration of overall health.[1–3]

Efforts to modify human food with nutritional ingredients for better health, disease prevention, and management have led to many dietary theories and healthy eating guidelines, such as low-carbohydrate diets, high-protein diets, or combined diets like the 'Atkins diet', etc.[1,4] Furthermore, a concept of optimal diet was also postulated, having an ideal balance of micro- and macronutrients required for maintaining the ideal health.[1,5] These postulates have helped medical professionals in setting standard parameters for medical care for specific diseases and different stages of life. Laboratory and clinical research data are vital on nutrition in the pathogenesis of chronic diseases, including metabolic syndromes. The nutrient analytical report paved the way for doctors to prescribe a specific diet including the fruits that influence the whole-body physiology at the molecular and cellular levels.[6] On a global level, nutrition analytical data influences public health policy and food standards, including the economic sustainability and benefits of traditional dietary practices. These analytical data have **helped develop** evidence-based dietary guidelines and recommendations for benefiting individual health status, preventing disease, and fostering well-being for future generations. The proverbs 'You have to know the past to understand the present' and 'We are not makers of history, we are made by history' describe the key historical incidents in the development of current nutrition principles and policy.[7]

NUTRIENT ANALYSIS AND DISCOVERY OF INGREDIENTS

The 20th century has witnessed the identification and synthesis of many vitamins and minerals in the first half, including their use to check and cure deficiency-related disorders such as beriberi, scurvy, rickets, pellagra, nutritional anemias, and xerophthalmia. Casimir Funk (1913) postulated a 'vital amine' in food that protected chickens from a beriberi-like condition when fed unprocessed rice hulls,[7] and this compound (vital amine, later 'vitamin') was first isolated in 1926, named thiamine, and synthesized in 1936 as vitamin B_1. In 1932, vitamin C was isolated and described for the first time to be useful to cure scurvy,[7] nearly 200 years after when a ship's surgeon James Lind used lemons to treat scurvy among sailors,[7] and by the mid-20th century, all major vitamins had been identified and synthesized. Detailed investigations on these vitamins in animals and humans have established their nutritional importance and deficiency symptoms. The resulting knowledge was adopted to tackle anemia, beriberi, rickets, pellagra, scurvy, pernicious anemia, etc. This understanding was later synthesized into supplements and, finally, developed into multivitamins to protect against deficiencies, giving rise to the entire vitamin supplement industry.[7]

Currently, there are low-cost processed staple foods fortified with vitamins and minerals on the market that have raised cases of diet-based non-communicable body ailments such as heart disease, dental caries, hypertriglyceridemia, and cancer. Analytical results have revealed that low-fat, low-cholesterol, and low-sugar diets are good for a healthy physique.[7,8] And these theories relied on a nutritional model to establish and extract the pure ingredient. Additionally, the impact of the pure phytochemical has been studied on physiology, and optimal intake quantity to prevent disease. Additionally, metabolic syndromes such as type 2 diabetes mellitus, obesity, and cancer have risen, though the coronary mortality cases were reduced. The dietary guidelines to avoid too much saturated fat, cholesterol, and fatty foods with adequate starch and fiber were recommended. The reduced quantity of sugars and salt,[7,9] along with the ample presence of major micronutrients such as different minerals (iron, zinc, calcium, etc.), vitamins, and iodine, are the salient features of the dietary guidelines drafted from 1970

DOI: 10.1201/9781003512868-3

to 1990. An enhanced quantity of vitamin A supplements along with iodine and different minerals in foods under the WHO umbrella has resulted in reduced cases of child mortality from measles and prevented night blindness, goiter, hearing loss, etc.[7,9,10]

Most important scientific studies, including randomized clinical trials, observational cohorts, and genetic consortiums, have revealed a range of foods, nutrients, diet patterns, and diversity in health outcomes. Additionally, the clinical trials for a particular effect of an isolated supplement in a specific diet pattern of a highly vulnerable age group population are more informative. The genetic consortiums decipher the potential of genetic influences on gene-diet interactions affecting disease risk factors and dietary choices, though there are many limitations.[7,11] They conclude that the single nutrient theory is inadequate for explaining the effects of diet on non-communicable diseases, as the higher-dose vitamin A supplements can also be toxic.[7] The possible complexity of higher doses of food supplements is due to nutritional limitations for general well-being versus treatment of specific conditions.[12] The diet composition has proven more beneficial because of the effects of different foods on overlapping pathways such as liver function, glycemic response, satiety, and microbiome.[7,13] Over the long term, some foods may have neutral effects on weight, while others can disrupt weight regulation pathways or enhance the body's ability to maintain a healthy weight. This understanding is crucial in anti-obesity efforts, as it shifts the focus from simply losing weight to avoiding foods that contribute to long-term weight gain in individuals with obesity.In long-term use some foods may have relatively neutral effects, others may impair pathways of weight homeostasis, and others may enhance the integrity of weight regulation, a long-term impact relevant to anti-obesity, a shift from weight loss in people with obesity using avoidance of the foods of long-term weight gain.[14] There is a need for strange nutritional specifications for different foods and food supplements, indicating the load of pesticides, heavy metals, and microbial contents, including aflatoxins, residual solvents, and preservatives, along with basic parameters, guided by failures in the past, for accelerated social acceptance.[7]

NON-NUTRITIVE PHYTO-INGREDIENTS

The fruits of wild origin have been reported to have better protective properties and nutritional value compared to their cultivated counterparts.[15] In recent years, there has been a high focus on quality-oriented variants for a better health output and more revenue-generating options in nutraceutical and pharmaceutical applications. Research literature screening has revealed that phytochemical and pharmacological investigations on wild fruiting species have been limited to the isolation and characterization of compounds, along with a few pharmacological characteristics, even though these species may be more significant to scientific and industrial utilization.[15–17]

Mostly, cereals and legumes have high amounts of micronutrients and macronutrients, along with, though rarely, antinutritional factors such as phytic acid, saponins, tannins, lectins, gossypol, amylase inhibitors, goitrogens, and protease inhibitors. These ingredients combine with nutrients, resulting in reduced nutrient bioavailability. Other factors such as phytates and trypsin inhibitors are present mainly in cereals and legumes, resulting in reduced mineral absorption and protein digestibility and causing micronutrient malnutrition along with mineral deficiencies. There are various traditional procedures and techniques used to reduce the quantity of these anti-nutrients, such as debranning, fermentation, autoclaving, germination, soaking, etc., which are used to reduce the anti-nutrient contents in herbals.[18,19] These components, if in excess, interfere with the nutritional value of foods by reducing protein digestibility and mineral absorption and causing toxicity and health disorders. Phytic acid forms complexes with bivalent metallic elements, resulting in reduced biological absorption and deficiency (e.g., calcium, zinc, etc.) in the body. The high concentration of saponins alters the integrity of intestinal epithelial cells and affects the absorption of vitamins A and E along with lipids. The excess of phenolic compounds in the food chain resulted in loss of appetite, body weight, and cardiac and breathing complications. Lectins and hemagglutinins in excess have resulted in hyperplasia, hypertrophy, impaired growth, and reduced nutrient absorption. Proteinases have diverse roles in improving the functional and nutritional properties of various protein molecules through different pathways. Cereal seeds mainly have plant serpins, the protease inhibitor, and are also termed 'suicide inhibitors', which generally inhibit chymotrypsin and trypsin and limit the enzyme activity by protein-protein interactions.[18,20]

ANALYTICAL VALIDATION AND PRODUCT SPECIFICATION

Food and nutritional security is one of the key concerns around the world, and by the time insufficient food intake and its poor availability are unresolved issues globally. The wild edible fruiting species have been reported to be richer in nutrients compared to their cultivated variants,[15] and their use in daily diets for food and nutrition purposes is beneficial in preventing age-related and chronic diseases, while also supporting biodiversity conservation and the sustainable utilization of these species.[21] The use of wild edible fruits as food has additional ingredients (flavonoids, anthocyanins, carotenoids, dietary glutathione carotenoids, vitamins, phenols, tannins, and flavonoids) that have higher antioxidant activities with free radical scavenging molecules. Vitamins and gut microbiota-friendly compounds protect the human body against oxidative stress, cardiovascular problems, cancer, and other age-related degenerative diseases.[22]

The oral use of whole seed extract of *Syzygium cumini* (L.) Skeels collected from India is reported to increase serum insulin levels within 30 minutes of ingestion in streptozotocin-induced diabetic rats and inhibit the activity of insulinase, but the fruits of Brazilian origin do not have any such biological reaction.[16] *Moringa oleifera* Lam., leaves have been reported for the richness of anti-diabetic compounds along with antinutritional ingredients, which develop a slight dullness and are not used in traditional practices to normalize blood glucose levels in diabetic patients.[16] The use of *Tribulus terrestris* Linn. in India, China, and Bulgaria is for different body ailments;[23] these properties are due to the presence of certain bioactives that vary with geo-environmental conditions and are influenced by the abiotic and biotic stress of the concerned plant at its origin, though the species is the same.[23] The analytical results are also expressed from the geographical indicator of the origin of plant material. Additionally, detailed analytical results are necessary to develop the material safety data sheet of the product, a regulatory requirement for global trade. Compounds, namely, β-carotene, ascorbic acid, β-sitosterol, stearic acid, isoleucine, iso-quercetin, palmitic acid, kaempferol, oleic acid, tocopherols, quercetin, etc., are common in wild fruiting plant species, and their therapeutic potential, role in maintaining good health, and methods of analysis are already established, but the information on the quantity of each ingredient is a requirement to be addressed by different agencies before their use as modern green medicine or a food supplement.

Several studies have revealed a direct link between the dietary intake of fruits and reduced rates of cardiac disease, cancers, aging, and degenerative diseases.[24] Researchers are concerned with the compositional analysis and biological properties of various types of wild edible fruiting plants globally. Except for very few, comprehensive investigations are lacking on their nutritional values,[25] but available analytical results decipher that these species are relatively rich in nutritionally essential ingredients, e.g., carbohydrates, proteins, sugars, etc.[26]

ANTIOXIDANT POTENTIAL AND ANALYSIS

Wild edible fruits are highly potent nutraceuticals and a natural source of bioactive compounds for functional foods or dietary supplements and are focused on due to increased social and industrial demand.[27] The protective and nutritional attributes against many diseases are due to the presence of several antioxidant phyto-ingredients, especially polyphenols and others, e.g., vitamins [ascorbic acid, α-tocopherol, and β-carotene (provitamin A)]. There is a strong consensus that polyphenols are responsible for much of the antioxidant activity of fruits and vegetables.[28] These antioxidants combat the causes of many diseases, such as neurodegenerative disorders, diabetes, aging, and cardiovascular diseases.[29] Polyphenols and vitamins in fruiting plants are responsible for such antioxidant activity, mainly due to the presence of many phenolic groups, biologically the most active site within the molecule.[30] Natural antioxidants are an alternative to synthetic ones because of their potential health benefits.[31] Therefore, the determination of phenolic compounds and related antioxidant activity in fruits and other plant parts has been of growing interest.[32,33] Different parts of widely fruiting edible plants, including their fruits after proper cleaning, are subjected to analysis as per standardized and validated methods, such as determination of the water content, acid-insoluble ash, water-soluble ash, total ash, total soluble solids, crude protein, crude fiber, crude fat, total carbohydrate, organic matter, foreign materials, etc.

EXTRACTION OF PLANT MATERIAL FOR ANALYSIS

Extraction is the process of obtaining or removing the targeted compounds from the parental material. The solvents used for the extraction of plant ingredients can be categorized into green solvents [e.g., water, acetic acid, glycerol, ethanol, fatty oils, ionic liquids, supercritical CO_2, isopropanol, natural deep eutectic solvents (NADEs), deep eutectic solvents, etc.] and other organic solvents such as hexane, acetone, cyclohexane, butanol, benzene, chloroform, ethyl acetate, methanol, methyl acetate, etc. The green solvents are recyclable, biodegradable, nontoxic, and renewable, and have a high flash point, with water being a universal solvent and highly used. It is a non-selective solvent and is used to extract hydrophilic substances, such as phenolics, saponins, polysaccharides, etc. The extraction efficiency of water may be enhanced by superheating, as it decreases the dielectric constant of water and imparts better penetration into cells. Superheated water is also a preferable solvent for the extraction of essential oils, as the polarity of water decreases significantly between 100°C and 374°C. Ethanol is used as a solvent to extract triterpenes and polyphenols, and its extraction effectiveness can be altered by adding water and acid. Glycerol (boiling point 290°C) has high thermal stability and is used as an extraction solvent above 60°C or with other co-solvents. It is only a selective solvent for polyphenolic extraction. Hydrophobic phytochemicals (e.g., coumarins, carotenoids, flavonoids, tocopherols, etc.) are extracted with fatty oils (e.g., almond, soybean, sunflower, olive, etc.). The acetic acid buffer is preferred to extract anthocyanins and phenolics. n-hexane is substituted by isopropanol, a green alternative solvent used to extract alkaloids, oils, natural resins, and gums. Supercritical CO_2 is used to extract anthocyanins, lignans, and essential oils.[19,34]

Ionic liquids have low or negligible vapor pressure, low flammability, and are non-volatile salts with low melting points (below 100°C). They have high thermal stability, high conductivity, and high heat capacity, and are used to extract a wide range of inorganic and organic compounds (e.g., alkaloids, flavonoids, lignans, saponins, etc.). The deep eutectic solvent is a mixture of two or more pure compounds (such as choline chloride and urea in a 1:2 combination, or choline chloride and zinc chloride in a 1:2 combination) having a eutectic point temperature below that of an ideal liquid mixture, and may be used for the extraction of saponins, flavonoids, phenolics, and alkaloids.[19,35] NADEs are mainly composed of hydrogen bond donors (such as citric acid, carboxylic acid, urea, and malic acid) and hydrogen bond acceptors (like betaine, choline chloride, etc.), which melt at a certain molar ratio at a temperature well below the individual components to form a transparent liquid. These solvents have a low melting point, low volatility, and a broad polarity range. These solvents can be used to extract the poorly water-soluble compounds.[19,36]

Acetone has low toxicity among organic solvents and is an appropriate solvent to extract terpenoid oils, alkaloids, etc. Ethyl acetate, a non-toxic organic solvent, is used to extract total phenolics, flavonoids, etc. Chloroform and methanol have inherent toxicity. Chloroform with other solvents such as fatty acids and ethanol is used for the extraction of anthocyanins and alkaloids, while methanol is used to extract flavonoids, saponins, tannins, etc. n-Butanol is mainly used for the fractional purification and isolation of pure phytochemicals. n-hexane has a low acute toxicity and is used for the extraction of fatty compounds from carbohydrates, saponins, and flavonoids. Benzene is a potentially dangerous solvent and is rarely used for extraction purposes. Cyclohexane is used for the extraction of oils, waxes, and fats.[19,37]

The extraction efficiency may be enhanced by optimizing extraction parameters such as temperature, extraction period, and choice of solvent. The extraction process starts with cell breakdown, resulting in an extract, followed by the separation of the solvent, and the isolation and purification of fractions/ingredients from the extract. Different techniques (e.g., TLC, 2-D-TLC, HPTLC, HPLC, GLC, etc.) are used to separate bioactive compounds from the mixture, and for authentication, hyphenated techniques such as LC-MS, GC-MS, NMR, UV-Vis., FTIR, etc., are used.[19]

Different plant parts are reduced into small pieces, then dried under shade and ground to a coarse powder, and the phyto-ingredients present in these parts were extracted using conventional methods such as percolation, decoction, maceration, Soxhlet extraction, reflux extraction, etc. Dried and powdered plant parts are first defatted with hexane or petroleum ether, and then separately and exhaustively extracted at room temperature with ethyl acetate (EtOAc), acetone, organochlorine solvent, methanol, and aqueous methanol by shaking at a regular interval until a discolored solvent is obtained, indicating completion of extraction. After distillation, the resulting extract is dried, and the percentage yield is calculated.

QUALITATIVE ANALYSIS

The chemical composition of each fraction is performed to establish a profile of different classes of phytochemicals. Qualitative chemical tests of petroleum ether, EtOAc, acetone, organochlorine solvent, MeOH, and aqueous MeOH extracts are carried out to detect the presence and/or absence of the various phyto-ingredients such as alkaloids, coumarins, phenols, steroids, flavonoids, tannins, saponins, terpenoids, etc., according to the standard protocols.[38] Either change in color and/or formation of precipitate with the addition of specific detecting reagents to the test solutions of various plant part extracts are observed, and results are recorded, after three subsequent analyses, as present (+) or absent (–) based on the observations.[39]

ANTIOXIDANT POTENTIAL

The antioxidant capacity of each fraction of the plant extract is determined by the five different ***in vitro*** protocols [2, 2-diphenyl-1-picrylhydrazyl (DPPH) free radical scavenging assay, 2,2-azino-bis-3-ethylbenzothiazoline-6-sulphonic acid radical scavenging assay, ferric reducing antioxidant power (FRAP) assay, nitric oxide scavenging capacity assay, and hydrogen peroxide scavenging assay].[39,40]

STATISTICAL DATA

Statistical analysis is a component of data interpretation used to decipher trends and patterns and is helpful in statistical modeling and studies. All the qualitative tests and quantitative measurements are generally repeated in three replicates. The statistical mean of all measurements is calculated with standard deviation (SD). Results are expressed as means ± SD.[38,39]

The *Aegle marmelos* (L.) Corr., (Hindi: Bael) plant is dedicated to Lord Shiva as per Hindu religion and is mostly cultivated around Hindu temples. Each part of the plant has medicinal values and has been extensively studied with analytical evidence. The unripe fruits are associated with more medicinal value compared to ripe fruits. The fruits, leaves, and bark of the species have been reported to have anti-diabetic properties. In folk medicine, the oil prepared from the unripe fruit after being soaked in sesame oil (also known as gingelly oil, cold-pressed sesame oil, or til ka tel) for a week is used to cure and remove the peculiar burning sensation in the soles but has not been analytically deciphered by the time.[16,41] Though the species is globally recognized for therapeutic properties, it still requires more exploration to identify its phytoconstituents and their unidentified therapeutic and pharmacological properties. Jamun (*Syzygium cumini* L.), an extremely perishable fruit with a 1–2-day shelf life under ambient conditions, delicate and petite, accepted as medicine in both traditional and modern molecular practices, remains one of the most underused commercially despite its many therapeutic properties, and there is no organized farming.[42] Its fruit or juice is consumed by diabetics and does not raise blood sugar levels. The value-added products of the species are available as OTC (over-the-counter) products globally, in the form of ready-to-serve beverages, syrup, squash, jam, etc., with acceptable sensory properties. Analytical parameters for quality assurance have revealed that total sugars increase with storage, but acidity, total phenolic, and anthocyanin contents decline in these products as a common trend.[42] The application of analytical data, even at the post-harvest and post-market stages, is equally important for health advantages and for encouraging the faith for consumption of various products from wild edible fruiting plants globally.

CONCLUSION

Wild edible fruit plants have been eaten since time immemorial by the tribals, and nearby populations to forests. Many of these species, however, are still underutilized due to a lack of biological importance. The research data of wild edible fruiting plants (mentioned in Section II of the present text) regarding their potential use as foods, food supplements, and for medicinal values, along with information on total soluble solids, total sugar, and acidity, will develop innovative ideas among the youth. Wild edible fruits have a potent scope to be used as supplementary raw material in the fruit processing industries. The high antioxidant ingredients, such as total phenolic content, ascorbic acid, total flavonol, total flavonoid, FRAP reducing power, and DPPH-free scavenging capacity of these plant species, suggest their potential as sources of bioactive compounds, and these analytical data can be used to extract attractive natural colors and to make high-value processed products such as wine, pickles, jams, and squash. Furthermore, the identification of an endophyte and the exploitation of its fungus for commercial purposes require research data for its growth optimization as well as its bio-culture conditions. This data may be useful to enhance the possible utilization of the endophytes without harvesting the wild fruiting plants from nature. Research data on various metabolic, antimicrobial, and bacteriostatic activities mitigating oxidative stress may be a potential source of cost-effective green herbal medicines to improve human health and cure chronic and acute diseases.

REFERENCES

1. Tanaka HT. 2017. Dietary tradition, nutritional theories, and science. *Mathews Journal of Nutrition & Dietetics*. 2 (1): 1–3.
2. Swinburn BA, Sacks G, Hall KD, McPherson K, Finegood DT, Moodie ML, Gortmaker SL. 2011. The global obesity pandemic: shaped by global drivers and local environments. *Lancet*. 378 (9793): 804–814.
3. Drewnowski A, Aggarwal A, Hurvitz PM, Monsivais P, Moudon AV. 2012. Obesity and supermarket access: proximity or price? *American Journal of Public Health*. 102 (8): e74–80.
4. Buchholz A, Schoeller D. 2004. Is a calorie a calorie? *American Journal of Clinical Nutrition*. 79 (5): 8995–9065.
5. Anderson A, Bryngelsson S. 2007. Towards a healthy diet: from nutrition recommendations to dietary advice. *Scandinavian Journal of Food & Nutrition*. 51(1): 31–40.
6. Norheim F, Gjelstad IM, Hjorth M, Vinknes KJ, Langleite TM, Holen T, Jensen J, Dalen KT, Karlsen AS, Kielland A, Rustan AC. 2012. Molecular nutrition research: the modern way of performing nutritional science. *Nutrients*. 4(12): 1898–1944.
7. Mozaffarian D, Rosenberg I, Uauy R. 2018. History of modern nutrition science-implications for current research, dietary guidelines, and food policy. *BMJ*. 13: 361: k2392. doi: 10.1136/bmj.k2392.
8. Johns DM, Oppenheimer GM. 2018. Was there ever really a "sugar conspiracy"? *Science*. 359: 747–50. https://doi.org/10.1126/science.aaq1618
9. World Health Organization. 2003. Food and Agricultural Organization. Diet, nutrition and the prevention of chronic diseases: report of a joint WHO/FAO expert consultation (report 916). World Health Organization-2003.
10. Sommer A, West KPJ. 1996. *Vitamin A Deficiency: Health, Survival, and Vision*. New York, NY: Oxford University Press. https://doi.org/10.1093/oso/9780195088243.001.0001
11. Mente A, de Koning L, Shannon HS, Anand SS. 2009. A systematic review of the evidence supporting a causal link between dietary factors and coronary heart disease. *Archives of Internal Medicine Research*. 169: 659–669. https://doi.org/10.1001/archinternmed.2009.38
12. Hall KD, Chen KY, Guo J, Lam YY, Leibel RL, Mayer LE, Reitman ML, Rosenbaum M, Smith SR, Walsh BT, Ravussin E. 2016. Energy expenditure and body composition changes after an isocaloric ketogenic diet in overweight and obese men. *The American Journal of Clinical Nutrition*. 104: 324–333. https://doi.org/10.3945/ajcn.116.133561
13. Gardner CD, Trepanowski J F, Del Gobbo LC, Hauser ME, Rigdon J, Ioannidis JP, Desai M, King AC. 2018. Effect of low-fat vs low-carbohydrate diet on 12-month weight loss in overweight adults and the association with genotype pattern or insulin secretion: the DIETFITS randomized clinical trial. *JAMA*. 319:667–79. https://doi.org/10.1001/jama.2018.0245
14. Mozaffarian D, Forouhi NG. 2018. Dietary guidelines and health, is nutrition science up to the task? BMJ .360: k822. https://doi.org/10.1136/bmj.k822
15. Martins D, Barros L, Carvalho AM, Ferreira ICFR. 2011. Nutritional and in vitro antioxidant properties of edible wild greens in Iberian Peninsula traditional diet. *Food Chemistry*. 125: 488–494.
16. Joshi DD, Deb L, Somkuwor BG, Rana VS. 2023. Relevance of Indian traditional tisanes in the management of type 2 diabetes mellitus: a review. *Saudi Pharmaceutical Journal*. 31:626–638. https://doi.org/10.1016/j.jsps.2023.03.003
17. Joshi DD, Changkija S, Sujata W, et al. 2017. Nutraceutical from *Capsicum chinense* fruits in shelf-stable herbal matrix. *Innovative Food Science & Emerging Technologies*. 42: 130–137. https://doi.org/10.1016/j.ifset.2017.06.006
18. Samtiya M, Aluko RE, Dhewa T. 2020. Plant food anti-nutritional factors and their reduction strategies: an overview. *Food Production, Processing and Nutrition*. 2: 6. https://doi.org/10.1186/s43014-020-0020-5
19. Kumar APN, Kumar M, Jose A, Tomer V, Oz E, Proestos C, Zeng M, Elobeid TKS, Oz F. 2023. Major phytochemicals: recent advances in health benefits and extraction method. *Molecules*. 28(2): 887. https://doi.org/10.3390/molecules28020887
20. Otlewski J, Jelen F, Zakrzewska M, Oleksy A. 2005. The many faces of protease–protein inhibitor interaction. *The EMBO Journal*. 24(7): 1303–1310.
21. Delang CO. 2006. Not just minor forest products: the economic rationale for the consumption of wild food plants by subsistence farmers. *Ecological Economics*. 59: 64–73.

22. Si H, Liu D. 2014. Dietary antiaging phytochemicals and mechanisms associated with prolonged survival. *Journal of Nutritional Biochemistry*. 25: 581–591.
23. Joshi DD, Uniyal RC. 2008. Different chemo-types of Gokhru (*Tribulus terrestris*): a herb used for improving physique and physical performance. *International Journal of Green Pharmacy*. 2(3): 138–141.
24. Eyre H, Kahn R, Robertson R M. 2004. Preventing cancer, cardiovascular disease, and diabetes: a common agenda for the American Cancer Society, the American Diabetes Association, and the American Heart Association. *CA: A Cancer Journal for Clinicians*, 54: 190–207.
25. Mahapatra AK, Mishra S, Basak UC, Panda PC. 2012. Nutrient analysis of some selected wild edible fruits of deciduous forests of India; An explorative study towards non-conventional bio-nutrition. *Advance Journal of Food Science and Technology*. 4(1): 15–21.
26. Hegazy AK, Al-Rowaily SL, Faisal M, Alatar AA, El-Bana MI, Assaeed AM. 2013. Nutritive value and antioxidant activity of some edible wild fruits in the Middle East. *Journal of Medicinal Plant* Research. 7(15): 938–946.
27. Egea I, Sanchez-Bel P, Romojaro F, Pretel MT. 2010. Six edible wild fruits as potential antioxidant additives or nutritional supplements. *Plant Foods for Human Nutrition*. 65: 121–129.
28. Pietta PG. 2000. Flavonoids as antioxidants. *Journal of Natural Products*. 63: 1035–1042.
29. Riboli E, Norat T. 2003. Epidemiologic evidence of the protective effect of fruit and vegetables on cancer risk. *American Journal of Clinical Nutrition*. 78: 559–569.
30. Leja M, Mareczek A, Ben J. 2003. Antioxidant properties of two apple cultivars during long-term storage. *Food Chemistry*. 80: 303–307.
31. Trichopoulou A, Costacou T, Bamia C, Trichopoulos D. 2003. Adherence to a Mediterranean diet and survival in a Greek population. *The New England Journal of Medicine*. 348, 2599–2608.
32. Nayak J, Basak UC. 2015. Antioxidant potential of some lesser-known wild edible fruits of Odisha. *The European Journal of Experimental Biology*. 5(8): 60–70.
33. Shan S, Huang X, Shah MH, Abbasi AM. 2019. Evaluation of polyphenolics content and antioxidant activity in edible wild fruits. *BioMed Research International*. ID1381989. https://doi.org/10.1155/2019/1381989
34. Shikov AN, Mikhailovskaya IY, Narkevich IA, Flisyuk EV, Pozharitskaya ON. 2022. Methods of extraction of medicinal plants. In *Evidence-Based Validation of Herbal Medicine*. Elsevier, Amsterdam, Netherlands. Pulok K. Mukherjee (Ed.) pp. 771–796. https://doi.org/10.1016/B978-0-323-85542-6.00029-9
35. Yang Z. 2018. Natural deep eutectic solvents and their applications in biotechnology. In *Application of Ionic Liquids in Biotechnology; Advances in Biochemical Engineering/Biotechnology Series*. Itoh T., Koo Y. M. (Eds.) Springer, Cham, Germany; New York, USA. Vol. 168 pp. 31–59. https://doi.org/10.1007/10_2018_67.
36. Hikmawanti N, Ramadon D, Jantan I, Mun'im A. 2021. Natural deep eutectic solvents (NADES): phytochemical extraction performance enhancer for pharmaceutical and nutraceutical product development. *Plants*. 10, 2091.
37. Kim SK, Wijesekara I. 2017. Role of marine nutraceuticals in cardiovascular health. In *Sustained Energy for Enhanced Human Functions and Activity*. Academic Press, Cambridge, MA. Debasis Bagchi (Ed.) pp. 273–279. https://doi.org/10.1016/B978-0-12-805413-0.00017-X.
38. Raaman N. 2006. *Phytochemical Techniques*. New India Publishing Agency, New Delhi.
39. Joshi DD. 2011. *Herbal Drugs: Quality and Chemistry*. Studium Press, LLC. USA. ISBN-13: 978-1933699882
40. Rymbai H, Verma VK, Talang H, Assumi SR, Devi MB, Vanlalruati, Sangma RHCH, Biam KP, Chanu LJ, Makdoh B, Singh AR, Mawleiñ J, Hazarika S, Mishra VK. 2023. Biochemical and antioxidant activity of wild edible fruits of the Eastern Himalaya, India. *Frontiers in Nutrition*. 10: 1039965. https://doi.org/10.3389/fnut.2023.1039965
41. Choudhary S, Choudhary G, Kaurav H. 2021. *Aegle marmelos* (Bael Patra): an ayurvedic plant with ethnomedicinal values. *International Journal of Research in Ayurveda and Pharmacy*. 12 (3): 147–156. https://doi.org/10.7897/2277-4343.120392
42. El-Safy S, Khalifa AM, Almashad AA, Mohamed Khalil AM, Hammad EM, Sami R, Aljahani AH, Pareek S, Helal M, Alharthi S, Taha IM. 2023. Utilization of Jamun Fruit (*Syzygium cumini* L.) for value added food products. *Journal of Food Quality*. https://doi.org/10.1155/2023/5460642

Section II

Description

3 *Aesculus indica* (Indian Horse Chestnut)

INTRODUCTION

Aesculus indica (Wall. ex Cambess.) Hook., (family: Hippocastanaceae) is known as Indian horse chestnut. It is a large, deciduous tree with a short, straight, cylindrical bole and spread crown, distributed in the Himalayas from west Nepal to Kashmir, at 900–3,600 MSL in shady ravines, forests, and watercourses.[1,2] It sheds leaves in winter and blooms fully during May and June with multi-colored buds. After fertilization, these buds produce a huge number of seeds, which are consumed as a stag in hilly areas like Himachal Pradesh, Kashmir, and Uttarakhand in India.[3] Genus *Aesculus* L. has 12 species of deciduous trees, including shrubs, in the northern hemisphere, mainly in eastern Asia and the eastern hemisphere.[4–7] *Aesculus* spp. is cultivated as medicinal crops to produce standardized therapeutic extracts. In European countries, its bark, leaves, seed extract, and aescin (a mixture of saponins) have been used to treat chronic venous insufficiency, postoperative edema, and hemorrhoids.[8–12] In China, the seeds of *A. chinensis* are utilized as a stomachic and analgesic to treat distention and pain in the chest and abdomen, malaria, and dysentery.[13] The tablets made from the seeds are used to treat heart diseases.[14] The insect *Cameraria ohridella* attacks the leaves of plants; it is also known as the 'horse-chestnut leaf miner'.[15] The main host of the leaf miner is the horse chestnut plant at the flowering stage, and it affects the quality of seeds but has no effect on the number of seeds that have been recorded.[16] About 100 varieties of *Aesculus* have been reported. As per the report, a total of 210 compounds from seeds of different species of the genus have been isolated.[17]

TRADITIONAL APPLICATIONS

In Himachal Pradesh (HP), India, *A. indica* plants are used as medicine, fodder, and timber in hilly areas. The tree bears huge numbers of seeds every year, and after drying, seeds are ground into flour. The flour is known as 'Tattwak Ahar', which is used for making Halwa (porridge). Tattwak Ahar (local word; in English, a diet rich in nutritious ingredients) is bitter, and there is a folk method to treat it before utilizing it.[18]

In the Chawar Valley of Mandi district (HP), India, the seeds are dried and ground into flour, which is known as Tattwak Ahar. Ripened fruits of *A. indica* are collected during October, and seeds are separated from the fruits and crushed into smaller pieces to facilitate the quick removal of bitter content. The crushed seeds are kept in big bamboo baskets, which are placed under running water in a stream or under tap water. The crushed seeds kept in baskets are stirred daily to enhance the cleaning process and to prevent the rotting of seeds. The stirring process is continued for 5–7 days, and then the crushed seeds are dried, cleaned, and stored in gunny bags for making flour. The flour (Tattwak Ahar) is usually prepared in local water flour mills known as 'Gharat'. This bitter flour is used for making Halwa (porridge), especially during marriages, and mixed with wheat flour to prepare Chapatis. The Tattwak Ahar flour is available in the local market in Chawar Valley and Sunder Nagar Tehsil of Mandi District. Bitterness is one of the major characteristics of seeds; hence, the cleaning process is extensively followed, and even flour prepared from the seed is washed two to three times before making halwa or mixing it with wheat flour. The bitter component gets dissolved in water and is removed when the water is decanted.[18] The processed flour becomes gluten-free. It is vital for patients experiencing celiac disease.[19] Tattwak Ahar is used as phalahar (non-cereal food) during fasts in Himachal Pradesh.[20]

Shoots and leaves of *A. indica* are lopped and used as cattle fodder. The crushed fruits, after steeping in water, are fed to cattle and mixed with wheat flour to improve the quality and quantity of cattle milk. The crushed seeds are used as soap to clean clothes. Seeds are processed by striking them with a stone to use as natural soap. The hot water extract of de-coated seeds is concentrated into a cake, the *Aesculus* soap. These cakes are used as washing soap. The seeds are rich in saponins (aescin) and contain oil, which is used in rheumatism and applied to wounds. The wood is used for making water troughs, tea boxes, packing cases, and decorative articles.[18]

A. indica whole plant has remarkable medicinal properties to cure diabetes. *A. indica* fruits are used to treat colic problems. Fruits are highly effective to counter complaints associated with vein ailments such as varicose veins, hemorrhoids, and ulcers. Traditionally its fruits are used to treat effusions of blood, migraines, limb complaints, and frostbite. The seed oil is used to cure skin diseases, rheumatism, and headaches.[18] The fruits/seeds are used to treat horses suffering from colic problems. The nuts are used to cure obstinate constipation and piles.[21] The seeds of *A. indica* are utilized as an astringent and nutritious substance, while roots are used in leucorrhea management.[22]

In folk medicine, *A. indica* extract and its value-added products are used for the management of cardiac venous insufficiency, pain, swelling and heaviness of the lower limbs, hemorrhoids,[23] burns, epidermis abrasion, diarrhea, phlebitis, fever, and to treat enlargement of the prostate gland.[24,25] In China, ß-escin is traditionally used as

DOI: 10.1201/9781003512868-5

a flatulence reliever, antiseptic, analgesic, antioxidant, anorexia, antiaging, and antipyretic agent.[26] ß-escin is used topically in the cosmetic industry and to treat infections of the ear, nose and throat regions.[27] It is reported to treat gastric ulcer,[28] venous congestion, brain trauma, hemorrhoids, stroke, thrombophlebitis,[29] cardiac vein insufficiency, epidermis abrasion, burns, frostbite, and skin inflammation.[30,31] ß-escin is used to reduce cellulite and hematoma, treat diarrhea and postoperative edema, and enhance the oxidative defense system.[32] An *A. indica* tree is a natural source of non-edible starch and timber.[33,34]

The seeds of *Aesculus turbinate* (Japanese horse chestnut) have traditionally been used since ancient times in Japan as a confectionery ingredient in rice cakes and rice balls.[35] The seed extract mixed with spirits has a folk application to treat bruises and sprains in a few regions of Japan.[36] In traditional Chinese medicine, its seeds are termed 'Sha Luo Zhi' and are used as a stomachic and analgesic in the treatment of distention and pain in the chest and abdomen, malaria, and dysentery.[13] Additionally, tablets made from seeds are used to cure heart diseases.[14]

'Horse chestnut', the common name of the plant, may have originated from its seeds being used by Greeks and Turks to treat overexertion or coughs in horses.[32] Horse chestnut has been in practice to treat fever since the early 18th century.[8] In Europe, its bark and leaves are used as an astringent to treat diarrhea and hemorrhoids.[9]

PHYTO-PHARMACOLOGY

Fruits and seeds of *Aesculus* have been used for medicine in Eurasia and North America since prehistoric times. *Aesculus* species is a storehouse of therapeutic ingredients, as more than 210 compounds have been isolated and identified from it.[17] These compounds include triterpenoids, triterpenoid glycosides (saponins), flavonoids, coumarins, carotenoids, long fatty chain compounds, etc. The plant contains a mixture of saponins, usually known for its medicinal properties. The seeds have ingredients of pharmacological value as antioxidant, antiviral, immunemodulatory, and anti-inflammatory properties.[37] The oil from seeds of *A. indica* has a composition of arachidic acid (5.67%), myristic acid (1.3%), palmitic acid (8.77%), oleic acid (57.49%), linoleic acid (16.91%), and linolenic acid (7.92%).[37] The fruit has about 50.5% moisture content, total sugars (5.58%), reducing sugars (4.59%), and non-reducing sugars (0.94%).[38] Seeds of Indian horse chestnut are a natural source of starch.[39] The bitter taste is due to saponins, which makes the fruits unsuitable for direct human consumption.[40] The studies have been conducted to remove its bitterness by different pre-treatments together with conventional techniques. Seeds are de-hulled, crushed/grated into a mass, and prepared for treatments, such as soaking, blanching, open-air cooking, cooking under pressure, and standardization separately.[41] After processing, the flour is edible and reported as not toxic. It is used as a sacred food during fasts, which are locally known as falahar.[17,18]

Hitherto, researchers have reported about 210 phyto-ingredients from *Aesculus*.[17] The main chemical classes are carotenoids, coumarins, glycosides (saponin types), triterpenoids, flavonoids, long fatty chain compounds, etc. *A. indica* has been reported to contain a mixture of saponins (aescin), a crystalline compound, and a hydroxyl-coumarin glycoside that absorbs ultraviolet rays in the bark of the branch.[3]

The horse chestnut seed extract (HCSE) is used to treat hemorrhoids, chronic venous insufficiency, and postoperative edema.[12] A mixture of saponins (aescin), also known as β-escin, is the major active fraction in HCSE. Its use has been clinically proven for chronic venous insufficiency, hemorrhoids, and postoperative edema. The therapeutic profile of aescin, along with its pharmacology and pharmacokinetics, has been investigated in detail[8] and reported for wider acceptance as an effective therapy for venous disorders and edema in the United States.[8]

The major ingredients of *Aesculus* species are escin, esculetin, esculin, scopoletin, and fraxetin, some of which are reported for their marked efficacy, such as escin (aescin, or β-escin), and are used for their anti-carcinogenic properties against various cancers.[42–44] The other secondary metabolites have a protective effect either alone or in the extract form. Molecular investigations have established the antibacterial and anti-inflammatory properties of escin.[45]

Zhu et al. have reported that escin is a potent chemotherapeutic moiety. The research was conducted to investigate the therapeutic effect of escin on osteosarcoma in an orthotopic model, and the result confirmed that escin can inhibit induced apoptosis, osteosarcoma proliferation, and autophagy. Apoptosis has been confirmed by increased expression of caspase-related proteins and the formation of apoptotic bodies, while autophagy has been identified by the increased level of LC3, ATG5, ATG12, Beclin expression, and autophagosome formation.[46]

HCSE has anti-edematous, anti-inflammatory,[18] hypoglycemic, antithrombotic,[31] anti-vagotonic,[47] and antibacterial activity toward *Streptococcus mutans*, *Staphylococcus aureus*, and *Escherichia coli*.[48]

SCOPE AND OPPORTUNITIES

Though the genus *Aesculus* has 12 species, only *A. indica* (common horse chestnut) and *A. chinensis* (Chinese horse chestnut) are officially recognized sources of herbal medicine in traditional healing systems. HCSE (aescin-rich fraction) from *A. indica* has been proven for its clinically significant activity in hemorrhoids, chronic venous insufficiency, and postoperative edema. It is due to its anti-inflammatory properties, which are well demonstrated by in vitro and in vivo assays. However, the mechanism of action in the case of Chinese horse chestnut is poorly understood and requires additional investigations. The poly-hydroxylated triterpenoid glycosides (saponins) in *Aesculus* extract are the major active principles, though other constituents may also have some bioactivity. The chemical differences due to geo-climatic conditions and the impact of biotic and abiotic factors reveal a chemotaxonomic significance among the species.[49,50] Detailed investigations on the saponins from the seeds of other *Aesculus* species have not been conducted in terms of phytochemical screening. There is a need to fully understand the chemical profile of the genus *Aesculus*. The biological and molecular activities of HCSE, aescin, and individual ingredients from the genus *Aesculus* have received much interest in recent years due to anti-inflammatory, antitumor, antiviral, antifungal, anti-obesity, antioxidative, antigenotoxic, and antiangiogenic (vascular protection) properties. The most unique and interesting property is the antitumor activity of some novel saponins isolated recently, which have potent cytotoxicity and inhibition of TOP1 in in vitro assays.[50,51] Furthermore, detailed animal studies are required to evaluate the potential of these saponins for the treatment of cancer.

REFERENCES

1. Anonymous. 1985. *The Wealth of India: A Dictionary of Raw Materials and Industrial Products, Raw Materials.* Publications and Information Directorate, New Delhi. Vol. 1. pp. 195–197.
2. Chowdhery HJ, Wadhwa BM. 1984. *Flora of Himachal Pradesh; Analysis.* Botanical Survey of India, Howrah.
3. Kumar S. 2014. The importance of antioxidant and their role in pharmaceutical science. *The Asian Journal of Research in Chemistry and Pharmaceutical Sciences.* 1 (1): 27–44.
4. Hardin JW. 1957. A revision of the American Hippocastanaceae. *Brittonia.* 9: 145–195.
5. Hardin JW. 1960. Studies in the hippocastanaceae, V. Species of the old world. *Brittonia.* 12: 26–38.
6. Xia NH, Thurland NJ, Gadek PA. 2010. Hippocastanaceae. Flora of China. Vol. 12: 1–4. 'eFloras. loras.org/florataxon. aspx?flora_id=2&taxon_id=10412, as on 18th June 2025.
7. Xiang QY, Crawford DJ, Wolfe AD, Tang YC, DePamphilis CW. 1998. Origin and biogeography of *Aesculus* L. (Hippcastanaceae): a molecular phylogenetic perspective. *Evolution.* 52 (4): 988–997.
8. Sirtori CR. 2001. Aescin: pharmacology, pharmacokinetics and therapeutic profile. *Pharmacological Research.* 44: 183–193.
9. Bisset NG. 1994. *Herbal Drugs and Phytopharmaceuticals.* Medpharm Scientific Publishers, CRC Press, Stuttgart, Germany. pp. 268–272.
10. Bielanski TE, Piotrowski ZH. 1999. Horse-chestnut seed extract for chronic venous insufficiency. *The Journal of Family Practice.* 48: 171–172.
11. Kahn SR. 2006. Review: horse chestnut seed extract is effective for symptoms of chronic venous insufficiency. *ACP Journal Club.* 145 (1): 20.
12. Persson IAL, Persson K. 2010. Horse chestnut (*Aesculus hippocastanum* L.). *Recent Progress in Medicinal Plants.* 28: 159–171
13. Jiangsu New Medical College. 1977. *Zhong Yao Da Ci Dian.* Shanghai People's Public Health Press, Shanghai. PR China. pp. 1961.
14. Institute of Materia Medica. 1984. *Chinese Academy of Medical Sciences.* Zhong Yao Zhi. People's Health Press, Beijing, PR China. Vol. 4. pp. 555.
15. Deschka GN, Dimic. 1986. *Cameraria ohridella* n. sp. aus mazedonien, jugoslawien (lepidoptera: lithocolletidae). *Journal of Acta Entomologica Jugoslavica.* 22: 11–23.
16. Thalmann C, Freise J, Heitland W, Bacher S. 2003. Effects of defoliation by horse chestnut leaf miner (*Cameraria ohridella*) on reproduction in *Aesculus hippocastanum. Journal of Trees.* 17: 383–388.
17. Zhang Z, Li S, Lian XY. 2001. An overview of genus *Aesculus* L. Ethnobotany, phytochemistry, and pharmacological activities. *Pharmaceutical Crops.* 1: 24–51.
18. Rajasekaran A, Singh J. 2009. Ethnobotany of Indian horse chestnut (*Aesculus indica*) in Mandi district, Himachal Pradesh. *Indian Journal of Traditional Knowledge.* 8 (2): 285–286.
19. Sood S, Mishra ML. 2014. Studies on physical attributes of Indian horse chestnut (*Aesculus indica*). *Indian Journal of Social and Natural Sciences.* 3: 68–73.
20. Parmar C, Kaushal MK. 1982. *Aesculus indica. Wild Fruits.* Kalyani Publishers, New Delhi, India. pp. 6–9.
21. Pal DK, Singh H, Kumar MA. 2012. Preliminary study on the *in-vitro* antioxidant activity of seeds of *Aesculus indica* and barks of *Populus euphratica. International Journal of Pharmacy and Pharmaceutical Sciences.* 4 (4): 249–250.
22. Kaur L, Joseph L, George M. 2011. Phytochemical analysis of leaf extract of *Aesculus indica. International Journal of Pharmacy and Pharmaceutical Sciences.* 3 (5): 232–234.
23. Kedzierskia B, Kocha WK, Widelskia J, Głowniak K. 2016. Impact of harvest time of *Aesculus hippocastanum* seeds on the composition, antioxidant capacity and total phenolic content. *Industrial Crops and Products.* 86: 68–72.
24. Srijayanta S, Raman A, Goodwin BLA. 1999. Comparative study of the constituents of *Aesculus hippocastanum* and *Aesculus indica. Journal of Medicinal Food.* 2: 45–50.
25. Makuch MD, Matlawska I. 2011. Flavonoids from the flowers of *Aesculus hippocastanum. Acta Poloniae Pharmaceutica - Drug Research.* 68: 403–408.
26. Patlolla JMR, Rao CV. 2015. Anti-inflammatory and anti-cancer properties of β-escin, a triterpenesaponin. *Journal of Current Pharmacology Reports.* 1: 170–178.
27. Marton G, Bakan A. 1995. Research and development of an integrated and waste free utilization of horse chestnut (*Aesculus hippocastanum*) seeds. *Journal of Bioresource Technology.* 54: 197–200.
28. Roy A, Geetha RV, Lakshmi T. 2011. Evaluation of the anti-mycotic activity of aqueous and ethanolic extracts of *Aesculus hippocastanum*-An *in-vitro* study. *The International Journal of Drug Development and Research.* 3: 335–338.
29. Braga AGS, Yilmaz S, Coruh N. 2012. Antioxidant capacity and cytotoxicity of *Aesculus hippocastanum* on breast cancer MCF-7 cells. *Journal of Food and Drug Analysis.* 20: 692–698.
30. Bombardelli E, Morazzoni P, Griffini A. 1996. *Aesculus hippocastanum* L. *Journal of Fitoterapia.* 67: 483–511.
31. Margină D, Olaru OT, Ilie M, Grădinaru D, Guțu C, Voicu S, Dinischiotu A, Spandidos DA, Tsatsakis AM. 2015. Assessment of the potential health benefits of certain total extracts from *Vitis vinifera, Aesculus hyppocastanum* and *Curcuma longa. Experimental and Therapeutic Medicine.*10:1681–1688.
32. Stajner D, Popovic BM, Calic D, Stajner M. 2014. Comparative study of antioxidant status in androgenic embryos of *Aesculus hippocastanum* and *Aesculus flava. Science World Journal.* 11: 1–8.

33. Castano J, Llamazares SR, Contreras K, Carrasco C, Pozo C, Bouza R, Franco CM, Giraldo D. 2014. Horse chestnut (*Aesculus hippocastanum* L.) starch: basic physico-chemical characteristics and use as thermoplastic material. *Carbohydrate Polymers*. 112: 677–685.
34. Jekkel Z, Gyulai G, Kiss J, Kiss E, Heszky LE. 1998. Cryopreservation of horse-chestnut (*Aesculus hippocastanum* L.) somatic embryos using three different freezing methods. *Plant Cell, Tissue and Organ Culture*. 52: 193–197.
35. Ogawa S, Kimura H, Niimi A, Katsube T, Jisaka M, Yokota K. 2008. Fractionation and structural characterization of polyphenolic antioxidants from seed shells of Japanese horse chestnut (*Aesculus turbinata* Blume). *Journal of Agricultural and Food Chemistry*. 56 (24): 12046–12051.
36. Sato I, Kofujita H, Tsuda S. 2007. Identification of COX inhibitors in the hexane extract of Japanese horse chestnut (*Aesculus turbinata*) seeds. *Journal of Veterinary Medical Science*. 69 (7): 709–712.
37. Sood S, Mishra M, Sood A, Thakur V. 2015. Hypoglycaemic and hypo-cholesterolimic efficacy of horse chestnut (*Aesculus indica*) using rat model. *Journal of Clinical Nutrition and Dietetics*. 1(1):1–8.
38. Majeed M, Khan MA, Bashir A, Hussain A. 2010. Nutritional value and oil content of Indian horse chestnut seed. *Global Journal of Science Frontier Research*. 10:17–19.
39. Uniyal SK, Singh KN, Jamwal P, Lal B. 2006. Traditional use of medicinal plants among the tribal communities of Chhota Bhangal, Western Himalaya. *Journal of Ethnobiology and Ethnomedicine*. 2: 14. https://doi.org/10.1186/1746-4269-2-14
40. Mishra ML, Sood S, Shukla UN. 2018. Phyto-nutritional and mineral composition of Indian Horse Chestnut (*Aesculus indica*) seeds. *Journal of Pharmacognosy and Phytochemistry*. 7: 2159–2162.
41. Thakur NS, Kumar P, Joshi VK. 2015. Improvement of traditional methods for the development of edible flour from Indian horse chestnut (*Aesculus indica*). *International Journal of Food and Fermentation Technology*. 5 (2): 169–176.
42. Ciftci GA, Iscan A, Kutlu M. 2015. Escin reduces cell proliferation and induces apoptosis on glioma and lung adenocarcinoma cell lines. *Cytotechnology*. 67: 893–904.
43. Huang GL, Shen DY, Cai CF, Zhang QY, Ren HY, Chen QX. 2015. Beta escin reverses multidrug resistance through inhibition of the GSK3beta/beta-catenin pathway in cholangiocarcinoma. *World Journal of Gastroenterology*. 21: 1148–1157
44. Petrova S, Yurukova L, Velcheva I. 2012. Horse chestnut (*Aesculus hippocastanum* L.) as a biomonitor of air pollution in the town of Plovdiv (Bulgaria). *Journal of BioScience and Biotechnology*. 1: 241–247.
45. Maghsoudi H, Hallajzadeh J, Rezaeipour M. 2018. Evaluation of the effect of polyphenol of escin compared with ibuprofen and dexamethasone in synoviocyte model for osteoarthritis: an in vitro study. *Journal of Clinical Rheumatology*. 37: 2471–2478.
46. Zhu J, Yu W, Liu B, Wang Y, Shao J, Wang J, Xia K, Liang C, Fang W, Zhou C, Tao H. 2017. Escin induces caspase-dependent apoptosis and autophagy through the ROS/p38 MAPK signaling pathway in human osteosarcoma cells in vitro and in vivo. *Cell Death & Disease*. 8. https://doi.org/10.1038/cddis.2017.488
47. Braga PC, Marabini L, Wang YY, Lattuada N, Calo R, Bertelli A, Falchi M, Dal Sasso M, Bianchi T. 2012. Characterisation of the antioxidant effects of *Aesculus hippocastanum* L. bark extract on the basis of radical scavenging activity, the chemiluminescence of human neutrophil bursts and lipo-peroxidation assay. *European Review for Medical and Pharmacological Sciences*. 16: 1–9.
48. Takahashi T, Tsurunaga Y, Schmidt WF, Yoshino K. 2017. Functional evaluation of horse chestnut seed and its application in the production of compounded paper for effective utilization of an untapped resource. *Journal of Wood Science*. 63: 484–495.
49. Forest F, Drouin JN, Charest RC, Brouillet L, Bruneau AF. 2001. A morphological phylogenetic analysis of *Aesculus* L. and *Billia Peyr*. (Sapindaceae). *Canadian Journal of* Botany. 79: 154–169.
50. Zhang ZZ, Li SY. 2007. Cytotoxic triterpenoid saponins from the fruits of *Aesculus pavia* L. *Phytochemistry*. 68 (15): 2075–2086.
51. Wang P, Ownby S, Zhang ZZ, Yuan W, Li SY. 2010. Cytotoxicity and inhibition of DNA topoispmerase I of polyhydroxylated triterpenoids and triterpenoid glycosides. *Bioorganic & Medicinal Chemistry Letters*. 20: 2790–2796.

4 *Amelanchier spicata* (Saskatoon Berry)

INTRODUCTION

The genus *Amelanchier* (family: Rosaceae) has about 25 species. These are distributed in North America and a few parts of Europe and Asia.[1] The plant can grow in soil of different pH and soil conditions and has been reported to survive at −60°C temperatures.[2] The genus *Amelanchier* has white flowers in the spring and produces red-purple berries during the summer. Its berries have a nutty almond flavor, are sweet in taste, and are available on the market either as fresh fruit or processed jam. Saskatoon berries are the second most important economically planted fruit produced in Canada, following strawberries.[3–5]

Amelanchier spicata (Linn.) K. Koch. (Saskatoon berry, Serviceberry, Juneberry) occurs naturally in North America (mostly in the USA). *A. spicata* is fully naturalized in Western Europe and is commonly found from England to Sweden.[6] It is a low bush (0.5–2 m) with numerous shrub-forming shoots. It has whitish or slightly pinkish flowers, up to 10 mm long, in thick clusters. The fruits are navy blue and white, juicy, and sweet. *A. spicata* is mainly an ornamental plant, but its fruits are also collected in some countries.[7] Fruits are eaten raw or processed and can be used to produce juices, jams, etc.[8] These berries are excellent sources of anthocyanins, flavonols, procyanidins, and phenolic compounds. Anthocyanins, along with other phenolics, have therapeutic interest due to their antioxidant properties and associated health benefits (including anti-inflammatory, anticarcinogenic, and antimicrobial activities), induced insulin availability in the body, and neuroprotective effects.[9] Berries are rich in dietary fiber, vitamin B group, and other mineral substances, especially potassium, as well as microelements such as cobalt and copper.[8,10] Fruits are a delicacy for birds. These plants are grown on a large scale in kitchen gardens and plantations.[11] Additionally, due to high frost resistance, a thick, bushy nature is used to establish wind protection belts.[12] The chemical composition of *A. spicata* berries has been deciphered as total anthocyanin (45–50 mg/100 g), carbohydrates (18 g), total dietary fiber (5.9 g), Ca (42 mg), iron (1.0 mg), vitamin C (3.6 mg), and vitamin A (35.7 IU).[13]

ETHNOPHARMACOLOGY

Historically, Saskatoon berries have been used for medicinal purposes. In the USA, prairies used the Saskatoon berry for disinfection, to prevent miscarriages, and additionally as a source of food.[14] The Blackfoot indigenous people were also using tea from leaves and twigs to cure diabetes.[15,16]

The Indigenous people in North America mix berries with animal fat and raw buffalo meat to make 'Pemmican', a preserved food. The dried 'Pemmican' is used as emergency food during long hunting trips by the natives.[2] The ripened Saskatoon berries are stored in the freeze-dried form to ensure off-season availability.[4]

PHYTOCHEMISTRY OF THE SASKATOON BERRIES

The Saskatoon berries are sources of antioxidants, fiber, essential elements, polyphenols, and vitamins. These berries contain high quantities of elements such as iron, manganese, potassium, vitamins (ascorbic acid, pantothenic acid, pyridoxine, riboflavin, thiamin, tocopherol, and folic acid), carotene, pectin, and different phenolic acids (3-feruloyl quinic acid, chlorogenic acid, and 5-feruloyl quinic acid).[4,17–19] The Saskatoon berries are rich in anthocyanins [mainly cyanidins (63% of all phenols and 94% of anthocyanins)][17,20] and flavonoids (such as avicularin, hyperoside, rutin, and quercetin).[4,17,19]

Young berries have a low content of anthocyanins, but they increase dramatically from stages 5 to 9 of the nine-stage maturation of berries.[5,19,21] The concentrations of anthocyanins vary in different cultivars of Saskatoon berry.[4] Hosseinian and Beta have reported that ripened Smoky Saskatoon berry has a comparable concentration of total anthocyanins to wild blueberry and a higher concentration than that in chokeberry, sea buckthorn, and raspberry.[22] In ripe Saskatoon berry, compounds like cyanidin 3-O-galactoside (C3Ga), cyanidin 3-O-arabinoside, cyanidin 3-O-glucoside (C3G), and cyanidin 3-O-xyloside are the most common and abundant anthocyanins.[4,20] In Saskatoon berry, the content of C3G (117.67 mg/100 g) is higher than in wild blueberry (27.48 mg/100 g), raspberry (35.88 mg/100 g), strawberry (9.53 mg/100 g), chokecherry (46.01 mg/100 g), and sea buckthorn (0.05 mg/100 g).[23] The primary flavonols of Saskatoon berries are derivatives of quercetin, including both di-glycosides (quercetin-3-O-rutinoside, quercetin-3-O-robinobioside, and quercetin-3-O-arabinoglucoside) and mono-glycosides (quercetin-3-O-galactoside, quercetin-3-O-glucoside, quercetin-3-O-arabinoside, and quercetin-3-O-xyloside).[24] The leaves, roots, and stems of the plant are a rich source of phenolic compounds (such as anthocyanins, proanthocyanidin, and quercetin). The composition of phenolics in other plant parts differs from that in the berries of Saskatoon. Chlorogenic acid, (−)-epicatechin, and quercetin 3-galactoside are the main phenolic ingredients present in the leaves, while catechins and hydroxybenzoic acids are present in the stem.[4,14]

DOI: 10.1201/9781003512868-6

PHYTOPHARMACOLOGY

Saskatoon berries are rich in polyphenols.[25] Polyphenols are the major bioactive ingredients of the species.[4] Phenolics are mainly flavonoids in Saskatoon berries, which encompass over 6,000 phenolic substances that are found in pigmented leaves, seeds, fruits, and their products like wine, jam, juice, tea, and soy.[4] The higher content of flavonoids is responsible for chemo-protective, antidiabetic, and anti-inflammatory effects.[5] Structurally, two aromatic rings (A and B rings) are linked by a 3-carbon chain with an oxygenated heterocyclic ring (C ring) in the flavonoids. There are seven subclasses of flavonoids [i.e. flavones, flavanols (proanthocyanidins), flavanones, isoflavones, flavonols, flavones, and anthocyanidins]. The distinction is due to different generic structures between subclasses of flavonoids, and each subclass characterized by specific hydroxylation and conjugation patterns.[26] Anthocyanidins in glycan form (anthocyanins) are highly water-soluble natural pigments in the plant kingdom. The red, blue, and violet colors of different fruits, vegetables, leaves, and seeds are due to anthocyanidins, which are strong natural antioxidants.[27] Other anthocyanidins include peonidin, delphinidin, malvidin, and petunidin. The red and purple colors of plants are due to cyanidin and pelargonidin, respectively, whereas delphinidin imparts the bluish colors in the plant kingdom. In botanicals, anthocyanins occur in either mono- or di-glycosylated forms of anthocyanidins (aglycones) and are generally linked to sugars such as arabinose, fructose, galactose, glucose, rhamnose, or xylose.[22] Saskatoon berries are rich in cyanidin-3-galactoside and cyanidin-glucoside.[17,20] Proanthocyanidins are known for their brown appearance and impart flavor and astringency to fruits.[19] The classification of proanthocyanidins depends on the degree of polymerization, the number of linked monomers, the presence of the hydroxyl groups in basic units, and the links between units. The individual oligomers are commonly known as dimers, trimers, tetramers, pentamers, hexamers, and heptamers.[28] Flavan-3-ol units compose proanthocyanidins, which are found widely in many types of fruits, nuts, seeds, and barks of pine.[15] The primary constitutive units are epicatechins and epigallocatechin, which form procyanidin and prodelphinidin structures, respectively.[15,28] Procyanidins represent the largest class of proanthocyanidins.[23] Flavan-3-ol units are often linked through B-type bonds, such as C4⟶C8, and to a lesser extent, C4⟶C6 linkages. Albeit less common, the flavan3-ol units can also be linked by an additional C2⟶O7 or C2⟶O5 linkage (double bond A-type). Proanthocyanidins are potent antioxidants and exhibit potential health benefits such as anticarcinogenic, anti-inflammatory, and vasodilatory activities. Their physical, chemical, and biological properties are based on their structures, particularly on their degree of polymerization.[28,29] Flavonols have a 3-hydroxy-flavone backbone, a subclass of flavonoids, and may have different positions of the phenolic-OH groups. These compounds are more common in apples, coriander, fennel, lovage, tea, pepper, radishes, berries, onions, and wine. The most common types of flavonols in human diets are quercetin, rutin, etc., and have antioxidant activities.[5,26]

Several studies have depicted that anthocyanins, proanthocyanidins, flavonols, phenolic acids, and phenolic derivatives have many protective functions, such as anticarcinogenic, anti-inflammatory, antioxidant, antiradical, potentially antidiabetic, vessel protecting, and neuroprotective in the biological system. These compounds have potential therapeutic effects on many body ailments, such as cardiovascular problems, inflammation, cancers, obesity, neurodegenerative pathologies, and muscular degeneration.[4,19]

Antioxidant effects: Saskatoon berries have a higher quantity of flavonoids (anthocyanin, flavonol, and proanthocyanidin), and flavonoids possess anti-inflammatory, antioxidant, antitumor, and antidiabetic properties. Studies have revealed that the total anthocyanin content is directly correlated to its antioxidant properties, and Saskatoon berries have a strong free-radical scavenging property.[29] Burns-Kraft et al. have reported that concentrated extract of Saskatoon berries inhibits nitric oxide production in activated macrophages and has a potential protective role against chronic inflammation.[14] Cyclooxygenase (COX, including COX-1 and COX-2) is an enzyme that helps form prostanoids, such as thromboxane, prostaglandins, and prostacyclins, from arachidonic acid. Inhibiting COX with drugs can alleviate symptoms such as inflammation, blood clotting, and pain. The findings reveal that the phenolic compounds in Saskatoon berry extracts have an effective protective role in the biological membranes to increase the resistance of low-density lipoprotein (LDL) to oxidation and metabolism, inhibit DNA damage, and influence lipid profile.[18,25]

ANTI-INFLAMMATORY EFFECTS

Anthocyanins are known to attenuate atherosclerotic cardiovascular diseases (CVDs). C3G and C3Ga are the common anthocyanins present in the Saskatoon berries.[22] Delphinidin-3-glucoside (D3G) is another type of anthocyanin that is higher in Saskatoon berries than in chokecherry, raspberry, wild blueberry, strawberry, and sea buckthorn.[22] These three glycosides interfere at multiple centers in the progression of CVD due to LDL. The high levels of glycated LDL (glyLDL) and oxidized LDL (oLDL) in type 1 and type 2 diabetic cases and coronary artery problems cause an elevation in the level of reactive oxygen species. Different investigations have revealed that the anthocyanins, namely C3G, C3Ga, and D3G, prevent glyLDL- and oLDL-induced upregulation.[22,30] Shen et al. have reported protective measures of C3G effects against *Streptococcus*.[31]

ANTITUMOR EFFECTS

C3G helps in the reproductive pathway and reduces tumors. Li et al. have reported that C3G has a protective function against cadmium-induced male reproductive dysfunction.[32]

Furthermore, studies have reported that C3G inhibited breast cancer-induced angiogenesis.[33] Harada et al. also evaluated the role of D3G on lipid accumulation and concluded that D3G inhibits the accumulation caused by palmitic acid.[34]

IMPACT ON THE GUT MICROBIOME

The gut microbiome has a vital role in the development of chronic inflammation, obesity, and finally diabetes. Zhao et al. reported the gut microbiota effect of mice using Saskatoon berry powder with a high-fat, high-sucrose diet for 15 weeks. The results deciphered that the high-fat, high-sucrose diet significantly increases the Firmicutes/Bacteroidetes ratio at the phylum level compared to the control diet group. The reason for the ratio increase was due to a decrease in the abundance of S24-7 in the feces of mice. There was a 40% increase in the abundance of S24-7 family bacteria in the gut upon supplementation of 5% Saskatoon berry extract, but this change was not significantly beneficial due to high-fat, high-sucrose diet. The availability of S24-7 family bacteria was negatively recorded with triglyceride, insulin, glucose, body weight, HOMA-IR, cholesterol, PAI-1, TNFα, and MCP-1.[35] The study concluded that the administration of 5% Saskatoon berry extract improves the gut microbiota profile by a relative increase in the presence of good bacteria and results in hypoglycemic, hypolipidemic, and anti-inflammatory effects in mice.

ANTIDIABETIC EFFECTS OF SASKATOON BERRY

Currently, the most common diabetes treatment is oral antihyperglycemic drugs and the biological use of insulin. Traditional/folk healing practices are equally useful, though they also have a few drawbacks. The ingredients of Saskatoon berries, especially phenolic derivatives, are useful for reducing blood glucose levels, regulating fat accumulation, and treating and preventing excess blood glucose levels.[25] Ethnopharmacological records and molecular biology research have revealed Saskatoon berries as a natural food and the best natural medicine to cure and check body sugar ailments. North American Indigenous people have used the plant to treat diseases such as inflammation, cancer, and diabetes as part of their traditional practices. Johnston has reported the use of leaves and twigs of the Saskatoon berry plant for making tea to prevent and cure diabetes in the Blackfoot Tribe of North America.[16] However, there is hardly any awareness beyond folklore about the impact of Saskatoon berries on diabetes treatment. Though one molecule closely related to diabetic complications (such as atherosclerosis, kidney disease, cataracts, neuropathy, and retinopathy) is 'aldose reductase' found in Saskatoon berries. It is used to prevent or delay the onset of diabetic side effects. Phyto-derived aldose reductase inhibitors are grouped as alkaloids, phenolics, flavonoids, and terpenoids. In a study focused on the antidiabetic activities of Saskatoon berries, Burns Kraft et al. reported 82% inhibition of aldose reductase by the nonpolar fraction of Saskatoon berries. The polar fraction of Saskatoon berries, rich in phenolic acids, anthocyanins, and proanthocyanidins, lowers the elevated blood sugar levels to normal and potentially reduces the expression of IL-1β and COX-2. Furthermore, it was reported that the Saskatoon berries can regulate lipid utilization in the body, thereby ameliorating biotic syndrome.[14]

Zhang et al. have demonstrated that leaf extract of Saskatoon berry and its sub-fractions strongly suppress mammalian α-glucosidase activity, delay or inhibit carbohydrates absorption, and significantly lower postprandial blood glucose levels in mice with high-fat diet-induced obesity and hyperglycemia.[15]

Moghadasian et al. have used Saskatoon berries powder in the diet of mice for different body ailments glucose levels. In type 2 diabetes animal model roughly a 30% decrease in blood and urine glucose levels was observed compared to the control model.[36]

Different scientists in different studies have concluded that Saskatoon berries have the potential to interfere with different biological pathways underlying hyperglycemia. Increased amounts of glyLDL or oLDL and concerned body toxicity (oxidative stress, apoptosis, mitochondrial dysfunction, etc.) are cured and prevented by Saskatoon berries.[37-39] Zhao et al. have described a study conducted in 24 male C57BL/6J mice, divided into three groups according to diet and fed for 15 weeks as control, high-fat/high-sucrose (HF+HS), and HF+HS+5% Saskatoon berries. The group with the high-fat/high-sucrose diet was reported to have increased plasma levels of glucose, cholesterol, triglycerides, etc., compared to the control group. The HF+HS+5% Saskatoon berries diet group showed a delayed increase in body weight and suppressed HF+HS plasma levels of glucose, cholesterol, triglyceride, etc., including the diet-induced disorders, compared to the high-fat/high-sucrose group.[2]

SCOPE AND OPPORTUNITIES

Chemical composition-related studies on *A. spicata* in Poland (case study-1) on three species of the genus *Amelanchier* revealed that each species has its unique ingredients and polyphenol content.[40]

CASE STUDY

In Poland, there are three species of *Amelanchier,* namely, *A. alnifolia*, *A. ovalis*, and *A. spicata*, which have close resemblances. Ochmian et al.[40] have conducted a study to characterize these three species of the genus *Amelanchier.* Plants of all three species were grown in the Research Stations (Danowo and Rajkowo), near Szczecin, Poland, and examined for the size and color of their leaves and fruit quality (firmness, chemical composition, size, and bioflavonoids). Saskatoon fruits were reported for low pH and vitamin C content. *A. ovalis* has the smallest fruit but the highest polyphenol content. *A. spicata* is characterized by the smallest but greenest leaves. Its fruits are relatively big, have higher extractive value, and have comparatively less polyphenolics than *A. ovalis*. During the experiment, all the cultivated plants of the genus *Amelanchier* did not indicate any frost damage, symptoms of disease, or pest infestation. Fruits were rich in polyphenols with a low content of organic acids and a mild flavor, which differentiated these from the chokeberries that have a similar appearance.

During the field experiment, each species was monitored differently from the others in terms of morphological features, quality, and chemical composition of fruits.[40,41] Furthermore, Saskatoon berries are not too familiar to the public for therapeutic purposes and are used primarily as bakery goods, jams, jellies, beers, pies, snack food, syrups, spreads, cereal, wines, cider, and ice cream.[2]

The folklore applications of the species are a clue for its future applications, as at present there is an increasing demand for green medicines due to their negligible or least side effects. Currently, oral use of antihyperglycemic compounds and insulin therapy is focused on the clinical treatments of diabetes patients, though there are many treatments. There are limitations and harmful side effects of each. So, there is a need for research into alternative treatments, as the number of diabetes patients is on the rise. There are limited studies on the therapeutic potential and benefits of the nutrients and other ingredients of Saskatoon berry and other parts of the plant species.

Furthermore, research on the health benefits of Saskatoon berries is mainly confined to animal models. Clinical studies on humans are required to verify the beneficial effects of Saskatoon berry and its products, especially for sugar management. Each plant part (buds, stem, stem bark, fruits, peels, and leaves), extracts, and its active compound(s) of the species responsible for therapeutic benefits are to be determined.

The berries have potent preventative and therapeutic impacts on diseases such as cancers, diabetes, inflammation, cardiovascular problems, obesity, neuro-disorders, muscular degeneration, etc. Research data on Saskatoon berries and diabetes are still not sufficient, and a long-term, large-population, randomized clinical study is needed. A variety of products with clinical data that are easily accessible to consumers on the market is a need of the hour, and Saskatoon berries may be one of the best modern green medicines for the prevention and treatment of diabetes in the future.

Saskatoon berry is a localized and seasonal crop. Its storage condition or a preferable form is to be optimized for using it as a functional food/-health supplement to overcome chronic diseases. Future studies on the safety and dose determination of Saskatoon berry products for common chronic diseases and the identification of active compounds are to be investigated. Furthermore, a detailed literature survey reveals confusion in the local names of species like Juneberry, Serviceberry, and Saskatoon. It is to be clear that Saskatoon, Serviceberry, and Juneberry are the same or different species.

REFERENCES

1. Adhikari DP, Francis JA, Schutzki RE, Chandra A. Nair MG. 2005. Quantification and characterization of cyclo-oxygenase and lipid peroxidation inhibitory anthocyanins in fruits of *Amelanchier. Phytochemical Analysis.* 16: 175–180.
2. Zhao L, Huang F, Hui A L, Shen G X. 2020. Review Article Bioactive components and health benefits of Saskatoon Berry. *Journal of Diabetes Research.* 2020: Article ID 3901636. 8 pages. https://doi.org/10.1155/2020/3901636.
3. St-Pierre RG, Zatylny AM, Tulloch HP. 2005. Evaluation of growth and fruit production characteristics of 15 Saskatoon (*Amelanchier alnifolia* Nutt.) cultivars at maturity. *Canadian Journal of Plant Science.* 85 (4): 929–932.
4. Lavola A, Karjalainen R, Julkunen-Tiitto R. 2012. Bioactive polyphenols in leaves, stems, and berries of Saskatoon (*Amelanchier alnifolia* Nutt.) cultivars. *Journal of Agricultural and Food Chemistry.* 60 (4): 1020–1027.
5. Jurikova T, Balla S, Sochor J, Pohanka M, Mlcek J, Baron M. 2013. Flavonoid profile of Saskatoon berries (*Amelanchier alnifolia* Nutt.) and their health promoting effects. *Molecules.* 18 (10): 12571–12586.
6. Binggeli P. 1988. Plants of the Pacific Northwest in Western Europe. *Botanical Electronic News* 195.
7. Kuusk V, Tabaka L, Jankeviciene R. 1996. *Flora of the Baltic Countries.* Eesti Loodusfoto AS, Tartu. pp. 372.
8. Mazza G. 2005. Compositional and functional properties of Saskatoon berry and blueberry. *International Journal of Fruit Science.* 5: 101–120.
9. Han X, Shen T, Lou H. 2007. Dietary polyphenols and their biological significance. *International Journal of Molecular Sciences.* 8: 950–988.
10. Mazza G. 1982. Chemical composition of Saskatoon berries (*Amelanchier alnifolia* Nutt.). *Journal of Food Science.* 47: 1730–1731.
11. Bakowska-Barczak A, Kolodziejczyk P. 2008. Evaluation of Saskatoon berry (*Amelanchier alnifolia* Nutt.) Cultivars for their polyphenol content, antioxidant properties, and storage stability. *Journal of Agricultural and Food Chemistry.* 56: 9933–9940.
12. Finn C. 1999. Temperate berry crops. In: *Perspectives on New Crops and New Uses.* Janick J. (Ed.) ASHS Press, Alexandria, VA. pp. 324–334.
13. Jagadeesha P M, Ravikumar B, Ramesh M H, Nagar D. 2014. Nutritional value of some unexploited fruit crops. 2nd International Conference on Agricultural & Horticultural Sciences, Tamil Nadu Agricultural University, India. *Agrotechnology.* 2: 4. https://doi.org/10.4172/2168-9881.S1.008
14. Burns Kraft T F, Dey M, Rogers R B, Ribnicky DM, Gipp DM, Cefalu WT, Raskin I, Lila MA. 2008. Phytochemical composition and metabolic performance-enhancing activity of dietary berries traditionally used by native North Americans. *Journal of Agricultural and Food Chemistry.* 56 (3): 654–660.
15. Zhang AJ, Rimando AM, Fish W, Mentreddy SR, Mathews ST. 2012. Serviceberry [*Amelanchier alnifolia* (Nutt.) Nutt. Ex . M. Roem (Rosaceae)] leaf extract inhibits mammalian α-glucosidase activity and suppresses postprandial glycemic response in a mouse model of diet-induced obesity and hyperglycemia. *Journal of Ethnopharmacology.* 143 (2): 481–487.
16. Johnston A.1987. Plants and the Blackfoot. *Lethbridge Historical Society.* 15: 1–68.

17. Lachowicz S, Oszmiański J, Pluta S. 2017. The composition of bioactive compounds and antioxidant activity of Saskatoon berry (*Amelanchier alnifolia* Nutt.) genotypes grown in central Poland. *Food Chemistry*. 235 (1): 234–243.
18. Lachowicz S, Oszmiański J. Seliga L, Pluta S. 2017. Phytochemical composition and antioxidant capacity of seven Saskatoon berry (*Amelanchier alnifolia* Nutt.) genotypes grown in Poland. *Molecules*. 22 (5): 853. https://doi.org/10.3390/molecules22050853
19. Jin AL, Ozga JA, Kennedy JA, Koerner-Smith JL, Botar G, Reinecke DM. 2015. Developmental profile of anthocyanin, flavonol, and proanthocyanidin type, content, and localization in Saskatoon fruits (*Amelanchier alnifolia* Nutt.). *Journal of Agricultural and Food Chemistry*. 63 (5): 1601–1614.
20. Prasain JK, Barnes S. 2014. Uptake and metabolism of dietary Proanthocyanidins. *Polyphenols in Human Health and Disease*. 1: 553–560.
21. Ochmian I, Oszmianski J, Skupien K. 2009. Chemical composition, phenolics and firmness of small black fruits. *Journal of Applied Botany and Food Quality*. 83: 64–69.
22. Hosseinian FS, Beta T. 2007. Saskatoon and wild blueberries have higher anthocyanin contents than other Manitoba berries. *Journal of Agricultural and Food Chemistry*. 55 (26): 10832–10838.
23. Marcano E. 2017. DFT study of anthocyanidin and anthocyanin pigments for dye-sensitized solar cells: electron injecting from the excited states and adsorption onto TiO_2 (anatase) surface. *Physical Sciences Reviews*. 2 (6): 9. https://doi.org/10.1515/psr-2017-0008
24. Ozga J A, Saeed A, Wismer W, Reinecke D M. 2007. Characterization of cyanidin- and quercetin-derived flavonoids and other phenolics in mature Saskatoon fruits (*Amelanchier alnifolia* Nutt.). *Journal of Agricultural and Food Chemistry*. 55 (25): 10414–10424.
25. Meczarska K, Cyboran-Mikolajczyk S, Wloch A, Bonarska-Kujawa D, Oszmianski J, Kleszczynska H. 2017. Polyphenol content and bioactivity of Saskatoon berry (*Amelanchier alnifolia* nutt.) leaves and berries. *Acta Poloniae Pharmaceutica-Drug Research*. 74 (2): 660–669.
26. Vinayagam R, Xu B. 2015. Antidiabetic properties of dietary flavonoids: a cellular mechanism review. *Nutrition & Metabolism*. 12 (1). https://doi.org/10.1186/s12986-015-0057-7
27. Bakowska-Barczak AM, Marianchuk M, Kolodziejczyk P. 2007. Survey of bioactive components in Western Canadian berries. [A selection of papers published in this special issue (part 2 of 2) on the Safety and Efficacy of Natural Health Products]. *Canadian Journal of Physiology and Pharmacology*. 85 (11): 1139–1152.
28. Hosseinian FS, Li W, Hydamaka AW, Tsopmo A, Lowry L, Friel J, Beta T. 2007. Pro-anthocyanidin profile and ORAC values of Manitoba berries, chokecherries, and sea buckthorn. *Journal of Agricultural and Food Chemistry*. 55 (17): 6970–6976.
29. Hellstrom J, Sinkkonen J, Karonen M, Mattila P. 2007. Isolation and structure elucidation of procyanidin oligomers from Saskatoon berries (*Amelanchier alnifolia*). *Journal of Agricultural and Food Chemistry*. 55 (1): 157–164.
30. Xie X, Zhao R, Shen GX. 2012. Influence of delphinidin-3-glucoside on oxidized low-density lipoprotein-induced oxidative stress and apoptosis in cultured endothelial cells. *Journal of Agricultural and Food Chemistry*. 60(7):1850–1856.
31. Shen X, Li G, Deng X, Wang J, Zhang P. 2019. Cyanidin 3-O-glucoside chloride attenuates Streptococcus suis-induced inflammation by inhibiting MAPK and NF-κB signaling pathways in murine macrophage J774 cells. *Journal of Microbiology and Biotechnology*. 19 (1). https://doi.org/10.4014/jmb.1904.04036
32. Li X, Guo J, Jiang X, Sun J, Tian L, Jiao R, Tang Y, Bai W. 2019. Cyanidin-3-O-glucoside protects against cadmium-induced dysfunction of sex hormone secretion via the regulation of hypothalamus-pituitary-gonadal axis in male pubertal mice. *Food and Chemical Toxicology*. 29: 13–21.
33. Ma X, Ning S. 2019. Cyanidin-3-glucoside attenuates the angiogenesis of breast cancer via inhibiting STAT3/VEGF pathway. *Phytotherapy* Research. 33 (1): 81–89.
34. Harada G, Onoue S, Inoue C, Hanada S, Katakura Y. 2018. Delphinidin-3-glucoside suppresses lipid accumulation in HepG2 cells. *Cytotechnology*. 70 (6): 1707–1712.
35. Zhao R, Khafipour E, Sepehri S, Huang F, Beta T, G. Shen X. 2019. Impact of Saskatoon berry powder on insulin resistance and relationship with intestinal microbiota in high fat–high sucrose diet-induced obese mice. *Journal of Nutritional Biochemistry*. 69:130–138
36. Moghadasian MH. 2019. The potential anti-diabetic effects of Saskatoon berry in experimental mouse models. *Austin Journal of Nutrition Food Sciences*. 7 (1). https://austinpublishinggroup.com/nutrition-food-sciences/fulltext/ajnfs-v7-id1111.php, as on 3rd October 2020.
37. Zhao R, Shen GX. 2007. Involvement of heat shock factor-1 in glycated LDL-induced upregulation of plasminogen activator inhibitor-1 in vascular endothelial cells. *Diabetes*. 56 (5): 1436–1444.
38. Zhao R, Le K, Moghadasian MH, Shen GX. 2013. Regulatory role of NADPH oxidase in glycated LDL-induced upregulation of plasminogen activator inhibitor-1 and heat shock factor-1 in mouse embryo fibroblasts and diabetic mice. *Free Radical Biology & Medicine*. 61: 18–25.
39. Xie X, Zhao R, Shen G. 2012. Impact of cyanidin-3-glucoside on glycated LDL-induced NADPH oxidase activation, mitochondrial dysfunction and cell viability in cultured vascular endothelial cells. *International Journal of Molecular* Sciences. 13 (12): 15867–15880.
40. Ochmian I, Kubus M, Dobrowolska A. 2013. Description of plants and assessment of chemical properties of three species from the *Amelanchier* genus. Dendrobiology. 70: 59–64.
41. Joshi DD, Uniyal RC. 2008. Different chemo-types of Gokhru (*Tribulus terrestris*): a herb used for improving physique and physical performance. *International Journal of Green Pharmacy*. 2(3): 138–141.

5 *Berberis aristata* (Kinmod)

INTRODUCTION

Berberis aristata DC. (Daruharidra,[1,2] Tree Turmeric,[1,2] Kinmod[3]), a spiny shrub native to the northern Himalayan region, is widely distributed from the Indian Himalayas to Bhutan and the hilly areas of Nepal.[1,2] It is also found in the Nilgiri hills in South India.[4] The family Berberidaceae consists of the most important natural wild fruits and comprises about 14 genera and 700 species.[5] *Berberis*, commonly known as barberry, is one of the genera of the family Berberidaceae.[6] As per geo-climatic conditions, barberry has different types of fruits, including seedless and seeded. The plants of the seeded type fruits are commonly found as natural vegetation in mountainous areas to protect soil against erosion or as decoration. The fruits of barberry are sometimes edible.[7] The seedless type of fruits is used as a food additive after drying in some countries, such as Iran.[6] Iran produces 95% of the world's seedless barberry fruits and is the largest producer globally.[8] Every year, Iran produces more than 5,000 tons of seedless barberry fruits.[9] South Khorasan, a province of Iran, has been reported to have the highest production of seedless barberry in the last 20 years, due to its suitable cultivation conditions, particularly the edaphic conditions favorable for the growth of the species.[10]

Recent concepts of food supplements or nutraceuticals have attracted the attention of many researchers toward unexploited barberry fruits. Literature reveals that barberry fruits are a good source of nutritional and therapeutic ingredients. These fruits have higher amounts of antioxidant components and low sugar, fat, protein, fiber,[11] and other ingredients of medicinal significance.[12] Barberry fruit and its bioactive components are used in the health and food industries.[13] In Persia, carbonated drinks, chocolates, marmalades, foods, sauces, jellies, and fruit nectars are made from barberry fruit. Fruit pigments are used as natural food colorants due to their attractive color.[14] Pigments of barberry fruits have health-promoting ingredients such as carotenoids, phenolic compounds, anthocyanins, and flavonoids.[15] These phyto-ingredients contribute to anti-mutagenic, anti-inflammatory,[16] and antioxidant activities; inhibit certain enzymes; prevent hepatitis; and protect food in the stomach from damage caused by free radicals, which are responsible for many chronic diseases.[17] *B. lycium* reduces blood cholesterol[11] and serum cholesterol and is effective as a growth promoter.[18]

The fruits of *B. aristata* are globose to ovoid and are usually covered with a bloom as in plums. Fruits are 7 mm long, 4 mm in diameter, weighing 227 mg, and 237 microliters in volume, with an aconite violet color (Figure 5.1). Seeds are 2 to 5 in number, varying in color as per age from yellow to pink, each weighing 25 mg and being 29 microliters in volume.[19]

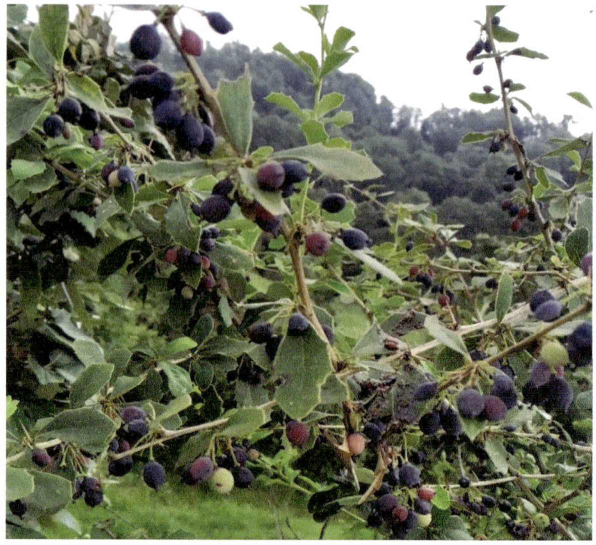

FIGURE 5.1 *B. aristata*: branch with mature fruits.

ETHNOPHARMACOLOGY

Barberry has a long history of use in Indian traditional medicines. The species of the genus have therapeutic roles in countries such as India, Iran, and Turkey. It has been used for treating eye diseases, fever, jaundice, gallbladder and kidney stones, rheumatism, vomiting during pregnancy, etc., in Asian and some European countries.[20] Traditional healing systems use barberry to cure different body ailments, especially internal wounds, bone fractures, and hepatitis.[21] It is also used as a tonic for the heart to prevent cardiovascular disease, control chronic bleeding, and reduce blood pressure.[14] It has a positive response to gallbladder treatment, neurological disorders, asthma, gout, kidney stones, prostate inflammation, and colon cancer.[22]

In traditional therapies, the extract of barberry is used to treat rheumatism and chronic inflammation.[23] In Europe, it is used to cure fever, biliary and liver diseases, and uterine bleeding.[24] In China, it is used as an antimicrobial, while in Japan, the bark of barberry is used as an antispasmodic, coolant, antiseptic, antipyretic, and to stop internal bleeding.[25] In folk medicine, the barberry plant is used as a painkiller, and its different parts are used in antibacterial, anti-fever, and itching treatments.[22,26] Currently, many pure phytochemicals from barberry are in use, and the most common is berberine, in the form of capsules, therapeutic creams, and complementary pills as over-the-counter

DOI: 10.1201/9781003512868-7

products globally. Chewing of *B. aristata* leaves results in a firmness of the gums. *Berberis* plants have an astringent property and reduce the side effects of vitamin C deficiency.[27] Barberry leaves are used to treat gastric ulcers and diarrhea problems. Leaves may be used either alone or mixed with other herbs.[10] Flowers of the species are used to treat rheumatism.[28] Barberry fruits have a sour and pleasant taste and unique applications in the food industry as food additives in sauces or food products such as desserts, beverages, jellies, and fruit rollers (Lavashak).[6] Barberry fruits are utilized in folk and traditional medicine against colitis,[29] treatment of acute and chronic inflammation,[30] effects on heart contractility,[31] treatment of high blood pressure and nervous problems such as seizure and epilepsy,[22] and for reducing cell viability.[10,32] In India, barberry fruits are used as an appetizing tonic and antimicrobial to treat injuries, and their dried extract is a throat disinfectant.[33,34] The barberry fruits have alkaloids, carotenoids, flavonoids, phenolics, anthocyanins, and minerals (Ca, Fe, K, P, and Na). Barberry fruits are a good source of K (~0.6–14.0 mg/g) along with other minerals.[35–37] Fruits have the highest quantity of phenolic compounds and chlorogenic acid. The pH of barberry fruits is between 2.5 and 3.9. The main components of fruits are proteins (9–103 mg/g), carbohydrates (162–248.5 mg/g), and fats (~5.2–29.6 mg/g).[38]

In Ayurvedic medicines, *B. aristata* is used to treat skin disease, jaundice, inflammation, wound healing, menorrhagia, infection of the eyes, and diarrhea. 'Rashut (Rasanjana or Rasavanti)', a valuable Ayurvedic medicine, is prepared from the *B. aristata* plant.[39,40] 'Rashut' is a thick, hot, aqueous concentrate made from the root bark, roots, and lower stem wood of *B. aristata*. The drug is a bitter tonic and is used as an antipyretic, cholagogue, laxative, diaphoretic, stomachic, and antiseptic. It is used in eye diseases, particularly in conjunctivitis, indolent ulcers, and hemorrhoids. *B. aristata* plant, either alone or in combination with other herbs, has efficacy against premature ejaculation, allergic conjunctivitis, fungal infection, acne vulgaris, viral hepatitis, and rheumatic pain. *B. asiatica* possesses antiperiodic, diaphoretic, astringent, and stomachic properties. Leaf extract has been reported to be hepatoprotective against paracetamol-induced liver damage in rats. The fruit, either fresh or in dried form, has cholesterol-lowering activity.[41] The whole plant extract is used as a cream, namely the 'Dermocept'. Dermocept is utilized to treat sarcoptic mange lesions. Additionally, the whole plant extract is used in an Ayurvedic formulation to inhibit *Salmonella typhi* in vitro. The whole plant extract, as an ingredient of a formulation, has anti-amoebic activity against *Entamoeba histolytica*. The whole plant extract is used to inhibit the activities of the aldolase, DNAse, alkaline phosphatase, RNAse, acid phosphatase, protease, and α-amylase.[42]

B. asiatica, as a drug, minimizes hepatic lesions due to paracetamol poisoning. In Nepal, a hot water extract from leaf-bud is used to treat eye inflammation and toothache.[43] Tea from its berries is used as a laxative, diuretic, appetizer, expectorant, and medicine to treat jaundice, hepatitis, diarrhea, and hemorrhages. It is also considered an antiseptic, diaphoretic, and astringent. The root bark tincture is used for arthritis, sciatica, and rheumatism. In the Chinese healing system of medicine, barberry is used to increase white blood cells and platelets after radiation or chemotherapy.[44]

PHYTOCHEMICAL SCREENING

Barberry flowers are rich in flavonoids, chlorogenic acid, palmatine, berberine, vitamins, and caffeic acid.[24,45] The roots, stems, shoots, flowers, and leaves of the barberry plant contain anthocyanins, berberine, berbamine, flavonoids, oxyacanthine, polyphenols, vitamins, and minerals. These compounds have therapeutic applications and have been widely applied in pharmaceutical industries.[46] Fruits of *B. aristata* have berbamine,[47] chlorogenic acid (86.3 mg/g), magnoflorine (1.8 mg/g), isocorydine (1.8 mg/g), glaucine (0.2 mg/g), jatrorrhizine (0.3 mg/g), tetrahydropalmatine (0.37 mg/g), tetrahydroberberine (0.1 mg/g), palmatine (0.01 mg/g), and berberine (3 mg/g).[48] *B. aristata* fruits have the highest amounts of anthocyanins in the genus *Berberis*, although all species of barberry have anthocyanins in fruits, which impart a fascinating color to them.[35] The concentration of anthocyanins is 4,684 mg/L in *B. asiatica*, the highest quantity in all barberry species. The astringent and bitter taste of fruits is due to the presence of tannins.[24]

Leaves of different barberry species have alkaloids, flavonoids, phenolic compounds, vitamins, and anthocyanins. Mazandarani et al. have reported that barberry leaves contain flavonoids (quercetin, 59.9 mg/g), anthocyanins (cyanidin-3-glucoside, 11.34 mg/g), and phenolic compounds (gallic acid, 29.4 mg/g).[46] Chlorogenic acid has a relatively higher amount in different species,[48] revealing the higher antioxidant properties of leaves. Leaves of *B. asiatica* have chlorogenic acid (38 mg/g) and berberine (1.9 mg/g).[48] Leaves of *B. asiatica* are used as a valuable source in the food and pharma industries for functional ingredients because of flavonoids and vitamin C.[48]

The stems of barberry have the lowest quantity of phenolic compounds. Chlorogenic acid is absent in stems of the *Berberis* genus except for *B. petiolaris* and *B. spseudoumbellata*.[48] There is also a very low concentration of flavonoid (quercetin, 8.2 mg/g) in the stems, and anthocyanins are absent altogether in the stems of the genus *Berberis*.[46] Tannins and fiber have been reported in *B. asiatica* stem bark.[49]

Berberine is one of the most potent therapeutic compounds in barberry. It occurs in different parts of the plant but is more common in the stem and roots. The highest amount of berberine is reported in the bark of *B. asiatica* and the shoot of *B. lyceum*. The assay of berberine is 102.3 and 158.5 mg/g, respectively.[48] Berberine is a pharmacopeial compound of many countries, including USP, BP, IP, JP, etc. Different studies reveal the therapeutic effects and functional properties of berberine, such as antimicrobial,[50] anti-inflammatory, antidiabetic, antioxidant, antidepressant, anticancer, antihypertensive, hepatoprotective, antidiarrheal, and hypolipidemic properties.[51] Berberine has been reported to decrease elevated fasting blood glucose and insulin levels, total cholesterol, and triglyceride levels.[52] Alzheimer's disease is cured using the stem/stem bark of the barberry plant because of the berberine.[53] Italian folk use barberry bark as an effective drug to treat spleen swelling, varicose veins, hemorrhoids, and rheumatism.[22] Phytochemical screening of barberry root has revealed the presence of the highest levels of alkaloids in the roots. The protoberberine and bis-benzyl-quinolones alkaloids are the main compounds having anti-inflammatory and immunosuppressive properties.[54] Due to this reason, most of the investigations are focused on the roots of the family. *B. lycium* has the highest amount of berberine (172.8 mg/g) in its roots, the highest quantity among all species.[48] Carbohydrates, phenolic compounds, flavonoids, saponins, and minerals are the main compounds found in barberry root. Ca and K are the main minerals in roots.[49] Vitamin C, fibers, and tannins have also been reported in the root of the genus *Berberis*.[49] Flavonoids are in higher concentration compared to phenolic compounds. In roots, chlorogenic acid and anthocyanins are absent.[46,48]

The root and root bark possess anti-inflammatory, anti-nociceptive, antipyretic, antibacterial, and antifungal activities, and the bark is useful for treating the liver disorders.[55,56] In Romania, roots and stem barks are used to treat hepatitis and kidney disease.[10] In Mexico, the roots of barberry are used to treat stomach and liver cancers, respectively. In China and Japan, the bark of *Berberis* roots is used as an anti-parasite and antiseptic and is used to treat fever, hepatic and cystic duct obstruction, jaundice, gallstones, and kidney stones.[28]

The global application of the genus *Berberis* in folk and traditional systems of medicine has resulted in considerable chemical screening of the plant and its ingredients. The phytochemical investigations have revealed more than 105 compounds with varying structures and therapeutic properties. Among these ingredients' phenolic compounds, alkaloids, anthocyanins, carotenoids, minerals, and vitamins are the major chemical classes. Berberine is the main therapeutic alkaloid of *B. aristata*, while other minor alkaloids are berbamine, jatrorrhizine, and palmatine. Glycosides, flavonoids, phenols, resin, and tannins are present in the fruits. *Berberis* fruits have a higher value of protein, fat, minerals, and fiber compared to cultivated fruits like apples. It is reported that 200 g of Berberis fruits have enough nutrients required by a person per day.[57]

SCOPE AND OPPORTUNITIES

B. asiatica plant is an important source of potentially useful compounds, which have clues for structure-related therapeutic activities. The structure-related clues are a silent guide for the development of new therapeutic agents, especially synthetic analogues/metabolites, even with a very short life span. Compounds with a very short life span may be stabilized in a nitrogen/inert environment, and the delivery mode may be selected as per the properties of the ingredients. The first step toward this goal is the in vitro and in vivo assay. The results of such studies lead to repeatability and reproducibility tests for clinical trials, a step in new drug development. New drug development is like nourishing a kid until the age of citizenship, a long and tiresome journey, so clues from folk are helpful in the reverse pharmacological drug development program.

Ethanolic extract of *B. asiatica* fruits shows significant activity against *Streptococcus pyogenes*, *Streptococcus aureus,* and *Bacillus cereus,* as well as against food poisoning bacteria and fungi. The in vitro antimicrobial studies of *B. asiatica* have considerable efficacy against various pathogenic bacteria. The study provides a scientific basis for the use of the plant as folk medicine.

The fruits of *B. asiatica* have a high level of essential nutrients, including minerals, carbohydrates, proteins, and lipids. Additionally, a few more advanced pharmacological and clinical studies would be required to investigate the in vivo mechanism of the nutraceutical effects of species. The chemo-compositional properties decipher the nutraceutical value due to the presence of ascorbic acid, anthocyanin, flavonoids, carotenoids, phenolic compounds, protein, total reducing and non-reducing sugar, fat, fiber, and minerals. In addition, further studies are required to determine the herb-herb interaction for a more effective multi-herbal formulation to support folklore utilizations.

Additionally, limited studies have been conducted on the plants of the barberry family seeded type, as the presence of seeds reveals chances of more valuable compounds compared to the seedless type.[35,36] Furthermore, abiotic conditions significantly affect the therapeutic composition of the plant. It is a matter of concern to chemically screen fruits of the species globally so that economical uses of fruits could be categorized as nutraceutical and pharmaceutical applications.

B. aristata (Daruharidra) is an Ayurvedic medicinal plant and is used as an astringent, antipyretic, antiperiodic, antidiabetic, and stomachic in the treatment of jaundice and eye infections. Due to its excessive harvesting by Ayurvedic/pharmaceutical industries, another species of *Berberis,* viz., *B. asiatica,* is being used as a substitute.[58] Rathi et al. have investigated anatomical similarities and differences between both species of *Berberis* (*B. aristata* and *B. asiatica*). Though both species have similarities mostly in external features, their microscopic and quantitative microscopic characters are quite different. The chemical and pharmacological work on both these plant species is fairly documented, but concrete comparative documentation is lacking, even though all the parts (root, stem, and leaf) of these two species are used in Ayurveda.[59]

REFERENCES

1. Anonymous. 2007. The Ayurvedic pharmacopoeia of India, Government of India, Ministry of health and family Welfare department of AYUSH, New Delhi. 2 (I): 34–36.
2. Anonymous. 1985. The Wealth of India Publications and Information Directorate CSIR. New Delhi. 2: 116–117.
3. Kumari P, Joshi GC, Tewari LM. 2011. Diversity and status of ethno-medicinal plants of Almora district in Uttarakhand, India. *International Journal of Biodiversity and Conservation*. 3 (7): 298–326.
4. Chauhan NS. 2006. *Medicinal and Aromatic Plant of Himachal Pradesh*. Indus Publishing Company, New Delhi. pp. 114–116.
5. Christenhusz MJM, Byng W. 2016. The number of known plants species in the world and its annual increase. *Phytotaxa*. 261 (3): 201–217.
6. Kafi M, Balandari A. 2004. *Barberry: Production and Processing*, 1st Edition. Ferdowsi University Publication, Mashhad.
7. Plants for a Future. 2019. Edible Shrubs: 70+ Top Shrubs, independently published. 2019. www.pfaf.org. ISBN-13: 978-1791954949.
8. Alemardan A, Asadi W, Rezaei M, Tabrizi L, Mohammadi S. 2013. Cultivation of Iranian seedless barberry (*Berberis integerrima* Bidaneh): a medicinal shrub. *Industries Crop Production*. 50: 276–287.
9. Sarraf M, Babaei AB, Naji-Tabasi S. 2019. Investigating functional properties of barberry species: an overview. *J Sci Food Agric*. 99: 5255–5269. https://doi.org/10.1002/jsfa.9804
10. Maskooki A, Mortazavi SA. 2013. *Extraction and Identification of Bioactive Compounds of Seedless Barberry Using Supercritical Fluid Carbon Dioxide and Subcritical Water Methods*. Project in Institute of Food Science and Technology. Mashhad, Iran.
11. Sood P, Modgil R, Sood M. 2010. Physicochemical and nutritional evaluation of indigenous wild fruit Kasmal *Berberis lyceum* Royel. *Indian Journal of Natural Products and Resources*. 1 (3): 362–366.
12. Gulfraz M, Qadir G, Nosheen F, Parveen Z. 2007. Anti-hyperglycemic effects of *Berberis lyceum* Royle in alloxan induced diabetic rats. *Diabetic Croatic*. 36 (3): 49–54.
13. Fallahi J, Rezvani P M, Nasiri M M. 2010. Effects of harvesting time on quantitative and qualitative properties of *B. vulgaris* fruit. *International Journal of Field Crops Research*. 8 (2): 225–234.
14. Ardestani SB, Sahari MA, Barzegar M, Abbasi S. 2013. Some physicochemical properties of Iranian native barberry fruits (Abi and Poloei): *Berberis integerrima* and *Berberis vulgaris*. *Journal of Food and Pharmaceutical Science*. 1: 67–74.
15. Giusti MM, Wrolstad RE. 2001. Characterization and measurement of anthocyanins by uv-visible spectroscopy. Unit F1.2. In: *Handbook of Food Analytical Chemistry*. Wrolstad R. E., Schwartz S. J. (Eds.) Wiley, New York. pp F1.2.1–F1.2.1.
16. Shamsa F, Ahmadiani A, Khosrokhavar R. 1999. Antihistaminic and anti-cholinergic activity of barberry fruit (*Berberis vulgaris*) in the guinea-pig ileum. *Journal of Ethno Pharmacology*. 64 (2): 161–166.
17. Svarcova I, Heinrich J, Valentova K. 2007. Berry fruits as a source of biologically active compounds: the case of *Lonicera caerulea*. *Biomed Pap Med Fac Univ Palacky Olomouc Czech Repub*. 151 (2): 163–174.
18. Chand N, Durrani FR, Qurashi MS, Durrani Z. 2007. Role of *Berberis lycium* in reducing serum cholesterol in broilers. *Asian-australian Journal of Animal Science*. 20 (4): 563–568.
19. Rashmi R, Rajasekaran A, Pant J. 2008. The genus *berberis* Linn: a review. *Pharmacognosy Review*. 2 (4): 368–385.
20. Srivastava SK, Srivastava M, Misra A, Pandey G, Rawat AKS. 2015. Review on biological and chemical diversity in *Berberis* (*Berberidaceae*). *EXCLIJ*. 14: 247–267.
21. Gulfraz M, Mehmood S, Ahmad A, Fatima N, Parveen Z, Williamson EM. 2008. Comparison of the antidiabetic activity of *Berberis lyceum* root extract and berberine in alloxan induced diabetic rats. *Phytotherapy Research*. 22 (9): 1208–1212.
22. Fatehi M, Saleh T, Fatehi M, Hassanabad Z, Farrokhfal KH, Jafarzadeh M, Davodi SA. 2005. A Pharmacological study on *Berberis vulgaris* fruit extract. *Journal of E*nthopharmacology.102: 46–52.
23. Zargari A. 1997. *Medicinal Plants*. Tehran University of Medical Sciences, Tehran.
24. Imanshahidi M, Hosseinzadeh H. 2008. Pharmacological and therapeutic effects of *Berberis vulgaris* and its active constituent, berberine. *Phytotherapy Research*. 22: 999–1012
25. Tang J, Feng Y, Tsao S, Wang N, Curtain R, Wang Y, 2009. Review; Berberine and coptidis rhizoma as novel antineoplastic agents: a review of traditional use and biomedical investigations. *Journal of E*thnopharmacology. 126: 5–17.
26. Kunwar RM, Nepal BK, Kshhetri HB, Rai SK and Bussmann RW, 2006. Ethnomedicine in Himalaya: a case study from Dolpa, Humla, Jumla and Mustang districts of Nepal. J Ethnobiol Ethnomed. 2: 44–45
27. Samsam SH. 1992. *Extraction of Effective Components from Medicinal Plants and Their Diagnostic and Evaluation Methods*. Mani Press, Esfehan, Iran. Vol. 1: pp. 8–20.
28. Javadzadeh SM, Fallah SR. 2012. Therapeutic application of different parts *Berberis vulgaris*. *International Journal of Agriculture and Crop Sciences*. 4: 404–440.
29. Minaiyan M, Ghannadi A, Mahzouni P, Jaffari-Shirazi E. 2011. Comparative study of *Berberis vulgaris* fruit extract and berberine chloride effects on acetic acid-induced colitis in rats. *Iranian Journal of Pharmaceutical Research*. 10: 97–104.
30. Kiasalari Z, Khalili M, Ahmadi P. 2011. Effect of alcoholic extract of *Berberis vulgaris* fruit on acute and chronic inflammation in male rats. *Journal of Babol University of Medical Sciences*. 13: 28–35.
31. Bhardwaj D, Kaushik N. 2012. Phytochemical and pharmacological studies in genus *Berberis*. *Phytochemistry* Reviews. 11: 523–542.
32. Hanachi P, Kua SH, Asmah R, Motalleb G, Fauziah O. 2006. Cytotoxic effect of *Berberis vulgaris* fruit extract on the proliferation of human liver cancer line (HepG2) and its antioxidant properties. *International Journal of Cancer Research*. 2: 1–9.
33. Shrinivas K, Kulkarni K, Dhir A. 2008. On the mechanism of antidepressant-like action of berberine chloride. *European Journal of* Pharmacology. 589: 163–172.
34. Kerry B. 2003. *A Clinical Guide to Blending Liquid Herbs: Herbal Formulations for the Individual Patient*, 1st Edition. Churchill Livingstone, St Louis, MO. Vol. 87.
35. Farhadi CM, Varidi M, Varidi MJ and Shahidi F. 2014. Evaluation of physical and chemical characteristics of three Iranian barberry species. *Journal of Food Research at University of Tabriz*. 24: 63–76.

36. Berenji AS, Sahari MA, Barzegar M, Abbasi S. 2013. Some physicochemical properties of Iranian native barberry fruits (abi and poloei): (*Berberis integerrima* and *Berberis vulgaris*). *Journal of Food and Pharmaceutical Sciences*. 1: 60–67.
37. Akbulut M, Sedat C, Marakog T, Coklari H. 2007. Some physic mechanical and nutritional properties of barberry (*Berberis vulgaris* L.) fruits. *Journal of Food and Science Technology*. 32: 497–511.
38. Wierzchowski Z, Budicz M. 1969. Carotenoids of the berries of *B. vulgaris*. *Lublin-Polpnia Sect C*. 14: 382–405.
39. Kurian A, Ssankar M. 2007. *Medicinal Plant Horticulture Sciences*. Ashe. Ed. Prof. KV Peter. Series foreword by Pushpangandan. New India Publishing Agency, New Delhi. Vol. 2: pp. 299–300.
40. Parmar C, Kaushal MK. 1982. *Berberis aristata*: *Indian: Wild Fruits*. Kalyani Publishers, New Delhi, India. pp. 10–14.
41. Gilani AH, Janbaz KH. 1995. Preventive and curative effects of *Berberis aristata* Fruit extract on paracetamol and CCl_4-induced hepatotoxicity. *Phytotheray Research*. 9 (7): 489–494.
42. Sohni YR, Kaimal P, Bhatt RM. 1995. The anti-amoebic effect of a crude drug formulation of herbal extracts against *Entamoeba histolytica in- vitro* and *in- vivo*. *Journal of Ethnopharmacology*. 45 (1): 43–52.
43. Doreswamy R, Sharma D. 1995. Plant drug for liver disorder management. *Indian Drugs*. 32(4): 139–154.
44. Foster S, Duke J. 2000. *Medicinal Plants and Herbs*. Eastern/Central Ed., Houghton Mifflin Co. New York.
45. Zarei A, Changizi-Ashtiyani S, Taheri S, Ramezani M. 2015. A quick overview on some aspects of endocrinological and therapeutic effects of *Berberis vulgaris* L. *Avicenna Journal of Phytomedicine*. 5: 485–497.
46. Mazandarani M, Ghasemi N, Bayat H. 2013. Investigation of secondary active compounds of medical plant *Berberis vulgaris* L. and its comparison among different part of the plant in southeast of Golestan Province. *Environmental Research*. 8: 59–70.
47. Mokhber-Dezfuli N, Saeidnia S, Gohari AR, Kurepaz-Mahmoodabadi M. 2014. Phytochemistry and pharmacology of *Berberis* species. *Pharmacognosy Reviews*. 8: 8–15.
48. Singh A, Bajpai V, Kumar S, Arya KR, Sharma KR, Kumar B. Quantitative determination of isoquinoline alkaloids and chlorogenic acid in *Berberis* species using ultra high-performance liquid chromatography with hybrid triple quadrupole linear ion trap mass spectrometry. *Journal of Separation Science*. 38: 2007–2013.
49. Patni S, Saha AN, Meena H, Pandey KH, Manchanda A. 2012. Physicochemical, phytochemical, and elemental analysis of stem bark and roots of *Berberis asiatica*. *Advances in Applied Science Research*. 3: 3624–3628.
50. Kosalec I, Gregurek B, Kremer D, Zovko M, Sankovic K, Karlovic K. 2009. Croatian barberry (*Berberis croatica* Horvat): a new source of berberine–analysis and antimicrobial activity. *World Journal of Microbiology and Biotechnology* 25: 145–150.
51. Amritpal S, Sanjiv D, Navpreet K, Jaswinder S. 2010. Berberine: alkaloid with wide spectrum of pharmacological activities. *Journal of Natural Products (India)*. 3: 64–75.
52. Wu D, Wen W, Qi CL, Zhao RX, Lu JH, Zhong CY, Chen YY. 2012. Ameliorative effect of berberine on renal damage in rats with diabetes induced by high-fat diet and streptozotocin. *Phytomedicine*. 19: 712–718.
53. Habtemariam S. 2011. The therapeutic potential of *Berberis darwinii* stembark: quantification of berberine and *in-vitro* evidence for Alzheimer's disease therapy. *Natural Product Communications*. 6: 1089–1990.
54. Si-Ying L, Li-Hua L, Teh BS, Seow WK. 1989. Anti-inflammatory and immuno-suppressive properties of the bis-benzylquinolones: in-vitro comparisons of tetrandrine and berbamine. *International Journal of Immunopharmacology*. 11:395–401.
55. Kupeli E, Kosar M, Yesilada E, Baser KHC, Baser C. 2002. A comparative study on the anti-inflammatory, antinociceptive and antipyretic effects of iso-quinoline alkaloids from the roots of Turkish *Berberis* species. *Life Sciene*. 72: 645–657
56. Duraiswamy B, Abraham M, Saritha GS, Nanjan MJ, Suresh B. 2002. Studies on the antimicrobial potential of *Berberis tinctoria* Lesch root and root bark. *Indian Journal of Pharmaceutical Sciences*. 64: 586–588.
57. Saklani S, Chandra S, Kandari AS. 2011. *Berberis asiatica* future based excellent fruit in nutritional profile, antimicrobial, and antioxidant ingredients. *IRJP*. 2 (12): 213–216.
58. Kumar EP, Elshurafa AA, Elango E, Subburaju T, Suresh B. 1998. Anti -tumour effect of berberis asiatica roxb. Ex. Dc. On dalton's lymphoma ascite. *Ancient Science of Life*. 17(4): 290–299.
59. Rathi B, Sahu J, Kaul S, Khosa RL. 2013. Salient features of *Berberis aristata* and *Berberis asiatica*: a comparative pharmacognostical study. *Der Pharmacia Le*ttre. 5: 40–42.

6 *Cassia fistula* (Amaltas)

INTRODUCTION

Cassia fistula Linn. (fam.: Fabaceae), a wild tree, is known for its whole-body medicinal properties.[1] The species is globally used in different folk and traditional medicines, such as Ayurveda, Chinese, and Unani, to cure and prevent diseases. *C. fistula* is native to South Asia but cultivated in other parts of the world.[1] It has different chemical classes of therapeutic ingredients, such as potassium, rhein, sugar, and triterpenes. Pharmacological studies based on animals have confirmed that *C. fistula* plays a vital and potential role in disease management via the modulation of biological activities. Investigations have revealed that it has antifertility[1] and antimicrobial properties.[2,3] *C. fistula* is a moderate-sized deciduous tree distributed throughout India, growing 8.5–24 m in height.[4] Its flowers are long, drooping, yellow racemes. The pod is cylindrical and pulpy, and the seeds are light brown, hard, and shiny.[5] Ayurvedic medicine recognizes seeds as an antibilious aperitif, carminative, and laxative. *C. fistula* is native to India and Sri Lanka and diffused in various countries, including Mauritius, South Africa, East Africa, Mexico, the West Indies, and China. It is a national tree of Thailand.[6,7] The flower of *C. fistula* is the state flower of Kerala and the national flower of Thailand.[8] Its flowers are of ritual importance in the worship of Lord Vishnu, a Hindu deity, especially in a festival in Kerala, India.[8]

ETHNOPHARMACOLOGY

C. fistula has several ethnomedicinal applications and is extensively used in Ayurveda to treat many diseases.[9] Traditionally *C. fistula* is used to treat leukoderma, metabolic disorders, heart disorders, pruritic, etc.[10] *C. fistula* is used as an antioxidant, for uterine and menstrual disorders, thoracic obstructions, skeletal features, curing burns, depression, dysuria, and pest control.[1,10] The root is utilized as a laxative and purgative. The plant is used to cure fever, migraine, dysentery, joint pain, chest pain, retained excretions, and hyperglycemia.[10] Leaves extract is applied for rheumatism, black wart fever, eczema, and ringworms. Leaves are also utilized as an antitussive, having anti-hypoglycemic properties, and as a wound healer.[10,11] Seeds are utilized to treat swollen throats, oral sores, and jaundice. Seeds have a slightly sweet taste and are used as a carminative, laxative, and cooling agent, as well as for treating swollen throats, skin diseases, and biliousness.[10,11] The bark is used for its antidiabetic, antioxidant, anti-inflammatory, and medicinal properties.[10–12] The pulp is used as a hepatoprotective, antiviral, antifungal, and anticandidal agent, and in the treatment of leprosy, diabetes, abdominal and urinary disorders, obstructions, and fever (antipyretic).[10–12] Pods of *C. fistula* are used as a laxative, antipyretic, and for the treatment of diabetes mellitus. Extract from fruits is used as an anti-estrogenic agent and has antifungal and purgative properties. *C. fistula* fruit extract is known as a killer of disease.[10,11]

The root is prescribed as a tonic, astringent, febrifuge, and strong purgative.[13–15] The leaf extract reduced mutagenicity in *E. coli*.[13] The leaves are laxative and used externally as emollient; a poultice is used for chilblains, insect bites, swelling, rheumatism, and facial paralysis.[13,14] Leaves have antiperiodic as well as laxative properties and are used to treat jaundice, piles, rheumatism ulcers, external skin eruptions, ringworms, and eczema. The leaves and bark mixed with oil are applied to pustules and insect bites.[14,15] The roots are used for chest pain, joint pain, migraine, and blood dysentery. The extract of the root lowered the blood sugar level by up to 30%.[16] Leaves and flowers are both purgative like the pulp.[17] Ashes from burnt pods mixed with a little salt and honey are taken 3–4 times to relieve cough.[18] The roots are useful in treating fever, heart diseases, retained excretions, and biliousness.[19] The fruits are used as cathartics and in the treatment of snake bites. The juice of the leaves is used for skin diseases.[20,21] Flowers and pods are used as purgatives, febrifuges, for biliousness, and as astringents. As per records of *The Wealth of India* and Kirtikar and Basu, the 50% ethanolic extract of pods has shown antifertility activity in female albino rats. The heated pods are applied to swellings on the neck caused by cold. The fruits are reported to be used for asthma.[14,17] The pulp is used to treat liver disorders. The fruit is used as an analgesic and antipyretic (including for malarial fever). Fruits are also used in the treatment of blood poisoning, anthrax, dysentery, leprosy, diabetes, and abdominal obstruction.[14] Extract from the flowers of *C. fistula* is used to inhibit ovarian function and stimulate uterine activity. Fruits are used to treat and reduce inflammation and body heat and are useful for chest complaints, throat troubles, liver complaints, eye diseases, and gripping.[17] Juice of the leaves is used as a dressing for ringworm, to relieve irritation, and to reduce dropsical swelling. The pulp of the fruit around the seeds is a mild purgative[16–18] and is also used in biliousness and diabetes. Externally, it is useful for evacuation in flatulent colic and as a dressing for gouty or rheumatic joints.[16–18] The pith is particularly useful if there is swelling in the stomach, liver, or intestine. Seeds are emetic, used to treat constipation, have cathartic properties,[16–18] and improve the appetite.[16,17] They are useful for skin diseases, swollen throat, biliousness, and jaundice. Dried seed produces marked hypoglycemic activity,[16] and seed powder is used to treat amoebiasis.[16]

DOI: 10.1201/9781003512868-8

Bark powder or decoction is used to treat jaundice, syphilis, heart diseases, and leprosy. The aqueous extract of root bark has been reported for anti-inflammatory properties. The root is used for cardiac disorders, rheumatic conditions, biliousness, ulcers, boils, hemorrhages, wounds, and various skin diseases.[16,22] The stem bark is used to treat chest pain, swellings, and amenorrhea.[13]

AYURVEDIC PREPARATIONS AND PHYTO-INGREDIENTS

C. fistula is an integral ingredient of an Ayurvedic formulation named 'Constivac' (a product of Lupin Herbal), used to relieve constipation and regulate bowel movements. Another Ayurvedic formulation has *C. fistula* as an active ingredient named 'Pilex' (a product of Himalaya), which is used to cure piles.[20] These Ayurvedic preparations are supported by the ingredients present in the plant parts used, as the pulp of the pod has anthraquinone glycosides, namely sennoside A, sennoside B, rhein and its glucosides, pectin, butyric acid, barbaloin, formic acid, aloin, oxalic acid, and tannins.[20,23] Seeds have free sugars, free amino acids, and galactomannan. Flowers are reported to have kaempferol, rhein, and cetyl alcohol. Leaves have free rhein and glycosides (sennoside A and sennoside B).[23] The pulp contains sugar, calcium oxalate, albuminous starch, tannic matter, and other important constituents. Leaves and flowers contain anthraquinone, tannin, oxyanthraquinone, volatile oils, and rhein.[18,21] The pulp consists of astringent matter, gluten, sugar, gum, coloring matter, and water.[20] Root barks have oxyanthraquinone substances, tannins, and phlobaphenes.[20] The plant contains rhein glucoside, rhein, fistulic acid, sennoside A, and sennoside B.[16]

PHYTOCHEMISTRY OF *C. FISTULA*

The whole plant of *C. fistula* contains anthraquinone, phenolic compounds, citronellol, free amino acids, linoleic acid, aloin, wax, free sugar, saponins, gum, cardiac glycosides, resins, alkaloids, tannins, *kaempferol*, emodin, rhein, galactomannan, phosphate, iron, calcium, steroids, terpenoids, sennoside A, sennoside B, and derivatives of flavan-3-ol.[1,23] However, *C. fistula* has a potential role in the prevention and treatment of diseases due to the presence of therapeutic ingredients. Among these ingredients, a few constituents have a role as antioxidants and antimicrobials, while others have different types of therapeutic implications, e.g., cancer prevention via a change in genetic pathways. Different parts of the plant, such as flowers, stems, and leaves, have different types of constituents and have proven therapeutic potential in health care. *C. fistula* stem bark is a chief source of ß-sitosterol, hexacosanol, and lupeol.[24,25]

Fruits and flowers of *C. fistula* are a source of valuable therapeutic ingredients for health management. The fruit pulp has derivatives of 1,8-dihydroxy-3-anthraquinone[25] and high concentrations of fructose, glucose, sucrose, and soluble sugar, as well as being a good source of microminerals, potassium, and calcium.[26]

Flowers have been reported to be rich in kaempferol, rhein, fistulin, and triterpenes.[25,27] Flowers of *C. fistula* have anthraquinone, oxyanthraquinone, volatile oil, tannins, isoflavonoids, glycosides, phenolic compounds, potassium, calcium, iron, and manganese, together with kaempferol, rhein, proanthocyanidins, catechins, tannins, fistulic acids, anthrones, sennosides, alkaloids, aurantiamide acetate, and ß-sitosterol, and *β-D-glucoside*.[28–30]

C. fistula seeds are rich in glycerides (oleic, stearic, linoleic, and palmitic acids) with traces of caprylic and myristic acids.[12] Other ingredients reported from the seeds are 5-(2-hydroxyphenoxymethyl)furfural, (2′S)-7-hydroxy-5-hydroxymethyl-2-(2′-hydroxypropyl)chromone, benzyl 2-hydroxy-3,6-dimethoxybenzoate, benzyl-2-β-O-d-glucopyranosyl-3,6-dimetho xybenzoate,5-hydroxy-methyl-furfural,(2′S)-7-hydroxy-2-(2'-hydroxypropyl)-5-methyl-chromone, two oxyanthraquinones (chrysophanol and chrysophanein),[31] and galactomannan.[32]

Leaves of *C. fistula* have heptacosanyl-5-hydroxypentadec2-enoate, octacosan-5, 8-diol,[11] and anthraquinones (rhein, chrysophanol, and physcion).[33]

In different studies, 27 compounds, including eight long-chain hydrocarbon derivatives (1-hexacosanol, palmitic acid, 1-octacosanol, stearic acid, oleic acid, linoleic acid, heptacosyl eicosanoate, and glyceryl-1-tetraeicosanoate), three sterols (ß-sitosteryl-3-O-Dglucopyranoside, ß-sitosterol, and stigmasterol), one triterpene (lupeol), eight anthraquinones (emodin, chrysophanol, citreorosein, physcion, ziganein, rhein, rhein methyl ester, and 1,4,5-trihydroxyanthraquinone), two coumarins (scopoletin and isoscopoletin), two chromones (2,5-dimethyl-7-hydroxychromone and 2,5-dimethyl-7-methoxychromone), and three aromatic compounds (vanillic acid, 2,4-dihydroxybenzaldehyde, and isovanillic acid) have been isolated and identified from the aerial parts of *Cassia fistula*.[28]

Roots of *C. fistula* have flavonoids, 7-methylphysicon, flavan-3-ol derivatives, ß-sitosterol, betulinic acid, 3-O-gentiobioside, and rhamnetin. The root bark of the *C. fistula* plant contains oxy-anthraquinone and phlobaphenes.[28,34]

The bark of *C. fistula* has flavanol glycosides, flavonoids, tannins, phenolics, and proanthocyanadins.[28,34] All 27 compounds previously described in aerial parts have also been reported and identified from the bark.[10]

C. fistula pollen has glutamic acid, phenylalanine, proline, methionine, carbohydrates, lipids, and free amino acids.[10] The dense inner part of the tree trunk, yielding the hardest timber (i.e., the heartwood), has fistucacidin, an optically inactive leucoanthocyanidin (3,4,7,8,4′-pentahydroxyflavan).[10] *C. fistula* fruit extracts, pulp, pulp powder, and pods have unique therapeutic properties, as they have rhein, 5,3,4-tri-hydroxy-6-methoxy-7-O-alpha-L-rhamnopyranosy-(12)-O-beta–D-galactopyranosoid,[34] along with eight other glycosides.[35] Polar compounds such as triacontane, sitosterol 5-nonatetracontanone, 16-hentriacontanol, 2-tetramer, aloin, hentriacontanone, and leucopelargonidin are also reported from *C. fistula* fruits.[11,36]

Flavonoids, phenolic compounds, proanthocyanidins, sennoside A, sennoside B, formic acid, barbaloin, butyric acid, aloin, ethyl ester, pectin, oxalic acid, and tannins have been reported.[28,37,38] The pulp of *C. fistula* has albuminous starch, calcium oxalate, gum, sugar, and coloring matter.[28] The pods contain 5-nonatetracontanone, 2-hentriacontanone, 3-beta-hydroxy-17-norpimar-8(9)-en-15-one, nonatetra contanone, 2-hentriacontanone, ß-sitosterol, quercetin derivatives, triacontane, 16-hentriacontanone, kaempferol, dihydrokaempferol, and different anthraquinone derivatives.[11]

PHYTOPHARMACOLOGY

The water extract of *C. fistula* fruit pulp has been reported to have a potent hepatoprotective activity.[36] Extracts from bark show significant radical scavenging by inhibiting lipid peroxidation initiated by CCl_4 and $FeSO_4$ in rat liver and kidney homogenates.[39] Senthil Kumar et al. studied the application of *C. fistula* for treating infected wounds and revealed that *C. fistula*-treated animals have better wound closure and improved tissue regeneration at the wound site.[40]

ANTIOXIDANT ACTIVITY

Antioxidants are compounds that neutralize the attack of free radicals and, therefore, reduce the risk of metabolic disorders, resulting in a vital role in the prevention and cure of various diseases. The rich sources of antioxidants in plants are flavonoids, tocopherol, and polyphenols, some essential amino acids, and all these constituents have a potential role in health care. Phenols, especially bioflavonoids, are a good source of antioxidants and have shown a valuable role as free radical scavengers. The importance of *C. fistula* in disease control has an ancient background due to its high antioxidant content. A recent study was conducted to evaluate the antioxidant potential and protective effect of *C. fistula* on H_2O_2-induced oxidative damage. This study confirmed that *C. fistula* ethanolic extract exhibits high antioxidant activity, providing more than 90% protection of erythrocytes. In comparison, the *C. fistula* aqueous extract showed 75% antioxidant and protective activity.[41] In another study, results have revealed that bark extracts from different age groups have high antioxidant activity.[42]

Results based on studies using albino rats to check the antioxidant activities of the water and methanolic extracts of the *C. fistula* barks have revealed that both extracts exhibited potent antioxidant activity in DPPH, nitric oxide, and hydroxyl radical-induced in vitro assay methods.[39] Many more studies on the antioxidant effect of different parts of *C. fistula* have also been conducted, and the results revealed that the *C. fistula* plant as a whole is a significant source of antioxidants.[43,44]

ANTI-INFLAMMATORY ACTIVITY

Inflammation is a normal physiological process in response to tissue injury, infection, metabolic disorders, and environmental factors that cause various pathological alterations. Flavonoids, an ingredient present in *C. fistula*, serve as safe and nontoxic remedies to prevent and treat the inflammatory process by modulating pro-inflammatory cytokines and other factors responsible for chronic inflammation. Flavonoids have been reported to play a vital role in inhibiting several enzymes that are activated in the inflammatory process.[45] *C. fistula* bark extracts have been found to have significant anti-inflammatory effects in both acute and chronic models.[39] The water extract of dried fruits of *Solanum xanthocarpum* and dried pulp of *C. fistula* in a 1:1 ratio (wt./wt.) at a dose of 500 mg/kg has showed maximum inhibition of 75%, which is comparable with the positive control, diclofenac sodium, which has been reported to have 81% inhibition.[46] Bhakta et al. have described that the anti-inflammatory effects of *C. fistula* were observed against all phlogistic agents, compared with phenylbutazone, using histamine-, dextran-, and carrageenan-induced paw edema in rats.[47]

Rajeswar et al. have reported that the anti-inflammatory properties of aqueous and alcoholic extracts of *C. fistula* bark in subacute models of inflammation confirmed that extracts have significant anti-inflammatory effects in both air pouch granuloma and cotton pellet granuloma models.[48]

ANTITUMOR ACTIVITY

C. fistula has an ancient history in cancer treatment via traditional medicine such as Unani, Ayurveda, and Chinese. Gupta et al. investigated the growth of Ehrlich cells and its impact on the survival period of tumor-bearing mice. They reported an increased lifespan, a decrease in tumor size, and a lower viable tumor cell count using the methanolic extract of C. fistula seeds.[49] Another study on the human colon adenocarcinoma cell line revealed that rhein has 40.59%, 58.26%, 65.40%, 77.92%, and 80.25% cytotoxicity at 200 μg/mL concentration for 6, 12, 24, 48, and 72 h incubation times, respectively.[50]

ANTIDIABETIC ACTIVITY

C. fistula has had a potential role in checking and treating diabetes mellitus since ancient times. Though the exact mechanism of action is not understood completely, it is considered to be due to an increase in insulin-stimulated glucose uptake. Results of a study have deciphered that *C. fistula* bark hexane extract at a dose of $0.15 \times 0.30 \times 0.45$ g/kg body weight for 30 days suppressed the elevated glucose levels in diabetic rats.[51] Methanol extract of bark and leaves at a 500 mg/kg dose showed more significant anti-hyperglycemic and anti-lipidemic activity than 250 mg/kg in the STZ nicotinamide-induced diabetic mellitus rats.[52] Results from another study concluded that the extract and its fractions evaluated for antidiabetic activity deciphered an appreciable decrease of glucose levels in the serum and other complications associated with diabetes.[53] A study based on gold nanoparticles to evaluate the hypoglycemic effects has revealed that *C. fistula* gold nanoparticles have promising antidiabetic properties.[54] Stem barks of *C. fistula* and *Tamarindus indica* were examined for anti-hyperglycemic effects in diabetic rats (alloxan-induced), and the results deciphered a significant decrease in blood glucose levels in the treated group of diabetic rats.[55] Oral administration of catechin (20 mg/kg b. wt.) isolated from *C. fistula* for 60 days produced a better glucose tolerance pattern in streptozotocin-induced diabetic male albino Wistar rats.[56]

ANTIBACTERIAL ACTIVITY

Diseases due to microbial infections are one of the major causes of morbidity and mortality worldwide, especially during the pandemic period. *C. fistula* has a vital role in the prevention and cure of infectious diseases via its inhibitory effect on various types of pathogens. The antifungal and antibacterial research data of hydro-alcoholic extracts of leaves of *C. fistula* against Gram-positive, Gram-negative, and fungal strains have revealed that there is a potent inhibition of bacterial growth against the organisms that were tested.[57] Other findings with different extracts from different plant parts revealed that the *C. fistula* plant has potent antibacterial activity.[10,58–61]

HEPATOPROTECTIVE EFFECT

Various chemicals, such as a high dose of paracetamol, anti-analgesic/antipyretic drugs, excess alcohol consumption, infections, and toxic materials, cause alterations in liver cells, mainly by lipid peroxidation, leading to hepatic disorders. *C. fistula* has been proven to have a potential role in the prevention and cure of liver diseases via detoxification and excretion of toxic materials through urine.[62–65] Methanolic extracts of *C. fistula* (200 and 400 mg/kg) have been reported to reverse the altered biochemical markers to normal levels in a dose-dependent manner.[66]

ANTIPYRETIC EFFECT

C. fistula and its constituents have a role as antipyretic, and it is supported by the results of animal model studies. The use of ethanol extract of *C. fistula* (250 and 500 mg/kg b. wt.) has been reported to reduce TAB vaccine-induced pyrexia after 60 min, and a dose of 750 mg/kg. b. wt. reduced the vaccine-induced elevated body temperature after 30 min of its use.[67] Another study examining the antipyretic activity of the pod of *C. fistula* has concluded that methanol extract has antipyretic activity, which is significantly higher than that of control animals.[36]

ANTI-INFERTILITY EFFECT

C. fistula plant and its constituents have been reported to play a role in reproduction and control of hormones involved in reproduction. It is supported by results of animal studies, as oral administration of aqueous extract of *C. fistula* seeds to mated female rats from day 1–5 of pregnancy at the doses of 100 and 200 mg/kg body weight resulted in 57.14% and 71.43% prevention of pregnancy, respectively, and 100% pregnancy inhibition was noted at 500 mg/kg bw.[1]

IMMUNOMODULATORY EFFECT

C. fistula has a significant stimulation of cell-mediated immunity and no effects on humoral immunity.[68]

LARVICIDAL AND OVICIDAL ACTIVITY

The methanol leaf extract of *C. fistula* has larvicidal and ovicidal properties against *Anopheles stephensi* and *Culex quinquefasciatus*.[69] In another study, the application and uses of larvicidal efficacy of different solvent extracts of flowers were assessed against *Anopheles subpictus, Culex tritaeniorhynchus*, and *Aedes albopictus*. The results concluded that crude extracts of flowers have excellent potential for controlling *C. tritaeniorhynchus*, *A. albopictus,* and *A. subpictus* mosquito larvae.[70] The activity of methanol extract of leaves was evaluated against *Anopheles* mosquitoes, and results confirmed that leaf extracts have a promising mosquitocidal efficacy against *A. stephensi*.[71]

WOUND-HEALING EFFECT

C. fistula plant has both wound-healing and wound-treatment properties. Senthil Kumar et al. have reported that *C. fistula*-treated animals showed better wound closure, improved tissue regeneration at the wound site, and supporting histopathological parameters related to wound healing.[40] Bhakta et al. studied the wound-healing effect of methanol extract in the form of an ointment in two types of wound models, namely excision and inclusion wound model rats. The results confirmed that ointment at two different concentrations responded significantly in both wound models tested.[72]

TOXICITY AND SAFE DOSE

Toxicity and safe dose of *C. fistula* have been evaluated to avoid the non-targeted effect on animal model testing. Akanmu et al. have reported that *C. fistula* infusion, when compared with the Senokot tablet, and the infusion of *C. fistula* pods, exhibited very low levels of toxicity. It has an LD_{50} of 6,600 mg/kg and did not show any pathological effects on the targeted organs.[73] The acute toxicity studies with the extracts of *C. fistula* and *T. indica* showed no signs of toxicity up to a dose of 2,000 mg/po.[55] Another study for acute toxicity showed no sign of toxicity at a dose of 2,000 mg/po.[39] Additional efforts have been made for safety, and different toxicity studies have been done by researchers who reported that different parts of the plant are nontoxic or very less toxic to humans (Table 6.1).[9]

TABLE 6.1
Toxicity Status of *Cassia fistula*[9]

Solvent Used	Plant Part	Results
Aqueous	Pods	Deciphered for very low levels of toxicity, and LD_{50} of 6,600 mg/kg, with pathological effects on organs.[73]
Alcoholic	Stem bark	No symptoms of toxicity up to a dose level of 2,000 mg/po.[55]
Aqueous and methanolic	Bark	Studies related to acute toxicity showed no symptoms of toxicity up to a dose level of 2,000 mg/po.[39]
Methanolic	Seeds	A high LC_{50} value indicates that the plant is not toxic to humans.[61]
Ethanolic	Fruit	*C. fistula* extract up to a dose of 5,000 mg/kg did not induce any mortality, and subacute studies have shown its doses of 250, 500, and 1,000 mg/kg to rats have not induced mortality.[74]

TABLE 6.2
A Few Therapeutic Ingredients from *Cassia fistula* Plants

Plant Organ	Active Ingredients/Isolated Compounds
Stem bark	Lupeol, βsitosterol, and hexacosanol.[24]
Fruit tissue	Source of calcium, iron, manganese, potassium, and 1,8-dihydroxy-3-anthraquinone derivative.[26]
Flowers	Leucopelargonidin tetramer, rhein, kaempferol, fistulin, and triterpenes.[27]
Leaves	Anthraquinones (chrysophanol, physcion, and rhein), and heptacosanyl-5-hydroxypentadec-2-enoate and octacosan-5, 8-diol[33]
Seed	Seeds have galactomannan,[32] stearic, oleic, linoleic, palmitic, caprylic, and myristic acids.[31]

SYNERGISTIC EFFECT

The herbal preparation with *Solanum xanthocarpum* and *C. fistula* has a synergistic effect,[46] even at very low concentrations, and has anti-inflammatory activity. *Cassia fistula,* 'Amoxy-Cassia' (*Amoxicillin* with the aqueous fruit solution of *Cassia* fistula), has been traditionally used to increase the immunity of the host.[12] *C. fistula* and fluconazole (an antifungal medicine) show a synergistic effect.[31]

SCOPE AND OPPORTUNITIES

Species *Cassia fistula* is used to treat common body ailments like constipation, leprosy, burning sensations, skin diseases, syphilis, and fever. A complete profile of phytochemicals of the *C. fistula* plant (root, stem, leaf, flower, and seed) has been investigated in detail, and a few important ingredients (Table 6.2) have been well-known biologically. It is an ornamental tree with golden yellow flowers, a dark-brown old stem, brownish-red roots, green pods, and ovate and brown seeds. The plant has biological potential as an antifungal, antibacterial, anti-inflammatory, antioxidant, antifertility, anticonvulsant, antiparasitic, etc., and has proven on a molecular basis to have these important therapeutic values. Drugs of synthetic origin have adverse effects and affect the various biological pathways, while alternative medicines have another window into health management due to their least side effects and cheaper market values. *C. fistula* is an ancient medicinal plant of Chinese and Indian systems of medicine for different diseases (e.g., antioxidant, anti-inflammatory, chemopreventive, and chemotherapeutic activity). The efficacy and safety of *C. fistula* as a medicine make it a potential candidate to treat and prevent various diseases. Recent studies (in vivo and in vitro) have confirmed that *C. fistula* has a role in disease inhibition by various physiological and biochemical processes, but the exact mechanism of action is not fully understood. Detailed studies based on molecular pathways are needed to understand the exact mechanism of action of *C. fistula* in the prevention and treatment of various diseases.

C. fistula has been used as an important curative plant for patients. It is a highly useful medicinal plant, and there is a need for further exploration to understand the molecular path of its therapeutic mechanisms. It has various pharmacological properties. The present text aims to mobilize researchers to investigate further to achieve lead molecules/compositions for potential health-friendly green medicines.

REFERENCES

1. Yadav R, Jain GC. 1999. Antifertility effect of aqueous extract of seeds of *Cassia fistula* in female rats. *Advances in Contraception*. 15: 293–301.
2. Vasudevan DT, Dinesh KR, Gopalkrishnan S, Sreekanthc SK, Shekar S. 2009. The potential of aqueous and isolated fraction from leaves of *Cassia fistula* Linn as antibacterial agent. *International Journal of Chemical Sciences*. 7: 2363–2367.
3. Panda SK, Padhi LP, Mohanty G. 2011. Antibacterial activities and phytochemical analysis of *Cassia fistula* (Linn.) leaf. *Journal of Advanced Pharmaceutical Technology and Research*. 2: 62–67.

4. Rajagopal PL, Premaletha K, Kiron SS, Sreejith KR. 2013. Phytochemical and pharmacological review on *Cassia fistula* Linn. the golden shower. *International Journal of Pharmaceutical, Chemical, and Biological Sciences.* 3: 672–679.
5. Neelam C, Ranjan B, Komal S, Nootan C. 2011. Review on *Cassia fistula. International Journal of Research in Ayurv eda and Pharmacy.* 2: 426–430.
6. Moshahid M, Rizvi A, Gamel IM, Hassadi EI, Younis BS. 2009. Review of bio-efficacies of *Cassia fistula. African Journal of Pharmacy and Pharmacology.* 3: 287–292.
7. Ajay K, Satish S, Ibrahim S, Karunakara H. 2017. Therapeutic uses of *cassia fistula*: a review. *International Journal of Pharma Sciences and Research.* 3: 38–43.
8. IndianLaburnum(*Cassiafistula*)–TheStateFlowerofKerala. https://organikos.net/2012/03/17/indian-laburnum-cassia-fistula-the-state-flower-of-kerala/#:~:text=Indian%20laburnum%20is%20also%20known,that%20attracts%20bees%20and%20butterflies, as on 11th September 2020.
9. Sanoria S, Qadrie ZL, Gautam SP, Barwal A. 2020. *Cassia fistula*; Botany, phytochemistry, pharmacological leverages-A Review. *International Journal of Pharmacy and Pharmaceutical Sciences.* 12 (6): 1–7.
10. Duraipandiyan V, Ignacimuthu S. 2007. Antibacterial, antifungal activity of *Cassia fistula* L.: An ethnomedicinal plant. *Journal of Ethnopharmacology.* 112: 590–594.
11. Sharma DK. 2017. Numerations on phytochemical, pharmacological and ethnobotanical properties of *Cassia fistula* Linn: yellow shower. *The Journal of Phytopharmacology.* 6 (5): 300–306.
12. Ali NH, Kazmi SH, Faizi S. 2008. Modulation of humoral immunity by *Cassia Fistula* and Amoxy-Cassia. *Pakistan Journal of Pharmaceutical Sciences.* 21(1): 21–23.
13. 2001. *Ayurvedic Pharmacopoeia of India*, Part 1. Government of India Publication, New Delhi. Vol. 5. pp. 8–9.
14. Anonymous. 2007. *The Wealth of India*. First Supplement Series (Raw Materials). National Institute of Science Communication and Information Resources, CSIR. Vol 3 (Ca-Ci). Pp. 340–342.
15. 2002. *Indian Herbal Pharmacopoeia*, revised new edition. Indian Drug Manufacturers Association Mumbai. pp. 106–113.
16. Anonymous. 2007. *The Wealth of India*. First Supplement Series (Raw Materials). National Institute of Science Communication and Information Resources, CSIR 1st Supplementary Series, New Delhi, Vol 1 (A-Ci). pp. 223–224.
17. Kirtikar KR, Basu BD. 2006. *Indian Medicinal Plants.* International Book Distributors. Vol. 2: pp. 856–860.
18. Gupta RK. 2010. *Medicinal & Aromatic Plants*, 1st Edition. CBS Publishers & Distributors. pp. 116–117.
19. Nadkarni KM. 2009. *Indian Materia Medica.* Bombay Popular Prakashan. Vol. 1. pp. 285–286.
20. Agarwal SS, Paridhavi M. 2005. *Clinically Useful Herbal Drugs.* Ahuja Publishing House. pp. 281–282.
21. Chopra RN, Nayar SL, Chpora IC. 2006. *Glossary of Indian Medicinal Plants.* National Institute of Science Communication and Information Resources. pp. 54.
22. Erik B, Wyk V, Michael W. 2009. *Medicinal Plants of the World.* Briza Publications. pp. 403
23. Khare CP. 2007. *Indian Medicinal Plants.* Springer. pp. 128.
24. Sen AB, Shukia YN. 1968. Chemical examination of *Cassia fistula. Journal of the Indian Chemical Society.* 45: 744.
25. Rahmani AH. 2015. *Cassia fistula* Linn: potential candidate in the health management. *Pharmacognosy* Research. 7 (3): 217–224.
26. Barthakur NN, Arnold NP, Alli I.1995. The Indian laburnum (*Cassia fistula* L.) fruit: an analysis of its chemical constituents. *Plant Foods for Human Nutrition.* 47: 55–62.
27. Kumar A, Pande CS, Kaul RK. 1966. Chemical examination of *Cassia fistula* flowers. *Indian Journal of Chemistry.* 4: 460.
28. Danish M, Singh P, Mishra G, Srivastava S, Jha KK, Khosa RL. 2011. *Cassia fistula* Linn. (Amulthus) – An important medicinal plant: A review of its traditional uses, phytochemistry and pharmacological properties. *Journal of Natural Product and Plant Resources.* 1: 101–118.
29. Jehangir A, Nagi AH, Shahzad M, Zia A. 2010. The hepato protective effect of *Cassia Fistula* (Amaltas) leaves in isoniazid and rifampicin induced hepatotoxicity in rodents. *Biomedica.* 26: 25–29.
30. Bhalodia NR, Nariya PB, Acharya RN, Shukla VJ. 2011. Evaluation of *in-vitro* antioxidant activity of flowers of *Cassia fistula* Linn. *International Journal of PharmTech Research.* 3(1): 589–599.
31. Bansal Y, Saini P, Bansal K. 2014. Synergism between *Cassia fistula* and Fluconazole, A new approach against candidiasis. *IJPSR.* 5(3):1000–1005.
32. Kulkarni A, Govindappa M, Ramachandra YL, Koka P. 2015. GC-MS analysis of methanol extract of *Cassia Fistula* and its *in-vitro* anticancer activity on human prostate cancer cell line. *Indo American Journal of Pharmaceutical Research.* 5: 937–944.
33. Sharma DM, Onkar DJM, Sharma DO. 1019. An overview of botanical and therapeutic aspects of Aragvadh-[*Cassia Fistula* Linn]. *World Journal of Pharmaceutical and Medical Research.* 5(3): 82–87.
34. Bahorun T, Neergheen VS, Aruoma O. 2005. Phytochemical constituents of *Cassia fistula. African Journal of Biotechnology.* 4 (13): 1530–1540.
35. Maheep B, Sunil V, Yogesh V, Durgesh S, Kanika S. 2010. Antioxidant activity of fruit pulp powder of *Cassia fistula. PHCOG Journal.* 2: 219–228.
36. Singh MP, Singh A, Alam G, Patel R, Datt N. 2012. Antipyretic activity of *Cassia fistula* Linn. Pods. *Journal of Pharmacy Research.* 5(5): 2593–2594.
37. Gracea MH, Lateganb C, Graziosec R, Smithb PJ, Raskinc I, Lilaa MN. 2012. Antiplasmodial activity of the ethnobotanical plant *Cassia fistula. Natural Product Communications.* 7 (10): 1263–1266.
38. Das S, Sarma G, Barman S. 2008. Hepatoprotective activity of aqueous extract of fruit pulp of *Cassia fistula* (AFCF) against carbon tetrachloride (CCl_4) induced liver damage in albino rats. *Journal of Clinical and Diagnostic Research.* 2: 1133–1138.
39. Ilavarasana R, Mallikab M, Venkataramanc S. 2005. Anti-inflammatory and antioxidant activities of *Cassia fistula* Linn bark extracts. *African Journal of Traditional, Complementary and Alternative Medicines.* 2: 70–85.
40. Senthil Kumar M, Sripriya R, Vijaya Raghavan H, Sehgal PK. 2006. Wound healing potential of *Cassia fistula* on infected albino rat model. *Journal of Surgical Research.* 131: 283–289.
41. Abid R, Mahmood R, Rajesh KP, Kumara Swamy BE. 2014. Potential *in-vitro* antioxidant and protective effect of *Cassia fistula* Linn. fruit extracts against induced oxidative damage in human erythrocytes. *International Journal of Pharmaceutical Sciences and Research.* 6: 497–505.

42. Lai TK, Liew KC. 2013. Total phenolics. Total tannins and antioxidant activity of *Cassia fistula* L. extracts of bark, stem, leaf and root under different age classes. *Asian Journal of Pharmaceutical Research and Health Care*. 5: 52–57.
43. Manonmani G, Bhavapriya V, Kalpana S, Govindasamy S, Apparanantham T. 2005. Antioxidant activity of *Cassia fistula* (Linn.) flowers in alloxan induced diabetic rats. *Journal of Ethnopharmacology*. 97: 39–42.
44. Bhalodia NR, Nariya PB, Acharya RN, Shukla VJ. 2013. In vitro antioxidant activity of hydro alcoholic extract from the fruit pulp of *Cassia fistula* Linn. *AYU*. 34: 209–214.
45. Kwon KH, Murakami A, Tanaka T, Ohigashi H. 2005. Dietary rutin, but not its aglycone quercetin, ameliorates dextran sulfate sodium-induced experimental colitis in mice: attenuation of pro-inflammatory gene expression. *Biochemical Pharmacology*. 69: 395–406.
46. Anwikar S, Bhitre M. 2010. Study of the synergistic anti-inflammatory activity of *Solanum xanthocarpum* Schrad and Wendl and *Cassia fistula* Linn. *International Journal of Ayurveda Research*. 1: 167–171.
47. Bhakta T, Mukherjee PK, Saha K, Pal M, Saha BP. 1999. Evaluation of anti-inflammatory effects of *Cassia fistula* (Leguminosae) leaf extracts o rats. *Journal of Herbs, Spic es & Medicinal Plants*. 6: 67–72.
48. Rajeswari R, Thejomoorthy P, Mathuram LN, Raju KV. 2006. Antiinflammatory activity of *Cassia fistula* Linn. bark extracts in subacute models of inflammation in rats. *Tamil Nadu Journal of Veterinary and Animal Sciences*. 2: 193–199.
49. Gupta M, Mazumder UK, Rath N, Mukhopadhyay DK. 2000. Antitumor activity of methanolic extract of *Cassia fistula* L. seed against Ehrlich ascites carcinoma. *Journal of Ethnopharmacology*. 72: 151–156.
50. Duraipandiyan V, Baskar AA, Ignacimuthu S, Muthukumar C, Al-Harbi NA. 2012. Anticancer activity of rhein isolated from *Cassia fistula* L. flower. *Asian Pacific Journal of Tropical Disease*. 2: S517–S523.
51. Nirmala A, Eliza J, Rajalakshmi M, Priya E, Daisy P. 2008. Effect of hexane extract of *Cassia fistula* barks on blood glucose and lipid profile in streptozotocin diabetic rats. *International Journal of Pharmacology*. 4: 292–296.
52. Einstein JW, Rais MM, Mohd MA. 2013. Comparative evaluation of the antidiabetic effects of different parts of *Cassia fistula* Linn, a Southeast Asian Plant. *Journal of Chemistry*. 2013. Article ID 714063. https://doi.org/10.1155/2013/714063.
53. Jarald EE, Joshi SB, Jain DC, Edwin S. 2013. Biochemical evaluation of the hypoglycemic effects of extract and fraction of *Cassia fistula* Linn. in alloxan-induced diabetic rats. *Indian Journal of Pharmaceutical Sciences*. 75: 427–434.
54. Daisy P, Saipriya K. 2012. Biochemical analysis of *Cassia fistula* aqueous extract and phytochemically synthesized gold nanoparticles as hypoglycemic treatment for diabetes mellitus. *International Journal of Nanomedicine*. 7: 1189–1202.
55. Agnihotri A, Singh V. 2013. Effect of *Tamarindus indica* Linn. and *Cassia fistula* Linn. stem bark extracts on oxidative stress and diabetic conditions. *Acta Poloniae Pharmaceutica*. 70: 1011–1019.
56. Pitchai D, Manikkam R. 2012. Hypoglycemic and insulin mimetic impact of catechin isolated from *Cassia fistula*: A substantiate in silico approach through docking analysis. *Medicinal Chemistry Research*. 21: 2238–2250.
57. Bhalodia NR, Shukla VJ. 2011. Antibacterial and antifungal activities from leaf extracts of *Cassia fistula* L.: an ethnomedicinal plant. *Journal of Advanced Pharmaceutical Technology and Research*. 2: 104–109.
58. Seyyednejad SM, Motamedi H, Vafei M, Bakhtiari A. 2014. The antibacterial activity of *Cassia fistula* organic extracts. *Jundishapur Journal of Microbiology*. 7: e8921.
59. Arulpandi I, Sangeetha R. 2012. Antibacterial activity of fistulin: a protease inhibitor purified from the leaves of Cassia fistula. *ISRN Pharmacology*. 2012: 584073.
60. Lachumy SJ, Zuraini Z, Sasidharan S. 2010. Antimicrobial activity and toxicity of methanol extract of *Cassia fistula* seeds. *Research Journal of Pharmaceutical, Biological an d Chemical Sciences*. 1: 391–398.
61. Yadava RN, Verma V. 2003. A new biologically active flavone glycoside from the seeds of *Cassia fistula* (Linn.). *Jou rnal of Asian Natural Products Research*. 5: 57–61.
62. Parthasarathy G, Prasanth V. 2008. Hepatoprotective activity of *Cassia fistula* Linn. Bark extracts against carbon tetra chloride induced liver toxicity in rats. *Internet Journal of Pharmacology*. 6: 67–70.
63. Pradeep K, Mohan CV, Anand KG, Karthikeyan S. 2005. Effect of pretreatment of Cassia fistula Linn. leaf extract against subacute CCl_4 induced hepatotoxicity in rats. *Indian Journal of Experimental Biology*. 43: 526–530.
64. Bhakta T, Banerjee S, Mandal SC, Maity TK, Saha BP, Pal M. 2001. Hepatoprotective activity of *Cassia fistula* leaf extract. *Phytomedicine*. 8: 220–224.
65. Wasu SJ, Muley BP. 2009. Hepatoprotective effect of *Cassia fistula* Linn. *Ethnobotanical Leaflets*. 13: 910–916.
66. Chaudhari NB, Chittam KP, Patil VR. 2009. Hepatoprotective activity of *Cassia fistula* seeds against paracetamol-induced hepatic injury in rats. *Archives of Pharmaceutical Sciences and Research*. 1: 218–221.
67. Gobianand K, Vivekababdan P, Pradeep K, Mohan CV, karthikeyan S. 2010. Anti-inflammatory and antipyretic activities of Indian medicinal plant *Cassia fistula* Linn. (Golden shower) in Wister albino rats. *International Journal of Pharmacology*. 6: 719–725.
68. Jadhav SN. 2014. Evaluation of immunomodulatory activity of *Cassia fistula*. *International Journal of Chemical and Pharmaceutical Sciences*. 3: 291–293.
69. Govindarajan M, Jebanesan A, Pushpanathan T. 2008. Larvicidal and ovicidal activity of *Cassia fistula* Linn. leaf extract against filarial and malarial vector mosquitoes. *Parasitology Research*. 102: 289–292.
70. Govindarajan M. 2013. Larvicidal activity of *Cassia fistula* flower against *Culex tritaeniorhynchus* giles, *Aedes albopictus* skuse and *Anopheles subpictus* grassi (Diptera: Culicidae). *Journal of Pure and Applied Zoology*. 1: 117–121.
71. Mehmood S, Lateef M, Omer MO, Anjum AA, Rashid MI, Shehzad W. 2014. Adulticidal and larvicidal activity of *Cassia fistula* and *Piper nigrum* against malaria vector. *Sciece International (*Lahore*)*. 26: 331–334.
72. Bhakta T, Mukherjee PK, Mukherjee K, Pal M, Saha BP. 1998. Studies on *in- vivo* wound healing activity of *Cassia fistula* Linn. leaves (Leguminosae) in rats. *Natural Product Sciences*. 4: 84–87.
73. Akanmu MA, Iwalewa EO, Elujoba AA, Adelusola KA. 2004. Toxicity potentials of *Cassia fistula* fruits as laxative with reference to senna. *African Journal of Biomedical Research*. 7: 23–26.
74. Abid R, Mahmood R. 2019. Acute and sub-acute oral toxicity of ethanol extract of *Cassia fistula* fruit in male rats. *Avicenna Journal of Phytomedicine*. 9: 117–125.

7 *Carissa spinarum* (Karoda)

INTRODUCTION

Carissa spinarum L. (family: Apocynaceae) is known as 'Magic Shrub' in some African countries, as it is a source to treat various diseases and metabolic disorders.[1] *Carissa spinarum* L. (family: Apocynaceae)[2] is widely distributed in the tropical regions of Australia, Southern Asia, Africa, and the Indian Ocean countries. It is commonly called wild Karonda in India, referring to the related species karanda (*Carissa carandas*). It is often misidentified as *C. carandas* due to its physical similarities. All plants of the family Apocynaceae are used in the food and pharmaceutical industries as well as traditional/folk healing practices.[3]

Both species of the genus *Carissa* (*C. carandas* and *C. spinarum*) have similar medicinal properties.[4] All parts of these two species have been reported to have potent therapeutic properties. *Carissa* species are rich in terpenoids, glycosides, alkaloids, steroids, flavonoids, reducing sugar, tannins, saponins, etc. These chemical classes are attributed to the pharmacological activities of the species.[5]

ETHNOPHARMACOLOGY

C. spinarum fruits are commonly used as a condiment or additive to Indian pickles and spices. Its fruits are a good appetizer and are pickled before ripening. Ripe fruits have a high amount of pectin, so they are used in making squash, syrup, jelly, tarts, jam, and chutney. These items have a high demand in domestic as well as international markets.[6] The plant has bushes; hence, it is preferred for hedging in the kitchen gardens and is grown as an ornamental plant, as it has beautiful cherry-like fruits. The plant can be grown in a wide range of soils due to its drought tolerance, and hardy physiology. The species has been used as a traditional medicinal plant for thousands of years in the Homoeopathic, Unani, and Ayurvedic systems of medicine. Traditionally, the whole plant and its different parts have been used in the treatment of various diseases. Its fruits are eaten to counteract the putrefaction of blood, treat liver dysfunction, and cure fever, and roots are used to improve digestion. Its fruits are a very rich source of vitamin C and iron. In folk medicine, its fruits are used as an antiscorbutic, astringent, a remedy for biliousness, and to treat anemia. A decoction of leaves is used to treat earache, diarrhea, and fever, whereas a decoction of roots is used as an insect repellent, stomachic, remedy for itches, and vermifuge.[7]

C. spinarum is used to cure a myriad of diseases in African ethnomedicines. All parts of the plant (roots, bark, leaves, and even the fruits) are used for various remedies, which is why it is referred to as a 'magic herb' across African communities.[1] It is used to treat headache, chest complaints, sickle-cell anemia,[8] rheumatism,[8,9,10] gonorrhea, syphilis, rabies, herpes, malaria,[11] herniae, edema, toothache, cough, ulcer, worm infestation,[12] typhoid, jaundice,[13] male sexual disorders, and measles.[14] The decoction of the pounded root is used to treat epilepsy in some communities. In some communities, epilepsy patients are asked to inhale the vapors of the root infusion. The traditional birth attendants use the decoction of the dried leaves to increase labor and quicken childbirth when labor is difficult. A decoction from the barks, leaves, and roots of *C. spinarum* is used in many African traditional societies to treat and manage gonorrhea, breast cancer, headache, chest pains, cough, ulcer, lower blood pressure, fever, rheumatism, edema, syphilis, rabies, malaria, and to boost body immunity.[15] The plant is also used to treat chickenpox and other skin diseases.[16] Roots and root bark are used as snake repellent and anti-venom.[17,18]

PHYTOCHEMISTRY OF *C. SPINARUM*

Phytochemical screening of *C. spinarum* (**synonyms:** *C. edulis*)[19] fruits have revealed the presence of organic acids, sugars (including both the non-reducing sugars and reducing sugars), pectin, vitamin C, tannins, lupeol, citric, oxalic, malonic, tartaric, malic, and glycolic acids, phenyl alkaline, glycine, alanine, glucose, serine, galactose, etc.[20–24]

Roots of *C. spinarum* have carinol, odoroside H, glucose, carissone, carindone, D-digitalose, and digitoxigenin.[20–24] Seeds of *C. spinarum* have been reported to contain oleic acid, palmitic acid, arachidic acid, stearic acid, linoleic acid, etc.[20–24]

Leaves of *C. spinarum* have alcoholic triterpene and ursolic acid.[20–24] Flowers are reported to have canene, camphene, dipentene, myrcene, citronellal, dihydrojasmone, farnesol, β-ionone, nerolidol, geranyl acetate, and A-terpeneol.[20–24]

PHARMACOLOGICAL APPLICATIONS

C. spinarum has an extensive range of bioactive ingredients in its fruits, leaves, roots, and bark. These ingredients enhance the medicinal value of the plant. Based on ethnopharmacological knowledge, the pharmacological importance of the species has been evaluated by several scientists through in vitro and in vivo means, and they reported that the crude extract and its different fractions, as well as isolates, have therapeutic importance. A few findings are described below.

DOI: 10.1201/9781003512868-9

1. **Anthelmintic activity**: Harwansh et al. evaluated anthelmintic activity on adult Indian earthworms (*Pheretima posthuma*). The intestinal anatomy and physiology of earthworm and roundworm (a parasite of human beings) have a resemblance, so earthworm was selected for the study. The study was designed and conducted using three different doses (25, 50, and 100 mg/mL, respectively, in the distilled water) of each crude extract, methanolic, aqueous, and chloroform, as well as the standard medicine, piperazine citrate (PC). The study concluded that the methanolic (100 mg/mL) and chloroform (50 and 100 mg/mL) extracts have equivalent potency compared to PC (10 mg/mL) during both paralysis and death of *P. posthuma*. The reaction mechanism was postulated that an increased chloride ion conductance of muscles of worm membrane develops hyperpolarization and reduction in excitability that results in muscular relaxation and flaccid paralysis.[25]
2. **Antiarthritic activity**: Hegde et al. investigated the roots' ethanolic extract of *C. spinarum* for antiarthritic activity in rats. Arthritis in rats was induced by injecting 0.1 mL of Freund's adjuvant in the sub-plantar region and treated by using 100 mg/kg of phenylbutazone as a standard and 100, 200, and 400 mg/kg doses of ethanolic extract from roots of *C. spinarum*. The study has revealed that *C. spinarum* root extract had a potent and dose-dependent antiarthritic activity.[26]
3. **Anticonvulsant activity**: Yau et al. have concluded that *C. spinarum* (synonymous; *Carissa edulis*) hydroalcoholic extract of root bark has significant anticonvulsant activity in pentylenetetrazole (PTZ)-induced convulsion in mice and chicks for maximal electroshock-induced convulsion. Hydroalcoholic extracts of roots of *C. spinarum* (5, 10, and 20 mg/kg) were given through the IP route to rats for anticonvulsant screening. Naloxone and diazepam were used as standard drugs in PTZ-induced convulsion, while phenytoin was used as a standard drug in case of MEST-induced convulsion.[27]
4. **Antidiabetic activity**: EI-Fiky et al. investigated the effects of ethanolic extract of leaves of *C. spinarum* in streptozotocin-induced diabetic rats. A dose of 2.00 gm/kg extract was orally administered to animals previously given 40 mg/kg streptozotocin via the IP route. Blood samples for glucose levels were collected at 0, 1, 2, and 3 h from each animal. The study has concluded that *C. spinarum* extract has significant antidiabetic activity compared to metformin and glibenclamide.[28]
5. **Anti-inflammatory activity**: Beck and Namdeo have studied anti-inflammatory activity of alcoholic, aqueous, chloroform, and petroleum ether extracts of leaves of *C. spinarum* using a 200 mg/kg oral dose in albino rats in which inflammation was induced by formalin, and used Analgin (30 mg/kg) as the standard drug. The percentage inhibition observed was 17.04% for aqueous extract, 6.93 for both alcoholic and chloroform extracts, 4.76% for petroleum ether extract (4.76%), and 33.87% for the standard drug. The study report has concluded that *C. spinarum* leaves have a potent anti-inflammatory property at a dose of 200 mg/kg.[29] Woode et al. have studied carrageenan-induced paw edema in chicks to evaluate the anti-inflammatory activity of the extract of root powder and concluded that 70% ethanol extract potentially inhibits acute edema in the chick foot induced by carrageenan.[30]
6. **Antioxidant activity**: Sahreen et al. have studied the antioxidant potential of *C. spinarum* fruits using chloroform and aqueous fractions. The focus was on the wide application of the phenolic and flavonoid contents of *C. spinarum* fruits, and it was concluded that the extracts could be effectively and safe utilized as a source of antioxidants, although the antioxidant activities of the chloroform and aqueous fractions were lower compared to ascorbic acid and rutin. The study was also conducted on extracts prepared with butanol, chloroform, ethyl acetate, methanol, n-hexane, and water, respectively.[31] Rao et al. isolated carenone from *C. spinarum* and synthesized its various derivatives. All derivatives had been reported for potent antioxidant activity.[32] Woode et al. have studied the extract of root powder of *C. spinarum* with 70% ethanol for anti-inflammatory and antioxidant activity. Although *C. spinarum* roots are rich in phenolic content, the results were not as potent as in the case of the standard drug.[30]
7. **Antimicrobial activity**: Ibrahim et al. have reported that aqueous extracts of fruits and leaves of *C. spinarum* are more active on the Gram-positive (*Staphylococcus aureus* and *Bacillus subtilis*) compared to Gram-negative (*Pseudomonas aeruginosa* and *Escherichia coli*) organisms. The aqueous extract of leaves has more potent antimicrobial activity compared to its fruit extract, and both extracts have activity up to 1/10,000 dilution. Finally, it was concluded that the activity is due to tannins, saponins, and flavonoids. The different effects on Gram-negative bacteria and Gram-positive bacteria may be due to the structural difference between them.[33,34] Shahada et al. have investigated a cold extract of different parts of *C. spinarum* with various solvents and reported that extracts were more efficacious in Gram-positive bacteria compared to Gram-negative.[35]

Chandra et al. evaluated different extracts of *C. spinarum* fruits for antimicrobial activity (10 and 50 mg/mL). Ethanolic extract was reported to have the highest efficacy, followed by acetone, ethyl acetate extract, and water, respectively. The degree of inhibition was observed to be highest in *Bacillus cereus*, *S. aureus*, and *Streptococcus pyogenes*.[36] Ngulde et al. have studied various strains of microorganisms with ethanolic extract of *C. spinarum* root bark (25, 50, 100, and 200 mg/mL) using tetracycline (250 mg/mL) as a standard and reported that the extract has no action against *E. coli*, *P. aeruginosa*, *B. subtilis*, and *S. aureus*, but significant activity was noted on *Shigella dysenteriae, S. pyogenes typhi*, and *Salmonella* at doses of 100 and 200 mg/mL.[37]

8. **Antileishmanial activity**: Njau et al. have evaluated the antileishmanial potential of *C. spinarum* extracts on the promastigote form of *Leishmania major*. The results of the investigation have revealed that activity against promastigotes is not concerning to the polarity order of the extract ingredients. Extracts from less polar solvents were recorded for moderate activity, while extracts from polar solvents had weak activity. The activity of these extracts against the amastigote form of *L. major* has been reported to be dose-dependent. The higher dose of *C. spinarum* extracts has been noted to reduce the infection rate of macrophages. Extracts made by polar solvents (water, methanol, and ethyl acetate) were observed to be more active compared to extracts prepared by less polar solvents. At their highest concentrations (200 µg/mL), all extracts, except petroleum ether, had IR (infrared) values not significantly different from the standard reference drug pentostam at a concentration of 50 µg/mL ($p>0.05$).[38]
9. **Antinociceptive activity**: Maina et al. and Mworia et al. have reported that *C. spinarum* plant has antinociceptive potential.[39,40]
10. **Antiviral activity**: Tolo et al. have reported the antiviral activity of *C. spinarum* root bark aqueous extract against herpes simplex virus (HSV) using in vitro and in vivo studies at different parameters, such as cell cytotoxicity assay, plaque inhibition assay, and virus yield reduction assay, against Balb/C mice cutaneously infected with HSV. The plaque inhibition assay result reveals that the resistant strains of the virus are more susceptible to the extract than the wild-type strains. In a study for yield reduction, an assay of a 200 g/mL dose of the extract has reduced the virus yields of APr HSV-1 by 100%, HSV-2 by 99.5%, HSV-1 by 97.8%, and TK-HSV1 by 96.3%. In the animal experiments using Balb/C mice cutaneously infected with wild-type strains of HSV-1 or HSV-2 at 1×106 PFU/mouse, all the infected but untreated mice died, whereas those orally treated with the extract had some protection.[41]
11. **Cytotoxicity**: Doshi and Une have reported that *C. spinarum* extract has equivalent activity compared to the standard ADR for human breast cancer cell line MCF7. Further, mild progressive activity on human colon cancer cell line HCT15 and human leukemia cell line MOLT4 was also reported.[42]
12. **Diuretic activity**: Nedi et al. have reported the diuretic effect of the root bark and root wood of *C. spinarum* in albino Wistar rats with 80% methanol. The experiment was conducted at concentrations of 50, 125, 250, 500, and 1000 mg/kg of extract using hydrochlorothiazide (10 mg/kg) as a standard drug.[43]
13. **Hepatoprotective activity**: Hegde and Joshi have cited that ethanolic extracts of *C. spinarum* roots have hepatoprotective effects in pretreated animals with extract (100, 200, and 400 mg/kg), as well as with the standard drug (silymarin), in a dose-dependent manner.[44]
14. **Wound healing**: Sanwal and Chaudhary have studied the healing effect of *C. spinarum* root. An ointment of the methanolic extract of *C. spinarum* root was applied to the various stages of the healing process of mice. The study concluded with findings that the plant species have significant wound-healing activity.[45]

SCOPE AND OPPORTUNITIES

C. spinarum plant is used in Indian and Chinese traditional systems of medicine to cure various diseases. It has been used in the Ayurvedic medical system to cure liver, epileptic, microbial, cytotoxic, and viral diseases. The isolated metabolites and crude extracts of *Carissa spinarum* have wide pharmacological applications, including antioxidant, antimicrobial, antiviral, anticonvulsant, anticancer, antiarthritic, anthelmintic, and cytotoxic activity.

In an in-depth chemical screening of *Carissa spinarum,* 12 compounds were isolated (a coumarin, two cardiac glycosides, and nine lignans). These isolated compounds were evaluated for several biological activities, including antiherpetic, cytotoxic, antioxidant, and antibacterial effects. Pharmacological results have validated the use of *C. spinarum* in traditional medicines.

The root, stem, and leaf of *C. spinarum* have gained more attention in the era of the pandemic. The expansion of the research scope would provide more opportunities for the discovery of new bioactive principles from *C. spinarum*. The evergreen *C. spinarum* plant has cultural as well as medicinal value in day-to-day life. These properties are due to the presence of various chemical classes of phytochemicals. All parts of the species are used for medicinal and nutritional purposes throughout the world, especially in African countries. Ethnopharmacological studies have also strengthened the traditional applications of *C. spinarum* as a source to facilitate safe and effective treatments for body ailments. The present information on biology, ethnopharmacology, phytochemistry, and laboratory results on *C. spinarum* species serves as a valuable resource for the researchers in the future. The traditional and ethnomedicinal applications reveal its use as an effective and safe medicine to treat various ailments. The reverse pharmacological approach is the best one for natural drug discovery and can be followed to discover a potent and safe drug from *C. spinarum* for various chronic diseases.

In *C. spinarum,* different plant parts (root, leaf, and fruit) have much medicinal value to both humans and animals. Different parts of the plant are used for antimicrobial activity. *C. spinarum* plant has different chemical classes of phytochemicals in its barks, fruits, leaves, and roots, due to which it has medicinal value and antimicrobial properties that are still to be adequately explored.

The utilization of this plant species as complementary medicine is becoming prevalent and attaining worldwide popularity and demand. For further research, researchers must focus more on identifying the specific cellular and molecular targets of its various constituents, which exert specific therapeutic actions. The clinical potency and the toxicological studies of the species are required to be explored and documented. There is a need for standardized specifications for the different parts of *C. spinarum* to ensure their proper utilization as medicine.

Further, a detailed understanding related to herb-drug and food-drug interactions at the clinical level may help in searching out more potential drugs from the *C. spinarum* plant. The ethnopharmacological studies, which strengthen the concept of utilizing plants to cure human diseases, cultivation, and conservation strategy for further research on the *C. spinarum* plant, are the call of the hour.

REFERENCES

1. Sharma N, Kumar V, Gupta N, Shekhar P, Kaur PS. 2023. Traditional importance, phytochemistry, pharmacology, and toxicological attributes of the promising medicinal herb *Carissa spinarum* L. *Separations*. 10: 158. https://doi.org/10.3390/separations10030158.
2. Tropicos.org. 2018. Tropicos name-*Carissa spinarum* L. https://www.tropicos.org/name/1800028, as on 10th October 2021.
3. Worldagroforestry.org. 2018. Carissa edulis. https://www.worldagroforestry.org/treedb2/speciesprofile.php?Spid=443, as on 10th October 2021.
4. Alam F, Shahriar M, Bhuiyan MA. 2014. *In-vivo* pharmacological investigations of bark extracts of *Carissa carandas*. *International Journal of Pharmacy and Pharmaceutical Sciences*. 6: 180–185.
5. Mishra CK, Shrivastava B, Sasmal D. 2013. Pharmacognostical standardization and phytochemical identification of fruit and root of *Carissa carandas* Linn. *International Journal of Pharmacy and Pharmaceutical Sciences*. 5 (Suppl 3): 347–350.
6. Wani RA, Prasad VM, Hakeem SA, Sheema S, Angchuk S, Dixit A. 2013. Shelf life of Karonda jams (*Carissa carandas* L.) under ambient temperature. *African Journal of. Agricultural Research*. 8 (21): 2447–2449.
7. Malik SK, Chaudhury R, Dhariwal OP, Bhandari DC. 2010. *Genetic Resources of Tropical Underutilized Fruits in India*. NBPGR, New Delhi. pp. 178.
8. Bussmann R, Gilbreath G, Solio J, Lutura M, Lutuluo R, Kunguru K, Wood N, Mathenge SG. 2006. Plant use of the maasai of sekenani Valley, Maasai Mara, Kenya. *Jour nal of Ethnobiology and Ethnomedicine*. 2: 22. https://doi.org/10.1186/1746-4269-2-22
9. Giday M, Asfaw Z, Elmqvist T, Woldu Z. 2003. An ethnobotanical study of medicinal plants used by the Zay people in Ethiopia. *Journal of Ethnopharmacology* 85: 43–52.
10. Wambugu SN, Mathiu PM, Gakuya DW, Kanui TI, Kabasa JD, Kiama SG. 2011. Medicinal plants used in the management of chronic joint pains in Machakos and Makueni counties, Kenya. *Journal of E*thnopharmacology. 137: 945–955.
11. Addis G, Abebe D, Urga K. 2018. A survey of traditional medicinal plants in Shirka District, Arsi Zone, Ethiopia. *Ethiopian Pharmaceutical Journal*. 19: 30–47.
12. Burkill H, Dalziel J, Hutchinson J. 1985. *The Useful Plants of West Tropical Africa*. Kew: Royal Botanic Gardens.
13. Zafar M, Abbasi A, Khan M, Ahmad M, Khan H, Muhammad N, Sultana S. 2009. Medicinal plants used for the treatment of jaundice and hepatitis based on socio-economic documentation. *African Journal of Biotechnology*. 8: 1643–1650.
14. Wutthamawech W. 1997. *Encyclopaedia of Medicinal Plants*. Bangkok: Odeonstore Publishing. pp. 473.
15. Kokwaro J. 1976. *Medicinal plants of East Africa*, 2nd Edition. Nairobi: East African Literature Bureau. pp. 26.
16. Grade J, Tabuti J, Van Damme P. 2009. Ethnoveterinary knowledge in pastoral Karamoja, Uganda. *Journal of Ethnopharmacology*. 22: 273–293.
17. Pakrashi S, Datta S, Ghosh-Dastidar P. 1968. Indian medicinal plants- XVII.3 phytochemical examination of *Carissa Spp. Phytochemistry* 7: 495–496.
18. Chopra R, Nayar S, Chopra I. 1956. *Glossary of Indian Medicinal Plants*. Council of Scientific and Industrial Research, New Delhi. pp. 52.
19. Fatima A, Singh PP, Agarwal P, Irchhaiya R, Alok S, Verma A. 2017. Treatment of various diseases by Carissa spinarum L.-A promishing shrub. *IJPSR*. https://ijpsr.com/bft-article/treatment-of-various-diseases-by-carissa-spinarum-l-a-promising-shrub/?view=fulltext, as on 13th October 2021.
20. Dennis T, Sharma P, Yelne M. 2005. *Database on Medicinal Plants Used in Ayurveda*, 3rd Edition. Central Council for Research in Ayurveda & Siddha, New Delhi. pp. 369–377.
21. Bentley M, Brackett S, Chapya A. 1984. 2-hydroxyacetophenone: principal root volatile of the east African medicinal plant, *Carissa edulis*. *Journal of Natural* Produts. 47: 1056–1057.
22. Al-Youssef H, Hassan W. 2017. Chemical constituents of *Carissa edulis* Vahl. *Arabian Journal of Chemistry* 10: 109–113.
23. Achenbach H, Waibel R, Addae-Mensah I. 1983. Lignans and other constituents from *Carissa edulis*. *Phytochemistry*. 22: 749–753.
24. Achenbach H, Waibel R, Addae-Mensah I. 1985. Sesquiterpenes from *Carissa edulis*. *Phytochemistry*. 24: 2325–2328.

25. Harwansh R, Garabadu D, Rahman M, Garabadu P. 2010. *In-vitro* anthelmintic activity of different extracts of root of *Carissa spinarum. International Journal of Pharma Sciences and Research*. 1: 84–88.
26. Hegde K, Issac C, Joshi A. 2010. Antiarthritic activity of *Carissa spinarum* root extract in Freund's adjuvant induced polyarthritis in rats. *Pharmacology Online*. 2: 713–718.
27. Yau J, Yaro A, Abubakar M, Anuka J, Hussaini I. 2008. Anticonvulsant activity of *Carissa edulis* (Vahl) (Apocynaceae) root bark extract. *Journal of Ethnopharmacology*. 120: 255–258.
28. El-Fiky F, Abou-Karam M, Afify E. 1996. Effect of *Luffa aegyptiaca* (seeds) and *Carissa edulis* (leaves) extracts on blood glucose level of normal and streptozotocin diabetic rats. *Journal of E*thnopharmacology. 50: 43–47.
29. Beck N, Namdeo K. 2016. Evaluation of *in-vivo* anti-inflammatory activity of leaves extract of *Carissa spinarum* on formalin induced paw edema in albino rats. *UK Journal of Pharmaceutical and Biosciences*. 4: 36–40.
30. Woode E, Ansah C, Ainooson G, Abotsi W, Mensah A, Duweijua M. 2008. Anti-inflammatory and antioxidant properties of the root extract of *Carissa edulis* (forsk.) Vahl (Apocynaceae). *Journal of Science and Technology (Ghana)*. 27: 5–15.
31. Sahreen S, Khan M, Khan R. 2010. Evaluation of antioxidant activities of various solvent extracts of *Carissa opaca* fruits. *Food* Chemistry. 122:1205–1211.
32. Rao RJ, Kumar US, Reddy SV, Tiwari A, Rao JM. 2005. Antioxidants and a new germacrane sesquiterpene from *Carissa spinarum. Natural Product Research*. 19: 763–769.
33. Ibrahim H, Bolaji R, Abdurrahman E, Shok M, Ilyas N, Habib A. 2005. Preliminary phytochemical and antimicrobial studies of the leaves of *Carissa edulis* VAHL. *ChemClass Journal*. 2: 15–18.
34. Ibrahim H, Oyi R, Ehinmidu J, Musa K, Bright N. 2010. Antimicrobial activity of the water extracts of the leaves and fruits of *Carissa edulis* Vahl (Apocynaceae). *Journal of Medical Plants Research*. 4: 1028–1032.
35. Shahada F, Rubaka C, Ndakidemi P, Malebo H. 2014. Analysis of phytochemical and antibacterial activity of *Carissa spinarum* Linn crude extracts. *European Journal of Medicine* Plants. 4: 937–945.
36. Chandra S, Saklani S, Kandri A. 2011. Nutritional evaluation, antimicrobial activity and phytochemical screening of wild edible fruit (*Carissa opaca*). *International Research Journal of Pharmacy*. 2: 217–221.
37. Ngulde S, Sandabe U, Tijjani M, Barkindo A, Hussaini I. 2013. Phytochemical constituents, antimicrobial screening, and acute toxicity studies of the ethanol extract of *Carissa edulis* Vahl. root bark in rats and mice. *American Journal of Research Communication*. 1: 99–110.
38. Njau V, Maina E, Anjili C, Ingonga J, Koech J, Kariuki HW, Ngure PK. 2016. In vitro antileishmanial activity and phytochemical analysis of *Carissa edulis* against Leishmania major. *African Journal of Pharmacology and Therapeutics*. 5: 253–562.
39. Maina GS, Kelvin JK, Maina MB, Muriithi NJ, Kiambi MJ, Kelvin JK. 2015. Antinociceptive properties of dichloromethane: methanolic leaf and root bark extracts of *Carissa edulis* in rats. *Journal of* Phytopharmacology. 4: 106–112.
40. Mworia JK, Gitahi SM, Juma KK, Njagi JM, Mwangi BM, Aliyu U, Njoroge WA, Mwonjoria KJ, Mawia AM, Nyamai DW, Ngugi MP. 2015. Antinociceptive activities of acetone leaves extracts of *Carissa Spinarum* in mice. *Medicinal & Aromatic Plants*. 1: 1–4.
41. Tolo FM, Rukunga GM, Muli FW, Njagi EN, Njue W, Kumon K, Mungai GM, Muthaura CN, Muli JM, Keter LK, Oishi E. 2006. Anti-viral activity of the extracts of a Kenyan medicinal plant *Carissa edulis* against herpes simplex virus. *Journal of Ethnopharmacology*. 104: 92–99.
42. Doshi G, Une H. 2015. In vitro cytotoxicity studies on *Carissa congesta*, *Polyalthia longifolia*, and *Benincasa hispida* extracts by Sulforhodamine B assay method. *International Journal of Green Pharmacy*. 9: 157–161.
43. Nedi T, Mekonnen N, Urga K. 2004. Diuretic effect of the crude extracts of *Carissa edulis* in rats. *Journal of E*thnopharmacology. 95: 57–61.
44. Hegde K, Joshi AB. 2010. Hepatoprotective and antioxidant effect of *Carissa spinarum* root extract against CCl_4 and paracetamol-induced hepatic damage in rats. *Bangladesh Journal of* Pharmacology. 5: 73–76.
45. Sanwal R, Chaudhary A. 2011. Wound healing and antimicrobial potential of *Carissa spinarum* Linn. in albino mice. *Journal of Ethnopharmacology*. 135: 792–796.

8 *Cornus capitata* (Bamor)

INTRODUCTION

Cornus capitata Wall ex. Roxb. (fam.: Cornaceae) is an evergreen flowering (June to July) plant, and fruits ripen from September to November.[1] The genus *Cornus* includes about 58 morphologically heterogeneous plant species, mostly hermaphrodite shrubs or small trees.[2] The plant is native to the Himalayas and the Indo-China region. Though its hardiness varies, it cannot tolerate prolonged freezes in winter and therefore requires a sound irrigation system.[1] Its bark is rich in tannins and is used in folk remedies to treat injuries and arthritis.[3] Its inflorescences are composed of 80–100 perfect flowers contained within a capitulum, which is typically subtended by four large, showy white bracts that appear at the time of flower opening and persist for 5–7 days after anthesis. Each flower secretes minute amounts of nectar.[4] *C. capitata* fruits and leaves have anti-inflammatory, antioxidant, antidiabetic, analgesic, anticoagulant, and cytoprotective properties. The phenolic compounds, vitamins, and minerals are the main active ingredients of *C. capitata* plants.[5]

Its fruits are strawberry-like, fleshy (Figure 8.1), and edible, consisting of a high quantity of crude fiber and soluble carbohydrates.[6] The main constituents of *C. capitata* twigs and leaves are flavonoids, tannins, coumarins, etc.[1] The objectives of the present text are to collect the fragmented research information (including ethnobotanical, ethnopharmacological, nutritional, phytochemical, and pharmacological) to utilize the plant and its products, cultivate, and conserve the species.

ETHNOPHARMACOLOGY

In folklore, the *C. capitata* plant is known for its strong therapeutic activity and is widely used in traditional, modern, and veterinary medicine and pharmacy.[7,8] The fruits of *C. capitata* (Bamor) are widely used to treat dysentery and diarrhea.[9]

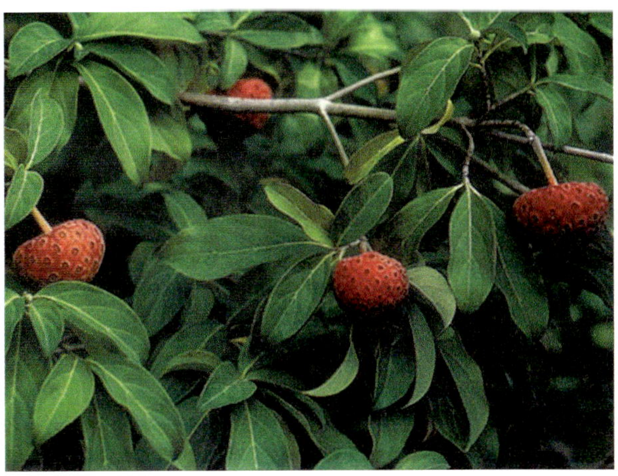

FIGURE 8.1 *C. capitata* (Bamor) branch with fruits.

PHYTOCHEMICAL SCREENING OF THE *C. CAPITATA* PLANT

Mishra et al.[2] have screened the *C. capitata* for nutritional, mineral, and phytochemical properties. The shade-dried fruits were powdered; 10.00 g of it was extracted with methanol (200 mL) at ambient temperature for 24 h, two times, filtered, mixed the filtrates, and distilled to dryness under vacuum at 40°C.

The moisture content of the fresh fruits was determined by the loss in weight of the original sample and expressed as percentage.[10,11] Protein content was determined by the Kjeldahl method, and the percentage of nitrogen was multiplied by 6.25 to obtain the value of the crude 170 protein.[12] The estimation of crude lipid was done by the Soxhlet extraction method.[13] Crude fibers and ash content were also determined.[12] The carbohydrate content was determined by subtracting the summed-up percentage compositions of moisture, protein, lipid, fiber, and ash contents from 100.[13] The mineral content (Ca, Mg, Zn, Na, K, Fe, P, Co, Cd, Se, and Mn) in the fruits of *C. capitata* was analyzed by ICP-MS using the internal standard method.[14]

The results of the study have concluded that the fresh, mature *C. capitata* fruits contain crude fiber (26.00%), carbohydrates (22.63%), crude protein (2.10%), ash (4.20%), crude lipid (1.32%), and moisture content (45.75%).[2] Saha et al. have reported a comparative study on the mineral contents of various wild edible species with the cultivated commercial fruit species, reporting a higher phosphorus content (0.77% ± 0.02) in *C. capitata* fruits.[15]

Total saponins (steroidal and triterpenoid saponins)[17] and total alkaloids[18] were determined using the gravimetric method.[17] The results showed that *C. capitata* fruits contained saponins (1.30%).[2]

Alkaloids have a specific role in the biological system, and their pharmacological effects are strictly controlled. Alkaloids in a higher quantity may cause harmful effects. The *C. capitata* fruits have a low concentration of alkaloids (1.20%),[2] indicating that there is no risk of harmful effects from eating these fruits.

The titrimetric method[19] was followed for the quantification of oxalate content. Oxalate binds with mineral elements, especially calcium and magnesium, forming oxalate crystals that are deposited as urinary stones associated with blockage of renal tubules.[20] Analytical results have revealed a low quantity of oxalate (0.47%, wt./wt.) in

DOI: 10.1201/9781003512868-10

TABLE 8.1
Phytochemical Screening of *C. capitata* Fruits[2]

Ingredient	[a]Value (%)	Ingredients	[a]Value (%)
Crude fiber	26.00±0.14	Moisture	43.75±0.10
Carbohydrate	22.63±0.12	Total saponins	1.30±0.05
Crude protein	02.10±0.25	Total alkaloids	1.20±0.10
Ash	04.20±0.15	Total oxalates	0.47±0.06
Crude lipids	01.32±0.20	Total tannins	0.30±0.25

[a] Each value is the average of three analyses (±=standard deviation)

TABLE 8.2
Phenolic Compounds of *C. capitata* Extracts[2]

Ingredients	Analytical Value[a]
Total phenolic content (mg GAE/g dry extract)	27.69±2.09
Flavonoid content (mg RUE/g dry extract)	5.18±0.09
Condensed tannins content (mg GAE/g dry extract)	21.29±0.54
Monomeric anthocyanins content (mg CGE/g)	10.7±0.01
Total anthocyanins content (mg CGE/g)	11.59±0.53

[a] Each value is the average of three analyses (±=standard deviation)

C. capitata fruits compared to spinach leaves (0.97%), the fresh weight.[16]

Mishra et al. have estimated tannins by spectrophotometric method[21] in the fruits of *C. capitata*. *C. capitata* fruits have been reported to contain 0.30% (± 0.25) total tannins (Table 8.1).[2]

Total phenolics content (Table 8.2) was assayed with the Folin-Ciocalteu method[5] and expressed in mg of gallic acid equivalents per gram of dried extract (mg GAE/g dry extract).[2] Total flavonoid content was determined using a spectrophotometric method that relied on the formation of a yellow complex[5] and expressed as rutin equivalents (mg RUE/g of extract). Furthermore, condensed tannins in the extract were determined according to the method described by Scalbert et al.[22] and expressed as the difference between total phenolic content and unprecipitated phenols, reported as gallic acid equivalents (mg GAE/g extract). Mishra et al. have determined the anthocyanin content by the pH-differential method[23] and expressed it on a cyanidin-3-glucoside basis as mg per gram of dried weight.[2]

C. capitata fruits have significant amounts of carbohydrates, protein, fat, fiber, and an appreciable quantity of minerals (K, Na, Ca, and Mg).[2]

PHYTOPHARMACOLOGY

The *C. capitata* plant has essential mineral elements, therapeutic ingredients, and antioxidant and antibacterial agents. These fruits are used as feed supplements and medicine in folklore to improve human health and growth performance. Species of the genus *Cornus* are very rich in phenolic compounds, and their folkloric applications are supported by molecular biologists based on the high nutritional and pharmacological properties of these phenolics.

Prieto et al. (2017) have studied the total antioxidant activity assay of *C. capitata* fruits by in vitro method,[24] and expressed as equivalents of ascorbic acid (AA) (mg/g of extract) using a standard curve. Scavenging activity on DPPH radicals was determined according to the spectrophotometric method with slight modification.[5] For ABTS+ radical scavenging activity of *C. capitata* fruits, the method of Re et al.[25] was adopted with slight modifications to study the lipid peroxidation inhibition activity (Table 8.3)[2] to inhibit the formation of Fe^{++} (ferrozine) complex.[26] Methanol extract of *C. capitata* fruits has 1201.1 μg/mL IC_{50} values of the ABTS assay, while in the case of DPPH assay, it was 234 μg/mL.[2]

Different phyto-compounds with antioxidant activity can inhibit lipid peroxidation via a chain reaction mechanism, which is an autocatalytic process.[27] The methanol extract of *C. capitata*, in an oil-in-water emulsion, does not inhibit 50% of lipid peroxidation at concentration lower than 4 mg/mL.

Phenolic compounds from plants are the most responsible for the chelation of iron ions. Mishra et al. have reported that the total phenolic content in *C. capitata* extract was low, and accordingly, the ability of plant extract to chelate metal ions and inhibit lipid peroxidation was significantly reduced. These results suggest that the extract may exhibit antioxidant activity via another mechanism.[2]

In bacteria, the Gram-negative *Escherichia coli* (MIC=2.5 mg/mL) has been reported as the most sensitive, followed by Gram-positive *Enterococcus faecalis* (MIC=5 mg/mL), in antimicrobial investigations against a panel of microorganisms using a methanolic extract of *C. capitata* dried fruits in in vitro studies. Due to different cell wall structures and permeability, Gram-negative and Gram-positive bacteria generally show different sensitivity. Shan et al. evaluated the antimicrobial activity of *C. officinalis* fruits and reported no inhibitory activity against *E. coli* bacteria.[28] Similar to the *C. officinalis*, extracts from fruits of *C. drummondii* do not inhibit the growth of *E. coli*

TABLE 8.3
In Vitro Antioxidant Activity of *C. capitata* Extract[2]

Ingredients	Analytical Value[a]
Total antioxidant capacity (mg AA/g of dry extract)	265.72 (±3.17)
ABTS • + scavenging activity (IC_{50}, μg/mL)	1,201.1 (±20.1)
Inhibitory activity toward lipid peroxidation (IC50, μg/mL)	>4,000
DPPH scavenging activity (IC_{50}, μg/mL)	234.00 (±2.11)
Metal chelating activity (IC_{50}, μg/mL)	>8,000

[a] Each value is the average of three analyses (±=standard deviation)

but have inhibitory activity against *Bacillus psychrophilus* and *Staphylococcus aureus*.[29]

The fruit extract of *C. capitata* was tested against a panel of seven microorganisms. All the bacterial strains were cultured overnight at 37°C in nutrient agar, and *C. albicans* was cultured on Sabouraud Dextrose Agar at 28°C for 48 h. The material obtained was suspended in sterile saline with a concentration of 5×10^5 CFU/mL for bacterial strains and 3×10^4 CFU/mL for fungi. The minimum inhibitory concentrations (MIC) of *C. capitata* extract against tested microorganisms were determined based on a microdilution method in 96 multi-well microtiter plates.[30] A change in color (colorless or purple to pink) has indicated bacterial growth. The lowest concentration for no color change was measured as the MIC value for bacterial strains, and the lowest concentrations without visible growth were noted as concentrations for complete inhibition of fungal growth (MICs).[2,30]

SCOPE AND OPPORTUNITIES

Fruits, rich in polyphenolic agar compounds (phenols, flavonoids, and anthocyanins), have long been regarded as a source of potential health benefits. Polyphenols are supposed to act as agents with bioactive properties. Fruits of *C. capitata* are rich in polyphenols, so there is scope for the development of value-added products with different functional properties, although there is not a single effort until the time, presenting opportunities for the food industry. The highly efficient antioxidants, usually with aromatic or phenolic rings (e.g., phenolic acids, flavonoids, tocopherols, and carotenoids), interrupt the free radical chain reaction, scavenge free radicals, inhibit Fe^{3+}/AA-induced oxidation, and act as reductants.[31]

C. capitata fruits have essential minerals, K (0.92), Na (170.62), Ca (5020.0), Mg (747.0), Mn (8.0), Zn (9.0), P (30.15), and Fe (100.32) in parts per million (ppm). Copper (0.2) and cadmium (0.1) have been reported in the least amount, whereas selenium was not detected. The presence of these essential nutrients and minerals implies that *C. capitata* fruits have the potential to be part of nutritional supplements and functional foods for human beings. Though these nutrients may not rocket medicine, they could be used in preventing diseases and malnutrition. High nutrient content (particularly crude fiber and carbohydrate) indicates that *C. capitata* can serve as a source of valuable edible nutrients. Furthermore, low anti-nutrient content, good mineral composition, and average moisture content may enhance nutritional status, availability of nutrients, and the possibility of application in fresh and processed conditions.

Minerals are very important in human nutrition and have been reported to be responsible for the repair of bones, teeth, and worn-out cells; the building of red blood cells; and regulating different body mechanisms. Further, potassium and calcium are essential to prevent diseases. A sufficient concentration of mineral elements is necessary for a healthy human diet to meet the recommended dietary allowance.[32] Fruits contain a group of natural antioxidants, and these compounds have multiple pharmacological activities (i.e., pleiotropic effects) in combination. The total antioxidant capacity varies considerably from one kind of fruit to another.[33]

Phenols act as reducing agents and hydrogen donors. Mechanisms for phenolic toxicity to microbes include enzyme inhibition by the oxidized compounds through specific or nonspecific interactions with proteins. Several properties of plants, such as the beneficial health effects or their potential antinutritional properties, are associated with the presence, type, and content of phenolic compounds.[34]

Saponins are known to reduce feed intake and are ascribed to a bitter/irritating taste, fight against cancer, and reduce blood cholesterol levels. These compounds help in the stimulation of a healthy immune system. Saponins have hemolytic properties and are used as a raw material for the synthesis of steroidal drugs like sex hormone stimulants, corticosteroids, and contraceptives.[32] Saponins are also used to treat viral diseases in folklore.[35] An excess quantity of saponins causes hypocholesterolemia as it binds cholesterol and makes it unavailable for absorption.[36] The formation of the saponins-protein complex reduces the protein digestibility.[37]

Tannins are astringent and bitter plant polyphenols, which can bind, precipitate, and shrink proteins, polysaccharides, and various organic compounds to form complexes with metal ions and with macromolecules. Tannins are known to have antiviral, antitumor, anti-inflammatory, and healing properties.[38,39] Dietary tannins are said to reduce feed efficiency and weight gain in chicks.[39]

The plant species *C. capitata* is widely used in both folk medicines and is to be utilized in modern green medicines. Its fruits and leaves have anti-inflammatory, cytoprotective, antioxidant, antidiabetic, analgesic, and anticoagulant activities. The phenolic compounds, vitamins, and minerals are the main active substances of the species, but the essence of flowers is to be chemically deciphered.

REFERENCES

1. Bhattarai K, Shrestha TM, Bajracharya R, Jain SC, Lamichhane J. 2010. Biological activities of three different medicinal plants from Himalayan Region of Nepal. *Nepal Journal of Science and Technology*. 11: 139–146.
2. Mishra A P, Saklani S, Stankovic M, Tiwari P, Jakovjevic D, Mihailovic V, Boroja T. 2017. Himalayan Dogwood (*Cornus capitata* Wall ex. Roxb.,) nutritional and bio-active properties. *Oxidation Communications*. 40(1-I): 168–177.
3. Li TSC, Schroeder WR. 1996. Sea buckthorn (*Hippophae rhamnoide* L.): a multipurpose plant. *Horticulture Technology*. 6: 370–380.
4. Song B, Niu Y, Stocklin J, Chen G, Peng DL, Gao YQ, Sun H. 2015. Pollinator attraction in *Cornus capitata* (Cornaceae): the relative role of visual and olfactory cues. *Journal of Plant Ecology*. 8 (2): 173–181.
5. Stankovic M, Topuzovic M. 2012. *In-vitro* antioxidant activity of extracts from leaves and fruits of common Dogwood (*C. sanguinea* L.). *A Bot Gall*. 159: 79–83.

6. Airi S, Rawal RS, Dhar U. 2005. Pre-sowing treatment effects on germination of *Cornus capitata* seeds. *Seed Science and Technology*. 33: 77–86.
7. Oskay M, Oskay D, Kalyoncu F. 2009. Activity of plant extracts against multi-drug resistant human pathogens. *Iranian Journal of Pharmaceutical Research*. 8: 293–300.
8. Rop O, Micek J, Kramarova D, Jurikova T. 2010. Selected cultivars of cornelian cherri (*Cornus mas* L.) as a new food source for human nutrition. *Academia Journal of Biotechnology*. 9 (8): 1205–1210.
9. Himachal Pradesh State Biodiversity Board. *Himachal Pradesh Council for Science, Technology & Environment (HIMCOSTE) Vigyan Bhawan, Bemloe, Shimla-1 Himachal Pradesh*. pp. 32. http://www.hpbiodiversity.gov.in
10. F.A.O. 1980. Compositional analysis methods. In: *Manuals of Food Quality Control*. Food Analysis, General Techniques, Additives, Contaminants and Composition of Food and Agricultural Organization of the United Nations, FAO, Rome, 203–232.
11. Chen C. 2003. Evaluation of air oven moisture content determination methods for rough rice. *Biosys Engineering*. 86: 447–457.
12. Ali A. 2011. Screening of less known two food plants for comparison of nutrient contents: Iranian and Indian Vegetables. *FFHD*. 10: 416–423.
13. Otitoju G. 2009. Effect of dry and wet milling processing techniques on the nutrient composition and organoleptic attributes of fermented yellow maize (*Zea mays*). *African Journal of Food Science*. 3: 113–116.
14. Yamanaka K, Fryer F. 2001. Measurement of macro and trace elements in plant digests using the 7500c ICP-MS System. *Agilent Technologies*. 1–6. Agilent Measurement of Macro Trace Elements in Plant Digests Using the 7500c ICP-MS System Manual PDF, as on 16th October 2020.
15. Saha D, Sundriyal M, Sundriyal RC. 2014. Diversity of food composition and nutritive analysis of edible wild plants in a multi-ethnic tribal land, Northeast India; An important facet for food supply. *Indian Journal of Traditional* Knowledge. 13 (4): 698–705.
16. Noonan SC, Savage GP. 1999. Oxalate content of food and its effect on humans. *Asia Pacific Journal of Clinical Nutrition*. 8 (1): 64–74.
17. Hudson BJF, El-Difrawi EA. 1979. The sapogenins of the seeds of four lupin species. *Journal of Plant Foods*. 3: 181–186.
18. Harborne JB. 1973. *Phytochemical Methods*. Chapman and Hall Ltd, London.
19. Day JRA, Underwood AL. 1986. *Quantitative Analysis*, 5th Edition. Prentice-Hall Publications, London.
20. Blood DC, Radostits OM. 1989. *Veterinary Medicine*, 7th Edition. Balliere Tindall, London. pp. 589.
21. Trease GE, Evans WC. 1989. *Pharmacognosy*, 13th Edition. Brailliere Tindall, London.
22. Scalbert A, Monties B, Janin G. 1989. Tannins in wood: comparison of different estimation methods. *Journal of Agricultural and Food Chemistry*. 37: 1324–1329.
23. Chang KG, Fechner GH, Schroeder HA. 1989. Anthocyanins in autumn leaves of Quaking aspen in Colorado. *Forest Science*. 35: 229–236.
24. Prieto P, Pineda M., Aguilar M. 1999. Spectrophotometric quantitation of antioxidant capacity through the formation of a phosphomolybdenum complex: specific application to the determination of Vitamin E1. *Analytical Biochemistry*. 269: 337–341.
25. Re R, Pellegrini N, Proteggente A, Pannala A, Yang M, Rice EC. 1999. Antioxidant activity applying an Iiproved ABTS radical cation decolorization assay. *Free Radical Biology and Medicine*. 26: 1231–1237.
26. Carter P. 1971. Spectrophotometric determination of serum iron at the sub-microgram level with a new reagent (ferrozine). *Analytical Biochemistry*. 40: 450–458.
27. Katanic J, Mihailovic V, Stankovic N, Boroja T, Mladenovic M, Solujic S, Stankovic MS, Vrvic MM. 2015. Dropwort (*F. hexapetala* Gilib.): potential role as antioxidant and antimicrobial agent. *EXCLI Journal*, 14: 1–20.
28. Shan B, Cai YZ, Brooks JD, Corke H. 2007. The in-vitro antibacterial activity of dietary spice and medicinal herb extracts. *International Journal of Food Microbiology*. 117: 112–119.
29. Post DM, James UE.1995. Antimicrobial activity of dogwood fruits (*Cornus drummondii*) from winter food caches of Eastern Woodrats (Neotoma floridana). *Journal of Chemical Ecology*. 21(4): 419–425.
30. Sarker SD, Nahar L, Kumarasamy Y. 2007. Microtitre plate-based antibacterial assay incorporating resazurin as indicator of cell growth, and its application in the *in-vitro* antibacterial screening of phytochemicals. *Methods*. 42: 321–324.
31. Oancea S, Grosu C. 2014. Protective effect of *Allium cepa* L. anthocyanin extract on the oxidative stability of sunflower oil. *Oxidation Communication*. 37(2): 474–482.
32. Dogan Y. 2015. Amino acid profile, nutrients content and yeal of chickpea (*Cicer arietinum* L.) Genotypes. *Oxidation Communication*. 38 (3): 1275–1285.
33. Wang H, Guohua C, Ronald P. 1996. Total antioxidant capacity of fruits. *Journal of Agricultural and Food Chemistry*. 44: 701–705.
34. Proestos C, Chorianopulos N, Nychas GJ, Komaitis M. 2005. RP-HPLC analysis of the phenolic compounds of plant extracts. Investigation of their antioxidant capacity and antimicrobial activity. *Journal of Agricultural and Food Chemistry*. 53: 1190–1195.
35. Sale JF, Maji JO. 2006. The phytochemical and antimicrobial screening of honey based (Ilesha Wonder Drug). In: *Proceedings of the 1st National Conference*, Faculty of Natural Sciences, University of Abuja, Nigeria.
36. So etan KO, Oyewole OE. 2009. The need for adequate processing to reduce the anti-nutritional factors in animal feeds: a review. *African Journal of Food Science*. 3 (9): 223–232.
37. Shimoyamada M, Ikedo S, Ootsubu R, Watanabe K. 1998. Effects of soyabeans saponins on chemotryptic hydrolyse of soybeans proteins. *Journal of Agricultural and Food Chemistry*. 46: 4793–4797.
38. Pasquale GD, Ostedgaard L, Vermeer D, Swaim WD, Karp P, Chiorini JA. 2012. Bovine AAV transcytosis inhibition by tannic acid results in functional expression of CFTR *in vitro* and altered biodistribution *in vivo*. *Gene Therapy*. 19: 576–581. https://doi.org/10.1038/gt.2011.138
39. Huang Q, Liu X, Zhao G, Hu T, Wang Y. 2018. Potential and challenges of tannins as an alternative to in-feed antibiotics for farm animal production. *Animal Nutrition*. 4: 137–150.

9 *Dioscorea bulbifera* (Air Potato)

INTRODUCTION

Dioscorea bulbifera Linn. is a traditional healing plant used in both Indian and Chinese traditional medicines. It is one of the most widely consumed aerial yams. The plant is characterized by considerable numbers of aerial bulbils.[1,2] The plant has been phytopharmacologically studied for its antidyslipidemic,[3] analgesic,[4] anti-inflammatory,[5] diuretic,[6] gastroprotective,[7] antioxidant,[8] antimicrobial,[9,10] antiviral,[11] antifungal,[11,12] anthelmintic,[13] neuropharmacological,[14] cardioprotective,[15] anorexiant,[16] anti-hyperthyroid,[17] antitumor,[18] and anti-HIV activities.[19] Different chemical classes of phytochemicals have been reported and isolated from the plant, such as flavonoids, glycosides, steroids, saponins, tannins, alkaloids, fatty acids, essential oils, etc. The plant is considered to have a broad spectrum of activity against several body ailments. Different parts of the plant have been explored for antiviral, diuretic, antitumor, anti-HIV, antidyslipidemic, analgesic, anti-inflammatory, antifungal, gastroprotective, antioxidant, antimicrobial, anthelmintic, neuropharmacological, cardioprotective, anorexiant, anti-hyperthyroid, and plasmid-curing activities.

D. bulbifera is commonly known as 'Varahikanda' in Ayurveda, the ancient Indian healing system. The species is native to the tropics of the Old World. It is common in the rainforests of the west coast of Africa and throughout India, ascending to 2,802 MSL in the Himalayas, but does not occur in the dried parts. Its wild form occurs in Australia, West Africa, South-Central America, Louisiana, Hawaii, Southeast Asia, Puerto Rico, Polynesia, and Texas.[1,2,20]

D. bulbifera is a long-stemmed perennial vine with non-spiny stems 20 M or more in length with vigorous twining and free branching. The internodes are round or slightly angled in cross-section and twine counterclockwise. Plants have two types of storage organs, the bulbils (aerial parts) and the tubers, beneath the ground. Tubers are likely small potatoes with a bitter taste. Conspicuous aerial tubers (called bulbils) are pale and round to globose in shape, which gives *D. bulbifera* the common name 'air potato'.[1,2] Bulbils are heavy and hard, dish-brown in color, and uniformly distributed with tubercle-like eyes. Bulbils are of different sizes and shapes and are abundant. In certain cultigens, tubers are suppressed in favor of rather large bulbils with all the reserve food. Small bulbils are, as a rule, warts but may be smooth when large (Figure 9.1). Tubers are usually small and round but may have a large size under cultivation (Figure 9.2). They weigh up to 1 kg. Tubers are toxic or edible depending on the variety; they are renewed annually. Their skin is purplish-black or earth-colored, usually coated with abundant small feeding roots, but smooth in some cultivated varieties, which have flesh ranging from white to lemon yellow, sometimes marked with purple flecks and very mucilaginous. A few roots and root scars are present on the tubers, with the outer surface being dark brown and the inner yellow to light brown.[1,2]

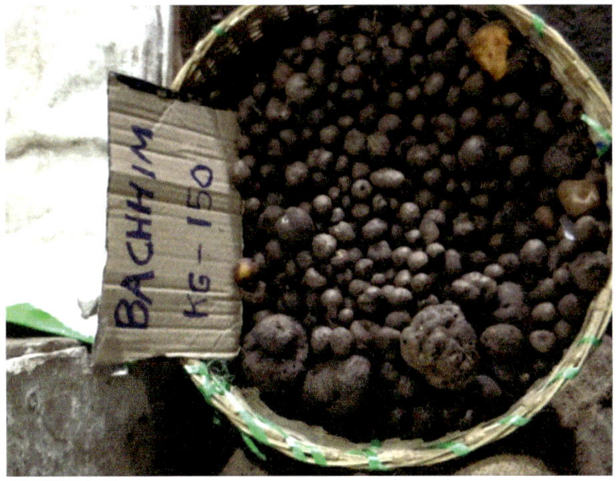

FIGURE 9.1 *D. Bulbifera* bulbils.

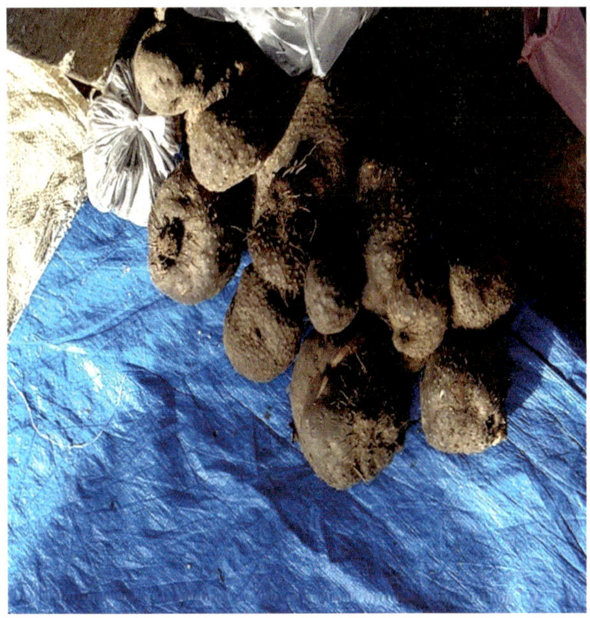

FIGURE 9.2 *D. bulbifera* tubers.

D. bulbifera is a unique plant among 600 species in the family Dioscoreaceae. It has healing applications throughout the world. The aglycones of its steroid saponins, such as diosgenin, have been used as precursors in the synthesis of fertility control compounds, sex hormones, corticosteroids, cardiotonic glycosides, and anabolic agents.[21]

DOI: 10.1201/9781003512868-11

ETHNOMEDICAL APPLICATIONS

D. bulbifera is used to improve appetite and complexion, as it is bitter and pungent. In Ayurveda, it is used to treat bronchitis, piles, dyspepsia, leukoderma, and tumors.[22] It is used to treat leprosy and tumors in Bangladesh, and sore throats and struma are treated in China.[23,24] Its infusion is applied on sores and cuts in Zimbabwe, while in Cameroon and Madagascar, it is used to treat boils, abscesses, and wound infections.[25] In Indian traditional medicine, it is utilized to treat inflammation, piles, and ulcers.[26,27] Modern and ancient literature on the bulbils of *D. bulbifera* deciphers its therapeutic applications as a rejuvenating tonic, diuretic, aphrodisiac, anthelmintic, de-flatulent, and purgative. Its uses to cure hematological disorders, general weakness, worm infestations, scrofula, diabetic disorders, hemorrhoids, skin disorders, polyurea, etc. in different folk healing practices have been observed. Decoction of the crushed tubers of *D. bulbifera* is emulsified into oil to treat infected ulcers and sinuses.[2,28] Both Indian and Chinese traditional practices use tubers to cure gastric cancer, carcinoma of the rectum, and goiter.[29]

The extracts of *D. bulbifera* are reported to be plasmid curing, antihyperglycemic, anti-hyperlipidemic, anorexiant, antitumor, analgesic, antioxidant, anti-inflammatory, and antidiabetic.[3,4,17,19,29–32] Dried yam is used to cure scrofula, purulent infections, and carbuncles and dissolve toxins. In Brazil and Java, it is considered a remedy against dysentery, diarrhea, and syphilis. In China, it is used against food poisoning, hepatic fibrosis, snakebites, and dog bites.[33] Further, the remedial potential of *D. bulbifera* against biliousness, dyspepsia, urinary discharges, leucoderma, jaundice, asthma, diabetes, bronchitis, and conjunctivitis has been reported in different research reports.[34]

D. bulbifera has been used to enhance memory and is an antiaging food supplement with laxative and antipyretic properties.[35] Its infusion is applied on sores and cuts for speedy healing of wounds in a flamed membrane.[36] In Madagascar and Cameroon, the pounded bulbils of *D. bulbifera* are applied on boils, wound infections, and abscesses.[37] Other medicinal applications of *D. bulbifera* include the treatment of piles, cough, sexual diseases, dysentery, syphilis, ulcers, diabetes, leprosy, tuberculosis, and its use as a contraceptive, but clinical significance depends on the mode of dosage and its administration (Table 9.1).

D. bulbifera has a higher nutritional value compared to other *Dioscorea* species.[36] *D. bulbifera* has the highest levels of minerals (sodium, calcium, zinc, and magnesium), vitamins (B1, B3, and C), and protein content among all the species. Despite the valuable medicinal applications and nutritional value *of D. bulbifera,* other yam species are generally preferred for their flavor. It is the best food for diabetic patients and people with other health ailments such as obesity, as these are more nutritious and less sweet.[44] Leaves of the plant are used as a staple food by hunter-gatherers living in the forest, such as the Abayanda in Uganda and Pygmies in Central Africa.[45]

PHYTO-CONSTITUENTS

The plant D. bulbifera contains polyphenolic organic acids and has potent antioxidant properties. Phytochemical screening of *D. bulbifera* reveals the presence of flavonoids, glycosides, polyphenols, tannins, saponins, sterols,[46] and steroidal saponins.[47] *D. bulbifera* has a bitter-salty taste and a faint odor. The bulbil of *D. bulbifera* has diosgenin, a steroidal phytochemical characterized for antifertility activity.[48]

The phytochemicals present in *D. bulbifera* plants vary with the biotic and abiotic factors of the location, the parts of a plant, and the solvents used for extraction.[49] Examples may be cited from the rhizome extract in 27% ethanol collected from China and subsequently re-extracted with ethyl acetate. The ethyl acetate soluble fraction has kaempferol-3,5-dimethyl ether, catechin, caryatin, quercetin-3-O-galactopyranoside, myricetin-3-O-glucopyranoside, and myricetin-3-O-galactopyranoside.[19] The extract prepared from the rhizomes of *D. bulbifera* collected from China, when extracted with 95% ethanol and subsequently re-extracted with ethyl acetate, has diosbulbisins (A, B, C, and D), diosbulbisides (A and B), and diosbulbiside C.

The aqueous methanolic extract of bulbs of *D. bulbifera* collected from India has 8-epidiosbulbin E acetate.[32] The chloroform extract has diosbulbin B as the main ingredient.[19] Carotenoids such as zeaxanthin, lutein, and neoxanthin are also prevalent in *D. bulbifera*.[50] Methanol extract of bulbils collected from Cameroon is rich in bafoudiosbulbins

TABLE 9.1
Ethnomedicinal Applications of Bubils of *D. bulbifera*

Plant Part	Processing	Application	Utility
Bulbil	Powdered dried bulbil, 10 mg is given once a day for 5 days, after menses	Oral	Contraceptive[38-40]
Bulbil	Bulbils are either roasted or cooked as a vegetable	Topical, oral	Dysentery, piles, ulcers, and syphilis[41]
Bulbil	Bulbils are cooked and roasted as a vegetable	Oral	Cough, diabetes, and leprosy[41]
Bulbil	Bulbils are boiled 2–3 times with ash	Oral	Tuberculosis[42]
Bulbil	Bulbils are boiled 2–3 times with ash	Oral	Sore throat and struma[42]
Bulbil	Bulbils are boiled	Oral	Sexual vigor food[2]
Bulbil	Bulbils are boiled	Oral	As wild food for HIV patients in Uganda[43]

(A, B, C, F, and G).[51] Bulbils collected from Nigeria and tubers from Bangladesh are rich in demethylbatatasin IV and diosbulbin D.[52] Flowers of *D. bulbifera* collected from Cameroon have dioscoreanosides (A, B, C, D, E, F, G, H, I, J, and K).[47]

D. bulbifera contains a steroidal saponin called diosgenin. Diosgenin is a principal raw material for the synthesis of estrogen, contraceptives, and corticosteroids.[53] *D. bulbifera* bulb is one of the ten important natural sources of steroids. Diosgenin is often prescribed as a medicine of herbal origin.[54] Diosgenyl saponins are abundant in the bulbils and used for several biological functions.[55] Diosgenin, a primary furostanol saponin, is found in *Dioscorea* species (yams), as well as in Trigonella *foenum-graecum* and *Costus speciosus*. This compound is useful to maintain healthy blood cholesterol levels,[56] has been reported to retard the progression of osteoporosis,[57] and is known for its potent anti-inflammatory property.[57] Diosgenin glycosides have been reported for myocardial mechanical activities through the modulation of extracellular calcium (Ca^{2+}) flux across the plasma membrane.[58,59] Diosgenin has been reported to ameliorate myocardial infarction by lipo-peroxidative action.[15,60]

A literature survey reveals that *D. bulbifera* tuber has alkaloids, terpenoids, cardiac glycosides, oxalates, phenolics, saponins, flavonoids, tannins, organic acids, and polysaccharides.[51] Polysaccharides are formed by the condensation of a large number of aldoses and ketoses, which have high molecular weight and structural complexity with inorganic compounds.[61] Natural polysaccharides are known to have antiviral, immunomodulatory, antioxidant, anticoagulant, anti-inflammatory, antitumor, antimicrobial, and hypoglycemic effects.[62]

Phytochemical screening of *D. bulbifera* revealed the presence of glycosides, sterols, polyphenols, alkaloids, proteins, fats, tannins, flavonoids, and saponins, which vary according to geo-climatic locations,[47] similar to their utilization for therapeutic purposes (Table 9.2). The micronutrients present in the *D. bulbifera* include Zn, Fe, Mo, B, Cu, Br, Mn, Co, Na, Cl, I, and V.[47]

PHARMACOLOGY

Ancient and modern applications and literature on *D. bulbifera*'s medicinal uses have ample evidence for its effectiveness in treating nervous excitability, hysteria, senility, infertility, syphilis, hemorrhoids, dysentery, diarrhea, hormonal deficiency, colic, abdominal pain, and cramps; promoting body weight; and soothing digestive organs.[64] *D. bulbifera* is commonly used in traditional African, Chinese, and Indian medicines to treat breast cancer,[65] sore throats,[42] and type 2 diabetes mellitus.[8,18] Clinical trials have revealed the effectiveness of *D. bulbifera* in treating subacute thyroiditis with its ethyl acetate fraction.[66]

TABLE 9.2
Traditional Applications of *D. bulbifera*[41,46,63]

Country/Region	Medicinal Uses
India	*D. bulbifera* is a staple medicinal food substitute in India. The rural and local people detoxify it before using it as food. Tubers are either left overnight in-stream and successively boiled or soaked overnight in water to remove the bitterness. The powdered form of tubers is prescribed with honey and milk for an antiaging effect; it rejuvenates cells and tissues, improving the sperm and semen quantity and efficacy. Infertility and impotence are cured by using tubers as a tonic for male/female reproductive organs. Tubers are used for improving voice, physical strength, immunity, and digestion by balancing Kapha and Vata in Ayurveda. Tubers are used to treat asthma, cough, tuberculosis, leprosy, cold, constipation, bone fracture, abdominal pain, contraception, indigestion, muscular pain, dysentery, sore throat, cuts, struma, wounds, boils, injury, carbuncle, and tumors, and are also used as a cooling agent to reduce body heat during summer. Tubers have properties such as aphrodisiac, purgative, rejuvenating, de-flatulent, and tonic anthelmintic, hemorrhoids, scrofula, general debility, and worm intestations. Decoction of the fresh tuber is used to cure laryngitis in children, goiter, fever, ringworm, and insect bites. Powdered roots are used as a local medicine to treat tuberculosis. It regulates kidney function and is used in diseases of the lungs and spleen.
Bangladesh	Body ailments such as tumors and leprosy are cured.
Latin America	Depression, diarrhea, conjunctivitis, body fatigue, and dysentery are treated using tubers of *D. bulbifera*.
Zimbabwe	An infusion of tubers is applied on cuts and sores.
Java, Brazil	Tubers are used to treat diarrhea, syphilis, and dysentery.
China	Hepatic fibrosis, sore throat, snakebites, dog bites, struma, food poisoning, gastric and rectum cancer, and goiter are treated.
Tanzania	Leaves and tubers are used for eye steam baths.
Africa	Bulbils are used as hunting poison and tubers as fishing poison. Externally bulbils are used as a medicine for skin diseases and boils.
Zaire	Infected wounds are covered by a grilled leaf with little palm oil.
Cameroon	A poultice remedy using tubers for abscesses boils and wound infections are in practice.
Congo	The juice of the whole plant is used to treat snakebite and eye inflammation.
Benin	Leaves juice is recommended to ease birth and reduce labor pain.
Madagascar	Wound infections, abscesses, and boils are treated using the pulp of pounded bulbils.

More recently, anti-HIV-1 integrase compounds have been reported from *D. bulbifera*. The ethyl acetate and water fractions of *D. bulbifera* bulbils were investigated using a molecular docking method. Catechol, galloyl, and sugar moieties from *D. bulbifera* bulbils were reported to successfully inhibit HIV-1.[67] The research supports the traditional use of *D. bulbifera* bulbils as anti-HIV medicine, and there is a high chance of having modern green medicine to treat HIV patients from *D. bulbifera* bulbils. Further, *D. bulbifera* bulbils are one of the natural foods recommended for HIV patients.[43] According to Kuete et al., the methanolic extract of *D. bulbifera* has an efficient antibacterial activity against multidrug-resistant bacteria like *Pseudomonas aeruginosa* PA124, *Enterobacter aerogenes* EA289, *Staphylococcus aureus*, *Klebsiella pneumoniae* KP63, and Mycobacteria strain with the lowest MIC (minimum inhibitory concentration) value.[9] Araghiniknam et al. have reported that *Dioscorea* supplementation is beneficial to elderly people, as it increases serum dehydroepiandrosterone sulfate and modulates lipid levels in humans.[68]

The literary study of Varahikanda (*D. bulbifera* L.) concludes its properties as Rasayana (immunomodulatory activity), Jeevaneeya (antioxidant activity), Pramehaghna (antidiabetic activity), Kushtaghna (antimicrobial activity), Balya and Vrushya (aphrodisiac activity), Raktapittahar (anticancer activity more focused on blood cancer), Udarshoolahar (anti-inflammatory and analgesic activity), Pravahikahar (antibacterial/viral), Nadivrunhar (wound healing activity), Medohar (dyslipidemic activity), and Krumiroghar (anthelmintic activity).[69]

TRADITIONAL DETOXIFICATIONS OF BULBILS

The main toxic ingredients of *D. bulbifera* are sapogenins and saponins (in species collected from India, South Africa, and Central America), polyphenols and tannins (in samples collected from the Indo-Chinese region), and furanoid and nor-diterpenes (of Chinese origin). Diosbulbin D is a major toxic compound (0.07 mg/g) in *D. bulbifera* varieties collected from Australia. Pre-treatment practices vary, from baking followed by overnight leaching of the sliced tubers for 12 h in running water, which results in a major loss of bitter and toxic compounds to a very low-level presence and a better taste threshold of the final palatable food.[70]

MOLECULAR KNOWLEDGE AND VALUE ADDITION

Numerous studies on drug-drug interactions with synergistic compatibility have been conducted using *D. bulbifera* bulbils.. Wang et al. studied a combination of *D. bulbifera* with other herbal medicines and reported that there was an improvement in therapeutic effects along with reduced toxic effects of bulbils.[71] The use of *Angelica sinensis* with *D. bulbifera* enhances the antitumor effect[71] and reduces renal[72–75] as well as kidney toxicity.[76] The combination of *D. bulbifera* with *Schisandra chinensis* has liver-healing properties.[77–79] The potential synergistic anticancer activity of *D. bulbifera* in combination with *Scutellaria barbata* is useful in the treatment of cancer.[80] The combination of *D. bulbifera* with *Glycyrrhiza uralensis* reduces liver damage and renal toxicity caused by *D. bulbifera*.[81] The co-administration of *D. bulbifera* and diosgenin reduces the harmful effects of diosgenin.[82]

SCOPE AND OPPORTUNITIES

D. bulbifera has been used since ancient times in different civilizations as folk medicine against several body ailments. Numerous studies on its therapeutic potential have deciphered *D. bulbifera* as a natural treasure of bioactive ingredients, which serve as useful principles for higher efficacy and biocompatibility with least side effects. The chemical composition of *D. bulbifera* depends on the geo-climatic factors of the plant, the part of the plant used, and the type of solvent selected for the extraction process.

The medicinal and food-related utilization of any plant species is greatly influenced by its conservation and sustainability. The conservation of *D. bulbifera* can be done by promoting the utilization of the species to encourage the farmers to cultivate it. The scientific cultivation will have real-time information on its germplasm and range of utilization, helping breeders select potential breeding stocks.

Finally, a trade based on the value-added products of *D. bulbifera* may have a sustainable source of income. There is a golden occasion to use tubers/bulbils in contraceptive capsules and tablets to treat the mentioned ailments. *D. bulbifera* has a variety of chemicals and may be used in a wide spectrum of biological activities, as shown in Table 9.2. The increased utilization and raised market demands will lead to *D. bulbifera* conservation and cultivation practices.

REFERENCES

1. Anonymus. 1998. *The Wealth of India. Raw Materials*. CSIR, New Delhi. Vol. 4: pp. 67–76.
2. Subasini U, Thenmozhi S, Sathyamurthy D, Vetriselvan S, Victor Rajamanickam G, Dubey GP. 2013. Pharmacognostic and phytochemical investigations of *Dioscorea bulbifera* L. *International Journal of Pharmaceutical and Life Sciences*. 4 (5): 2693–2700.
3. Ahmed Z, Chishti MZ, Johri RK, Bhagat A, Gupta KK, Gandhi Ram GR. 2009. Antihyperglycemic and antidyslipidemic activity of aqueous extract of *Dioscorea bulbifera* tubers. *Diabetologia Croatica*. 38 (3): 69–72.
4. Nguelefack TB, Dutra RC, Paszcuk AF, Andrade EL, Tapondjou LA, Calixto JB. 2010. Anti-nociceptive activities of the methanol extract of the bulbs of *Dioscorea bulbifera* L. varsativa in mice is dependent of NO-cGMP-ATP-sensitive-K+ channel activation. *Journal of Ethnopharmacology*. 128 (3): 567–574.
5. Tan XQ, Ruan JL, Chen HS, Wang JY, Wang JS. 2003. Study on anti-inflammatory constituents of *Dioscorea bulbifera* L. *Academic journal of Second Military Medical University*. 24: 677–679.

6. Omodamiro OD. 2015. Anti-inflammatory and diuretic activities of ethanol extract of *Dioscorea bulbifera* leaf. *AJDDT.* 2 (1): 029–038.
7. Balasubramanian J, Dhanalakshmi R, Jibnomen P, Manimekalai P. 2012. A preclinical evaluation on antioxidant and gastroprotective effect of *Dioscorea bulbifera* in wistar rats. *Indian Journal of Innovation Discovery.* 3 (1): 1–8.
8. Ghosh S, More P, Nitnavare R, Jagtap S, Chippalkatti R, Asok A, Kale S, Singh S, Shaikh ML. 2015. Antidiabetic and antioxidant properties of copper nanoparticles synthesized by medicinal plant *Dioscorea bulbifera. Journal of Nanomedicine and Nanotechnology.* S6: 007. https://doi.org/10.4172/2157-7439.S6-007
9. Kuete V, Teponno RB, Mbaveng AT, Tapoudjou LA, Meyer JJM, Barboni L, Lall N. 2012. Antibacterial activities of the extracts, fractions and compounds from *Dioscorea bulbifera. BMC Complement and Alternative Medicine.* 12: 228.
10. Teponno RB, Tapondjou AL, Gatsing D, Djoukeng JD, Abou-Mansour E, Tabacchi R, Tane P, Stoekli-Evans H, Lontsi D. 2006. Bafoudiosbulbins A, and B, two anti-salmonellal clerodane diterpenoids from *Dioscorea bulbifera* L. var sativa. *Phytochemistry.* 67: 1957–1963.
11. Cao RL, Sun ZY, Wang ZD, Yin XZ. 1957. The investigation of Chinese medicine decoction anti-fungal actvitiy *in vitro. Chinese Journal of Dermatology.* 5: 286–292.
12. Adetoun A, Ikotun T. 1989. Antifungal activity of dihydrodioscorine extracted from a wild variety of *Dioscorea bulbifera* L. *Journal of Basic Microbiology.* 29: 265–267.
13. Patel DM, Galani VJ. 2017. Evaluation of neuropharmacological activity of *Dioscorea bulbifera* using various experimental models. *Advances in Plants and Agriculture Research.* 7 (1): 00241.
14. Su L, Zhu JH, Cheng LB, Li YH. 2003. Experimental pathological study of sub-acute intoxication by *Dioscorea bulbifera* L. *Journal of Forensic Medicine.* 19: 81–83.
15. Vasanthi HR, Mukherjee S, Ray D, Jayachandran KSP, Lekli I, Das DK. 2010. Protective role of air potato (*Dioscorea bulbifera*) of yam family in myocardial ischemic reperfusion injury. *Food and Function.* 1: 278–283.
16. Song CS, Liu XF, Du YT, Zhao FZ, Wang SH, Ji DG, Cao HL. 1983. The experiment of heptatic and renal toxicity induced by *D. bulbifera. Bull Chin Mater Medica.* 8: 34–36.
17. Jindal MN, Kelkar VV, Doctor RB. 1969. The anorexient activity of Kalio-kund (*Dioscorea bulbifera* Linn.), methylphenidate and cocaine in rats: a preliminary study. *Indian Journal of Medical Research* 57: 1075–1080.
18. Ghosh S, Nitnavare R, Dewle A, Tomar GB, Chippalkatti R, More P, Kitture R, Kale S, Bellare J, Chopade BA. 2015. Novel platinum-palladium bimetallic nanoparticles synthesized by *Dioscorea bulbifera*: anticancer and antioxidant activities. *International Journal of Nanomedicine.* 10 (1): 7477–7490.
19. Gao HY, Kuroyanagi M, Wu LJ, Kawahara N, Yasuno T, Nakamura Y. 2002. Antitumor-promoting constituents from Dioscorea bulbifera L. in JB6 mouse epidermal cells. *Biological and Pharmaceutical Bulletin* 25 (9): 1241–1243.
20. Khare CP. 2016. *Ayurvedic Pharmacopoeial Plant Drugs-Expanded Therapeutics.* CRC Press, Boca Raton, FL, London, New York. pp. 227–228.
21. Culafic L, Savikin-Fodulovic K, Grubisic D, Neskovic M. 1999. *Dioscorea balcanica Kosanin and D. caucasica Lipsky: In Vitro Culture and Production of Diosgenin.* In: *Medicinal and Aromatic Plants XI. Biotechnology in Agriculture and Forestry.* Bajaj, Y.P.S. (Ed.) Springer, Berlin Heidelberg, New York. Vol. 43. pp. 85–102. https://doi.org/10.1007/978-3-662-08614-8_6
22. Kirtikar KR, Basu BD. 2007. *Indian Medicinal Plants Spp*, 2nd Edition. International Book Distributors. Vol. 4: pp. 2452–2456.
23. Murray RDH, Jorge ZD, Khan NH, Shahjahan M, Quaisuddin M. 1984. Diosbu lbin d and 8-epidiosbulbin e acetate, norclerodane diterpenoids from *Dioscorea bulbifera* tubers. *Phytochemistry.* 23: 623–625.
24. Komori T. 1997. Glycosides from *Dioscorea bulbifera. Toxicon.* 35: 1531–1536.
25. Mbiantcha M, Kamanyi A, Teponno RB, Tapondjou AL, Watcho P, Nguelefack TB. 2011. Analgesic and anti-inflammatory properties of extracts from the bulbils of *Dioscorea bulbifera* L. var sativa (Dioscoreaceae) in mice and rats. *Evidence-Based Complementary and Alternative Medicine.* 2011. Article ID 912935. https://doi.org/10.1155/2011/912935
26. Lather A, Gupta V, Garg S, Singh A, Sachdeva K. 2011. Pharmacological potential of the plants used in treatment of piles – a review. *Journal of Natura Conscintia.* 2: 255–265.
27. Gupta D, Singh J. 1989. p-Hydroxyacetophenone derivatives from *Dioscorea bulbifera. Phytochemistry.* 28: 947–949.
28. Tang Z, Zhou Y, Zeng Y, Zang S, He P, Fang Y. 2006. Capillary electrophoresis of the active ingredients of *Dioscorea bulbifera* L. and its medicinal preparations. *Chromatographia.* 63: 617–622.
29. Adeniran AA, Sonibare MA. 2013. In vitro potential anthelmintic activity of bulbils of *Dioscorea bulbifera* L. on earthworms and liver flukes. *Journal of Pharmacognosy and Phytotherapy.* 5: 196–203.
30. McKoy ML, Omoruyi F, Simon O, Asemota H. 2003. Investigation of the effects of a sapogenin-rich preparation from a Jamaican yam (*Dioscorea* sp.) on blood cholesterol levels in rats. *Proceedings of the Western Pharmacological Society.* 46: 156–159.
31. Bhandari MR, Kawabata J. 2004. Organic acid, phenolic content and antioxidant activity of wild yam (*Dioscorea* spp.) tubers of Nepal. *Food Chemistry.* 88: 163–168.
32. Shriram V, Jahagirdar S, Latha C, Kumar V, Puranik V, Rojatkar S, Dhakephalkar PK, Shitole MG. 2008. A potential plasmid-curing agent, 8-epidiosbulbin E acetate, from *Dioscorea bulbifera* L. against multidrug-resistant bacteria. *International Journal of Antimicrobial Agents.* 32: 405–410.
33. Williams C. 2013. Medicinal plants in Australia volume 4: an antipodean apothecary. *Rosenberg Publishing Science.* 552: 437–444.
34. Panduraju T, Bitra VR, Vemula SK, Reddy P, Reddy V. 2010. Wound healing activity of *Dioscorea bulbifera* Linn. *Journal of Pharmacy Research.* 3: 3138–3139.
35. Odugbemi T. 2008. *A Textbook of Medicinal Plants from Nigeria.* Lagos, Nigeria: University of Lagos Press.
36. Chinelo AE, Regina OA. 2018. Comparative analyses of phytochemical and nutritional compositions of four species of *Dioscorea. Acta Scientific Nutritional Health.* 2 (7): 90–94.
37. Cogne AL. 2002. Phytochemical Investigation of Plants Used in African Traditional Medicine: *Dioscorea* Sylvatica (Dioscoreaceae), *Urginea Altissima* (Liliaceae), *Jamesbrittenia Fodina* and *Jamesbrittenia Elegantissima* (Scrophulariaceae). 208. https://api.semanticscholar.org/CorpusID:202066454https://www.secheresse.info/spip.php?article81141, as on 31st July 2021.

38. Das B, Talukdar ADAS, Dutta Choudhury M. 2014. A few traditional medicinal plants used as antifertility agents by ethnic people of Tripura, India. *International Journal of Pharmacy and Pharmaceutical Sciences*. 6 (3): 47–53.
39. Kamble SY, Patil SR, Sawant PS, Sawant S, Pawar SG, Singh EA. 2010. Studies on plants used in traditional medicine by Bhilla Tribe of Maharashtra. *Indian Journal of Traditional Knowledge*. 9 (3): 591–598.
40. Swarnkar S, Katewa SS. 2008. Ethnobotanical observation on tuberous plants from tribal area of Rajasthan (India). *Ethnobotanical Leaflets*. 12: 647–666.
41. Dutta B. 2015. Food and medicinal values of certain species of *Dioscorea* with special reference to Assam. *Journal of Pharmacognosy and Phytochemistry*. 3 (4): 15–18.
42. Sharma LN, Bastakoti R. 2009. Ethnobotany of *Dioscorea* L. with emphasis on food value in chepang communities in Dhading District, Central Nepal. *Journal of Plant Science*. 6: 12–17.
43. Nabatanzi A. 2016. Wild food plants used by people living with HIV/ AIDS in Nakisunga sub-county, Uganda. *African Journal of Food Agriculture Nutrition and Development*. 16: 11310–11330.
44. Okeke EC, Eneobong HN, Uzuegbunam AO, Ozioko AO, Kuhnlein H. 2008. Igbo traditional food system: documentation, uses and research needs. *Pakistan Journal of* Nutrition. 7 (2): 365–376.
45. Byarugaba D, Ndemere P, Midgley J. 2007. The vulnerability and resilience of *Dioscorea* species in utilized and non-utilized zones of bwindi impenetrable national park. *African Journal of Ecology*. 45 (3): 258–264.
46. Ghosh S. 2015. Phytochemsitry and therapeutic potential of medicinal plant: *Dioscorea bulbifera*. *Medicinal Chemistry*. 5 (4): 160–172.
47. Tapondjou LA, Jenett-Siems K, Böttger S, Melzig MF. 2013. Steroidal saponins from the flowers of *Dioscorea Bulbifera* Var. Sativa. *Phytochemistry*. 95: 341–350.
48. Shajeela PS, Mohan VR, Louis Jesudas L, Tresina Soris P. 2011. Antifertility acitivity of ethanol extract of *Dioscorea esculenta* (L .) schott on male albino rats. *International Journal of PharmTech Research*. 3 (2): 946–954.
49. Jayachandran HS, Vasanthi, AHR, Gurusamy N. 2016. Steroidal saponin diosgenin from *Dioscorea bulbifera* protects cardiac cells from hypoxia-reoxygenation injury through modulation of pro-survival and pro-death molecules. *Pharmacognsy Magazine*. 12 (Suppl 1): S14–S20.
50. Ghosh S, Ahire M, Patil S, Jabgunde A, Dusane MB, Bimba N, Pardesi K, Jachak S, Dhavale DD, Chopade BA. 2011. Antidiabetic activity of gnidia glauca and Dioscorea bulbifera: potent amylase and glucosidase inhibitors. *Evidence-Based Complementary and Alternative Medicine*. 2012: 1–7.
51. Adeosun OM, Arotupin DJ, Toba OA, Adebayo AA. 2016. Antibacterial activities and phytochemical properties of extracts of *Dioscorea bulbifera* Linn (Air Potato) tubers and peels against some pathogenic bacteria. *The Journal of Phytopharmacology*. 5 (1): 20–26.
52. Adesanya SA, Ogundana SK, Roberts MF. 1989. Dihydrostilbene phytoalexins from Dioscorea bulbifera and D. dumentorum. *Phytochemistry*. 28 (3): 4–5.
53. Kamboj VP. 2000. Herbal medicine. General Article. *Current Science*. 78: 35–39.
54. Fowler MW, Mantell SH, Smith H. 1984. *Plant Biotechnology*. Cambridge University Press, Cambridge. pp. 3–37.
55. Francis G, Kerem Z, Makkar HP, Becker K. 2002. The biological action of saponins in animal systems: a review. *British Journal of Nutrition*. 88: 587–605.
56. Komesaroff PA, Black CV, Cable V, Sudhir K. 2001. Effects of wild yam extract on menopausal symptoms, lipids and sex hormones in healthy menopausal women. *Climacteric*. 4: 144–150.
57. Higdon K, Scott A, Tucci M, Benghuzzi H, Tsao A, Puckett A, Cason Z, Hughes J. 2001. The use of estrogen, DHEA, and diosgenin in a sustained delivery setting as a novel treatment approach for osteoporosis in the ovariectomized adult rat model. *Biomedical Sciences Instrumentation*. 37: 281–286.
58. Au AL, Kwok CC, Lee AT, Kwan YW, Lee MM, Zhang RZ, Ngai SM, Lee SM, He GW, Fung KP. 2004. Activation of iberiotoxin-sensitive, Ca^{2+}-activated K^+ channels of porcine isolated left anterior descending coronary artery by diosgenin. *European Journal of Pharmacology*. 502: 123–133.
59. Lísias GD, Azevedo CN, Karyne GP, Maria BF. 2007. Mechanisms involved in the vasodilator effect induced by diosgenin in rat superior mesenteric artery. *European Journal of Pharmacology*. 574: 172–178.
60. Jayachandran KS, Vasanthi HR, Rajamanickam GV. 2009. Anti-lipoperoxidative and membrane stabilizing effect of diosgenin, in experimentally induced myocardial infarction. *Molecular and Cellular Biochemistry*. 327: 203–210.
61. Le- Costaouëc T, Unamunzaga C, Mantecon L, Helbert W. 2017. New structural insights into the cell-wall polysaccharide of the diatom *Phaeodactylum tricornutum*. *Algal Research*. 26: 172–179.
62. Meng X, Liang H, Luo L. 2016. Antitumor polysaccharides from mushrooms: a review on the structural characteristics, antitumor mechanisms and immunomodulating activities. *Carbohydrate Research*. 424: 30–41.
63. Hans DN. 1996. *African Ethnobotany: Poisons and Drugs: Chemistry, Pharmacology, Toxicology*. Chapman & Hall GmbH, Heidelberg. pp. 423–424.
64. Uniyal RC. 1998. *The Ayurveda Encyclopedia Natural Secrets to Healing, Prevention & Longevity*, 1st Edition. Ayurveda Holistic Center Press, Bayville, NY, USA. pp. 108–109.
65. Anandpara RC, Tirgar PR. 2017. Investigation of therapeutics benefits of *Dioscorea bulbifera* in breast cancer. *Journal of Chemical and Pharmaceutical Research*. 9 (6): 313–326.
66. Hidayat A, Fadhlurrahman A, Chan CK, Mohamad J, Kadir HA. 2018. *Dioscorea bulbifera* induced apoptosis through inhibition of ERK 1/2 and activation of JNK signaling pathways in HCT116 human colorectal carcinoma cells. *Biomedicine and* Pharmacotherapy. 104: 806–816.
67. Chaniad P, Wattanapiromsakul C, Pianwanit S. 2016. Anti-HIV-1 integrase compounds from *Dioscorea bulbifera* and molecular docking study. *Pharmaceutical Biology*. 54 (6): 1077–1085.
68. Araghiniknam M, Chung S, Nelson-White T, Eskelson C, Watson RR. 1996. Antioxidant activity of *Disoscore*a and Dehydroepiandrosterone (DHEA) in older humans. *Life Sciences*. 59 (11). 8795709. https://doi.org/10.1016/0024-3205(96)00396-7
69. Galakatu SS, Surve PP, Ghotankar AM, Kharat RS. 2016. Review of Varahikand (*Dioscorea bulbifera*) for its pharmacological properties. *World Journal of Pharmaceutical Research*. 5 (4): 1738–1746.

70. Vijayakumar TM, Ilango K, Ramasamy MK, Agrawal A, Dubey GP. 2015. Effect of *Dioscorea bulbifera* and its major bioactive compound, diosgenin on CYP450 mediated drug metabolism. *Journal of Biologically Active Products from Nature*. 5 (5): 313–321.
71. Wang J, Xia XY, Peng RX, Li Y. 2003. Down regulated of *Angelica sinensis* polysaccharides cause the CYPE1 expression in rat Kufe cells induced by ethanol. *Chinese Journal of Clinical Pharmacology*. 20: 66.
72. Liu SM, Zhang L, Li Y, Luo MM. 2006. The effects of *D. bulbifera* combination with Angelica sinensis on the expression of rat's liver CYP1A2, CYP2E1 gens and mRNA. *Pharmacy and Clinics of Chinese Materia Medica*. 22: 97.
73. Tang Q, Liu SM, Wang JZ, Zhou Q, Liu TY. 2010. Effects of *Dioscorea bulbifera* rhizome and *Dioscorea bulbifera* rhizome plus *Angelica sinensis* root on expression of grp78 and bad genes in rat livers. *Adverse Drug Reaction Journal*. 12 (2): 91–95.
74. Liu SM, Cui LR, Yu DH, Jin Y, Dong WR. 2010. The protective effect of *Angelica sinensis* on liver structure damage induced by *D. bulbifera*. *Liaoning Journal of Traditional Chinese Medicine*. 37: 1823–1824.
75. Ding GM, Tang YX. 1992. The experimental observation of *Angelica sinensis* on *Dioscorea bulbifera* detoxification. *Chinese Traditional and Herbal Drugs*. 23: 192–199.
76. Yang H, Mou JZ, Yang C, Cui XQ, Li DJ, Wang YY, Yuan JC, Li JX. 2009. Toxic study of *Dioscorea bulbifera* L. on mice. *China Pharm*. 12: 706–709.
77. Liu GT, Bao TT, Wei HL, Song ZY. 1980. The induction effect of Schisandrin B on liver microsomal cytochrome P-450 in mouse liver cells. *Acta Pharmaceutica Sinica*. 15: 206–211.
78. Gao PJ, Piao YF, Guo XL, Ju DY, Ren B. 1996. Mechanism of hepato-protective effect of *Schisandra chinensis* polysaccharide. *Journal of Norman Bethune University of Medical Sciences*. 22: 23–24.
79. Niu CW, Sheng YC, Yang R, Lu B, Bai QY, Ji L, Wang Z. 2015. Scutellarin protects against the liver injury induced by diosbulbin B in mice and its mechanism. *Journal of Ethnopharmacology*. 164: 301–308.
80. Hua BC, Hu J, Wang RG, Li YC, Lin JM, Zheng LP, Lin RH, Chen XF. 2011. Experimental research of *Radix glycyrrhiza* on reducing hepatic toxicity induced by rhizome *Dioscorea bulbifera*. *World Journal of Integrated Traditional and Western Medicine*. 6: 24–27.
81. Fan JJ, Hua BC, Liu J, Huang ZF. 2014. Experimental study of rhizoma *Dioscora bulbifera* concerted *Radix glycyrrhiza* reducing renal toxiciy in rats. *Journal of Medial Researh*. 43: 31–33.
82. Suo Q, Cui LR, Liu SM, Yang TT, Liu XW. 2008. Study on the anti-tumor effect of the serum of *D. bulbifera* and its combination with *Angelica sinensis*. *Chinese Journal of Traditional Medical Science and Technology*. 15: 113–114.

10 *Diploknema butyracea* (Cheura)

INTRODUCTION

Diploknema butyracea (Roxb.) H. J. Lam. (Family: Sapotaceae) is distributed throughout Garhwal, Kumaon, Nepal to Sikkim, Darjeeling, Bhutan, and Arunachal Pradesh in the eastern Himalaya at an altitude of about 300–1,500 M.[1] Kureel et al. and Rajkumar and Parthasarathy have reported it from the Andaman Islands.[2,3] Interestingly, *D. butyracea* has not been reported from Mizoram, Manipur, Meghalaya, and Bangladesh,[4] a region between the Himalayan foothills and the Andaman Islands, but it was recently reported in the state of Tripura, India.[4] The associated species of *D. butyracea* in Tripura are *Diospyros* spp., *Castanopsis armata*, *Baccaurea ramiflora*, *Bombax ceiba*, *Cannabis indica*, *Engelhardia spicata*, *Garcinia acuminata*, *Saraca asoka,* and *Lithocarpus spicata*,[4] while the associated trees of *D. butyracea* in the north sub-Himalayan zone forest are *Artocarpus lakoocha*, *Bauhinia variegata*, *Blighia sapida*, *Bambusa nutans*, *Emblica officinalis*, and *Macaranga* spp.[5]

D. butyracea (Eng.: Indian butter tree) (Figure 10.1) grows up to a height of about 50 ft. Commonly, plants occur in wastelands near the villages, and the density inside the forest has been recorded as thin. Its fruits are sweet and scented. The average fruit yield has been estimated at 5–155 kg/tree across different girth class sizes. Its seeds are used to produce edible butter, used as medicine to treat gout, rheumatic conditions, and burns, and to produce candles without smoke and soaps.[6] The pulp of the fruit is juicy and sweet but has a short life span due to low keeping quality. Fruits are rich in nutrients and sugar.[6] The resulting cake after extraction of the fat has saponins, and it has toxic properties. The *D. butyracea* cake is used as a fish intoxicant.[6] The nectar from flowers is harvested either by honeybees or directly to produce jaggery, a highly prized food item in Uttarakhand, India.[7] It flowers during winter, and the fruit ripens between June and August. The ripened fruits are yellow in appearance. In one kilogram of weight, there are 100 fruits or 450–1,000 seeds.[8] The *D. butyracea* plant starts fruiting from 7 to 8 years after plantation and continues for 50–60 years on an alternate-year basis. The average seed yield is estimated at 70–80 quintals per hectare.[8]

Its leaves are used to prepare bowls and plates for eating food and fodder. Most of the trees are lopped for domestic purposes, which significantly reduces fruit productivity. Three different forms of fruit (from oval to round) have been noticed in different parts of the Sikkim Himalaya.[5]

D. butyracea is known as cheura in the Kumaon region of Uttarakhand and chiuri in Nepal, while the Sanskrit name 'Madhupushpa' translates into English as 'honey tree' or 'honey flower'. In Nepal, *D. butyracea* is found in 50 districts out of 75 districts of the country. The Chepang community of Nepal uses *D. butyracea* seedlings as dowries for daughters. It indicates the significance of the tree in the community and its social value as a means of livelihood.[9]

The population of *D. butyracea* in the Kumaun region of Uttarakhand is localized in the districts of Almora, Bageshwar, and Pithoragarh. In the Pithoragarh district, it is further localized to the areas bordering Nepal and the Champawat district.[10] The *D. butyracea* plant has medicinal and socio-economic importance to various ethnic communities in the western Himalayas. In Uttarakhand, a tribal

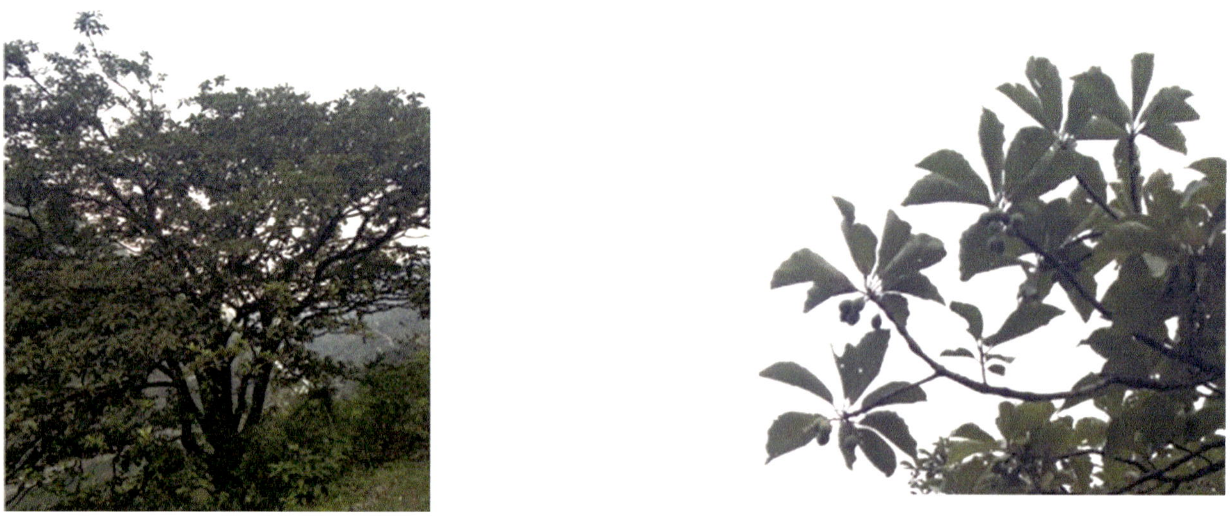

(a) (b)

FIGURE 10.1 (a) *D. butyracea* tree. (b) Fruit-bearing branch.

DOI: 10.1201/9781003512868-12

group (Van-Raji), one of the most ancient primitive vulnerable tribes (PVTs) of India with a population of around 700, traditionally uses *D. butyracea* for spiritual and cultural rites. A field survey conducted (2015–2017) by Joshi et al. to collect data on the availability and its uses by the tribal people in their nine hamlets in the Pithoragarh district of Uttarakhand reported that these tribal people use almost every part of the tree. It holds significant economic value in terms of food, fodder, timber, fuelwood, and other products used by the community to treat many diseases and body ailments (e.g., inflammation of tonsils, rheumatism, itching, ulcers, etc.).[10]

Naturally, the plant is found on steep and difficult slopes. Climbing on trees makes it difficult and risky to harvest fruits. In many instances, people fall from the tree and succumb to serious injury, and sometimes loss of life has also been observed. The harvesters place the doko (traditional basket) on one shoulder and pick fruits with the other hand, finally collecting them into the doko. Normally, the male climbs the tree, while women gather fruits that have fallen from the tree. Children also help in gathering the fruits.[11]

TRADITIONAL USES

The juice of cheura fruit is thermogenic and used to warm and intoxicate the body. The juice of the corolla is boiled to syrupy sugar for therapeutic purposes. The juicy pulp of fresh ripe fruits is used as a food supplement and sometimes as a substituted staple food. Juice of the bark (about 4 teaspoons) is used to treat indigestion and applied to treat rheumatic pain and boils. Seed oil is used to treat headaches, pimples, chapped skin, wounds, rheumatism, burns, and boils. The *D. butyracea* plant is an important source of pollen and nectar for bees. Leaves are used as plates and fodder. The resin of the tree is mixed with resins of Khirra (*Sapium insigne*) and Katahar (*Artocarpus lakoocha*) to make good quality glue used for trapping houseflies and birds. The pulp syrup is mixed with tobacco for smoking purposes in the Nargileh.[11]

COMMERCIAL USES

D. butyracea fat (Cheura ghee) is used to cook vegetables and Paratha (a value-added form of bread). The juice from fruits is consumed to quench thirst. It is used as an ingredient in preparation of different items such as confectionery, soothing cream for cracked skin, vegetable ghee, soap, and candles. Its oil (it is solid up to 55°C and is locally known as 'cheura ghee') is effective for rheumatism. The cheura ghee is also used to mix in animal ghee for better flavor and to enhance its therapeutic properties. The resulting cake after extracting seeds for oil/fat is used as manure, which has pesticide properties also. The cake is used on paddy and banana plantations, as an insecticide, nematicide, and rodenticide. It is rich in saponins and may be utilized as poultry feed after detoxification.[11]

PHYTOPHARMACOLOGY

The cheura tree (*D. butyracea*) is used in different ways; almost every part of it is used for some purpose. Seeds are brown and used to extract fatty acid oil (cheura ghee), a dense, white-colored mass. It is used as vegetable oil as well as for lighting lamps without any smoke. The yield of cheura ghee is 42%–47% of the weight of seeds.[10]

Traditionally, ripe cheura fruits are collected from *D. butyracea* trees and dried. After de-coating, the endosperm is crushed to obtain flour, which is then steamed in a perforated bamboo basket placed over a boiling metal pot. The steamed flour is squeezed while hot, and the fat in liquid form is collected. This traditional technique is very laborious and time-consuming, and the use of a modern press mill to extract fat has been rarely observed, though it may increase the yield and shorten the labor and process time. On average, a young tree yields 200 kg of seeds per season. One liter of cheura ghee is obtained from about 18 kg of seeds.[12] The main chemical constituents of cheura ghee/butter are triglycerides. Bushell and Hilditch[13] reported the triglyceride composition of Phulwara butter (Phulwara is a Nepali name for the *D. butyracea* tree). The fatty acid composition of triglycerides included linoleic acid (3.6%), oleic acid (36%), stearic acid (3.6%), and palmitic acid (57%). Additionally, Bushell and Hilditch have reported that the main ingredients of the glycerides are palmito-di-oleins (23%), oleo-di-palmitins (62%), tripalmitin (8%), and oleo-palmitostearins (7%).[13] Agarwal et al. and Sengupta and Choudhary reported a similar composition of Cheura ghee.[14,15] Further, Devkota et al. have reported a similar composition of Cheura ghee of Nepali origin.[16] Bandyopadhyay et al. have also published a similar report on the composition of different cheura ghee samples collected from India (Table 10.1). These studies have concluded that

TABLE 10.1
Chemical Composition of Fatty Acids (%) of Cheura Ghee of Different Origin

S. No.	Origin of Sample → Fatty Acid Ester	India[13]	India[14]	India[15]	Nepal[16]	India[17]
1	Palmitic acid methyl ester	57	55.86	55.6	58.4–66.0	56.8–64.1
2	Linoleic acid methyl ester	3.6	3.69	3.3	2.6–3.7	4.3–5.7
3	Steric acid methyl ester	3.6	1.63	5.2	2.4–2.9	2.4–3.5
4	Oleic acid methyl ester	36	38.55	35.9	28.9–35.2	28.0–31.3

cheura ghee has a high potential to be used in the cosmetics, confectionery, and pharmaceutical industries.[17] A few more investigations have also been carried out on fruits and seeds of the *D. butyracea* plant. For example, butyraceol,[18] MI-saponin A, 16α-hydroxy MI-saponin A, butyrosides A, B,[19] and butyrosides C, D have been reported from the seeds of *D. butyracea*.[20] β-sitosterol glucoside, α-spinasterol, α-amyrin acetate, and 3β-palmitoxy-olea-12en-28-ol have been isolated from fruit pulp and bark of *D. butyracea*.[21] Flavonoids, quercetin, and dihydroquercetin are reported from the nutshell.[22]

There are only a limited number of scientific investigations on the chemical composition and quality of cheura ghee/butter, and a few necessary chemical fingerprints for quality control of *D. butyracea* butter, based on infrared[23], ultraviolet[23], nuclear magnetic resonance spectroscopy,[23] and mass spectrometry,[23] have been developed.

HPTLC fingerprints: Seeds of *D. butyracea* have 60%–67% fat calculated on the kernel basis. After extraction, it is used for cooking, cosmetics, and manufacturing soaps. Traditionally, it is used as an ointment to treat sprains, rheumatism, and paralysis. The oil cake is rich in saponins and is used as fish intoxicant, fertilizer, detergent, and pesticide. The flowers are a rich source of sugars and are utilized for the preparation of jaggery-like products. The stem bark of the *D. butyracea* tree is used to treat ulcers, inflammation of the tonsils, rheumatism, itching and hemorrhage, diabetes, and leprosy.[24] HPTLC fingerprints are the main analytical data for the purity and authenticity of the Cheura ghee.

Rasmi and Sapna have studied the seeds of *D. butyracea* using high performance thin layer chromatography (HPTLC) to assess the quality and quantity of its main ingredients.[25] During the study, seeds were collected, shade-dried, and decorticated manually, and kernels were separated and coarsely powdered. The powdered material was extracted sequentially with the solvents of the eutrophic series, viz., chloroform, methanol, and aqueous solvent, by using the Soxhlet apparatus. Extraction was carried out until the extractives became colorless. The extracts were filtered using a cotton plug, followed by Whatman filter paper (no. 1). The filtrate was concentrated to dryness under reduced pressure by using a rotary evaporator. The percentages of each ingredient were calculated on an air-dried weight basis, and the yield of different extracts (chloroform, methanol, and aqueous form) was calculated.

All extracts were qualitatively studied for various phytochemical constituents. Major constituents were screened as per Sofowora's standard qualitative methods.[26] Tannins were analyzed by filtering 3 g of each seed extract in 6 mL of distilled water to which ferric chloride reagent was added. For cardiac glycosides, the Killer-Kiliani test was adopted (extract was added in acetic acid and H_2SO_4). Aqueous extract (0.5 g) was stirred with 5 mL of 1% HCl and filtered.[27] The filtrate was tested carefully with Mayer's reagent and resulted in a reddish-brown precipitate, proving the presence of alkaloids.[27,28] Saponins were identified by a frothing test. A hemolysis test on the frothed extracts in water has cross-verified the presence of saponins. The dried extract dissolved in ethyl acetate was shaken with dilute ammonia and then filtered. The appearance of yellow color deciphers the presence of flavonoids.[26] Further, the quantitative estimation of total terpenoids, flavonoids, and saponins content was carried out as per standard methods.[28–31]

Thin-layer chromatography analysis was carried out using 100% chloroform as a mobile phase.[28] Spots were developed by spraying with sulfuric acid, followed by heating at 100°C for 10 min. Spots were identified based on the color produced as a result of spraying. Chromatographic separation was carried out on an aluminum plate pre-coated with silica gel $60F_{254}$ (Merck) as the stationary phase for different extracts prepared.[25]

The qualitative analysis of the seed extracts reveals the presence of phytochemical constituents such as alkaloids, fixed oils, tannins, phenols, fats, glycosides, flavonoids, sterols, saponins, and terpenoids. The presence of flavonoids in the plant reveals its antioxidant and free-radical scavenging properties.[32] Steroidal compounds have biological importance and induce sexual activities. Saponins have antibacterial activity, and glycosides are linked with lowering blood pressure.[33] Due to the presence of these bioactive constituents, *D. butyracea* is considered an important medicinal plant and has been utilized in several ways in the pharmaceutical sector.

Tannins are widely distributed in almost all plant foods and are found to be effective in protecting the kidneys. Tannins have antiviral, antibacterial, and anti-parasitic effects.[34,35] Alkaloids are the most important class of natural products responsible for anti-plasmodial activity and are used in traditional practices for the treatment of malaria.[36] Further research on *D. butyracea* may help in the isolation of therapeutically potent compounds for studying pharmacological activities and conducting clinical trials to explore new pathways of utility. Devkota et al. analyzed the fat of seeds of *D. butyracea* in Nepal and reported methyl ester derivatives of palmitic acid, linoleic acid, stearic acid, and oleic acid as the main components.[16]

TRADITIONAL APPLICATIONS

The cheura ghee burns with a smokeless flame when used as an oil wick, so it can be used as eco-friendly biofuel, especially in generators, pump sets, etc.[37] It has industrial uses for making soaps, candles, and chocolates. The Cheura ghee is also used by the indigenous communities to cure common body ailments, such as rheumatic pains, itching, hemorrhage, ulcers, inflammation of tonsils, to relieve headaches, etc. During winter, it is applied on chapped hands and cracked heels. The oilcake, a residual product after the extraction of ghee, is used as manure. It has pesticidal properties. Further, it is used as a fish poison during fishing, and leech repellent in the rainy season to repel the leeches. The oilcake is considered toxic and not used as mulch for animals even after detoxification.[10]

Fruits are the second most important part of the *D. butyracea* tree. The fruit is a berry with an oval shape and contains three seeds. The pericarp has a thick, soft, and sweet pulp, which is used for making jaggery by crushing the fruit and boiling the juice into a thick syrup. The jaggery is reported to be tasty with therapeutic values and sold in the local market at highly remunerative prices. The residuals after squeezing the pericarp are mixed with fodder and used as animal feed. The fruit pulp is also edible. It is widely eaten by native villagers and by wild animals, many birds, and flies. Pulp juice is considered thermogenic but is not used during stomachaches, diarrhea, or coughing.[10]

The leaves of cheura are usually clustered at the apex of branchlets, obovate, alternate, and thinly coriaceous. The leaves of cheura remain green during the dry months of the year and are preferred by the cattle as fodder, especially for lactating cattle. Besides being a source of fodder, the leaves of cheura are used for making dona or thali (a sacred plate for food) locally, in various rituals by the natives of Uttarakhand. These plates are used for devoting edibles and other materials to the deities. Wild animals like Himalayan monkeys and macaque species love to feed on the leaves of the cheura plant.[10]

Flowering in cheura occurs from October to November, and the fruits ripen during the summer season. The inflorescence of cheura is colored and rich in sugar, which is traditionally considered good for foraging various pollinators, including birds, bats, and bees. The honey produced by the honeybees after foraging on cheura flowers is sold as 'cheura honey' by the natives at a high cost, thus being a good source of revenue. The nectar from the flowers is also collected directly to make 'cheura jaggery', a high-priced item in Uttarakhand.[10] The cheura nectar has a high medicinal and nutritional value and was used during the famine. Cheura honey is used to treat diabetes and asthma. The cheura flowers are used as a raw material for alcohol.[10] The roots have traditional uses as a tonic. After cleaning, the roots are mashed and soaked in water for a whole night or day, and the resulting juice is taken as a tonic.[10]

As per elders of the community, in the olden days, the stem bark of cheura was widely used in dyeing, but at present, this practice has been discontinued due to the availability of synthetic dyes.

The cheura tree stems are used as fuel and timber. The wood of cheura contains a resin and is considered best for fuelwood, as it does not allow it to extinguish fast and emits less smoke on burning compared to other types of fuelwood. The cheura wood is not very hard and durable and is used for making light furniture and other items, but not for making traditional storage bins.[10] The resin of the cheura tree is applied as an ointment for healing wounds and cuts by the 'Van-Raji', a tribal community in the Dharchula block of the Pithoragarh district, Uttarakhand, India.[10]

SCOPE AND OPPORTUNITIES FOR BIOTECH INTERVENTIONS

Observations from various reconnaissance surveys and field studies have concluded various factors contribute to decline in the abundance and distribution of the cheura tree, including the degradation of traditional knowledge and a lack of general awareness about the *D. butyracea* tree.[10] Lack of general awareness has resulted in low efforts for the preservation and conservation of the species, and threat levels are described as being at an all-time high because of relentless anthropogenic activities and the lack of focus by policymakers on the species.[10] It is a matter of urgent attention to save the habitat of this species to minimize further loss. The identification of potential areas for habitat restoration is important for the plantation programs of the species.

Professionally managed cultivation, utilization, and conservation of the cheura tree as a medicinal plant species, and for industrial use of its seed oil, may improve the economic and social status of the local inhabitants in the sub-Himalayan regions of Bhutan, Nepal, and India. Further, bioassay-guided scientific investigations using different plant parts may help in the development of modern green medicines. Similarly, a pool of knowledge on the altitude variation of components in seeds may help in selecting proper biological sources. Additionally, a specification-based 'cheura ghee' business, supported by its fingerprints for claims made (such as physiochemical properties, diffusion, washability, drug incorporation, and drug release potential ingredient), may boost a new era of its utilization in herbal medicine-related industries.

D. butyracea is a hard and tolerant species that has been adapted for the climactic ups and downs of local hill ecology and can be grown in infertile or degraded lands. Forests with rich populations of *D. butyracea* plants have the potential to improve the livelihood of forest-dwelling people, particularly tribal communities globally. As the *D. butyracea* plant is a tool to strengthen the economic condition of deprived communities, the natural pockets of cheura-grown localities are required to be identified, documented, mapped, and promoted with a geographical indication tag. Further, proper ex-situ and in situ conservation strategies and propagation by using tissue culture are the need of the hour, and nurseries at the block/village level may help promote wide plantation of the species in the region. Plantation at new suitable habitats in wastelands/panchayat lands may be more fruitful by involving the local communities with Govt. agencies in the region, even under the agroforestry schemes.

Though it is a localized species, there is a huge scope for studying its genetics to explore high-yielding races, mass production, and resistance to pests and diseases. The regeneration of the species is poor because the seeds are recalcitrant and quickly lose viability after dispersal.[38] The seeds rich in nutrition attract predators such as rove beetles, ants, and termites.[38] There have been several attempts at seed germination,[5,39] but none satisfactory. As per the Himalayan

Glaciation theory by Medlicott and Blanford, some of the Himalayan flora are regularly pushed southwards, resulting in discontinuities in the distribution of some tree species.[40] Puri et al. have reported ten types of the distribution pattern for important Indian trees, showing discontinuous distribution in Assam, the Andaman islands, the Eastern Ghats, Burma, the Western Ghats, and Sri Lanka. As *D. butyracea* is close to Bangladesh and the State of Mizoram (India), its occurrence in these territories is likely to be true.[41] *D. butyracea* has been described by different names in the taxonomic literature, and a chronological taxonomic study revealed that the species was prominently known as *Aesandra butyracea* before the current name *Diploknema butyracea*.[4]

REFERENCES

1. Brandis D. 1906. *Indian Trees: An Account of Trees, Shrubs, Woody Climbers, Bamboos, and Palms Indigenous or Commonly Cultivated in the British Indian Empire. Fifth Impression (1971).* Bishen Singh Mahendra Pal Singh, Dehradun, India.
2. Kureel RS, Gupta AK, Pandey A. 2008. *Cheura – A Wonder Tree Borne Oilseed.* National Oilseeds and Vegetable Oils Development Board, Ministry of Agriculture, Government of India, Gurgoan. Vol. 8: 1–8.
3. Rajkumar M, Parthasarathy N. 2008. Tree diversity and structure of Andaman giant evergreen forests, India. *Taiwania*. 53: 356–368.
4. Majumdar K, Datta BK, Shankar U. 2012. Establishing continuity in distribution of *Diploknema butyracea* (Roxb.) H. J. Lam in Indian subcontinent. *Journal of Research in Biology*. 2 (7): 660–666.
5. Sundriyal M, Sundriyal RC. 2003. Underutilized edible plants of the Sikkim Himalaya: need for domestication. *Current Science*. 85 (6): 731–736.
6. Mitra CR, Awasthi YC. 1962. Constituents of *Madhuca latifolia* and *M. butyracea* nuts. *Journal of Scientific and Industrial Research* 21 (D): 102–103.
7. Bahar N. 2011. Cheura [*Diploknema butyracea (*Roxb.) H. J. Lam.]: an important tree for poverty alleviation. *Indian Forester*. 137: 1344–1345.
8. Jackson JK. 1994. *Manual of Afforestation in Nepal*, 2nd Edition. Forest Research and Survey Center, Kathmandu, Nepal.
9. Shakya MR. 2000. Chepangs and Chiuri; The Use of Non-timber Forest Products in Nepal. ITFC. https://practicalaction.org/?id=food_chain, as on 24th May 2021.
10. Joshi NC, Chaudhary A, Rawat GS. 2018. Cheura (*Diploknema butyracea*) as a livelihood option for forest-dweller tribe (Van-Raji) of Pithoragarh, Uttarakhand, India. ESSENCE. *International Journal for Environmental Rehabilitation and Conservation*. IX (1): 134–141.
11. Dhakal BN. Development of Chyuri (*Diploknema butyracea*) Fruit Biomass Models (A case study from Piple Basaha Community Forest of Baglung, Nepal) A dissertation submitted for the partial fulfillment of the requirement of the degree of Master of Science in NRM&RD, Tribhuvan University, Institute of Forestry, Pokhara, Nepal.
12. Rastogi, R. 2008. *Let Us Identify the Useful Trees.* New Delhi Children Book Trust, New Delhi .
13. Bushell WJ, Hilditch, TP. 1938. Fat acids and glycerides of solid seed fats. IV. Seed fat of *Madhuca butyracea* (phulwara butter). *Journal of Society of Chemical Industry*. 57: 48–49.
14. Agarwal PN, Pandey SC, Sharma TR, Prakash O. 1963. The component fatty acids of the seed fat of *Madhuca butyracea. Journal Oil Technologists' Association India*. 18: 8–10.
15. Sengupta A, Roy Choudhary SK. 1978. Triglyceride composition of *Madhuca butyraceae* seed fat. *Journal of the American Oil Chemists' Society*. 55: 621–624.
16. Devkota HP, Watanabe T, Malla KJ, Nishiba Y, Yahara S. 2012. Studies on medicinal plant resources of the Himalayas: GC-MS analysis of seed fat of Chyuri (*Diploknema butyracea*) from Nepal. *Pharmacognosy Journal*. 4: 42–44.
17. Bandyopadhyay B B, Joshi L, Nautiyal MK. 2017. Relationship of the oil content and fatty acid composition with seed characters of *Diploknema butyracea. Academia of Agriculture Journal*. 2:1–4.
18. Mishra G, Banerji R, Nigam S K. 1991. Butyraceol, a triterpenoidal sapogenin from *Madhuca butyracea. Phytochemistry*. 30: 2087–2088.
19. Nigam SK, Li X, Wang D, Mishra G, Yang C. 1992. Triterpenoidal saponins from *Madhuca butyracea. Phytochemistry*. 31: 3169–3172.
20. Li X, Liu Y, Wang D, Yang C, Nigam S K, Mishra G. 1994. Triterpenoid saponins from *Madhuca butyracea. Phytochemistry*. 37: 827–829.
21. Awasthi YC, Mitra CR. 1968. *Madhuca butyracea*. Constituents of the fruit pulp and the bark. *Phytochemistry*. 7: 637–640.
22. Awasthi YC, Mitra CR. 1962. Flavonoids of *Madhuca butyracea* nut shell. *The Journal of Organic Chemistry*. 27: 2636–2637.
23. Devkota HP, Adhikari-Devkota A, Belwal T, Bhandari B R. 2019. Chapter 13: Chyuri (*Diploknema butyracea*) Butter. In: *Fruit Oils: Chemistry and Functionality*. Ramadan MF (Ed.) Springer Nature Switzerland AG. pp. 285.
24. Shakya MR. 2000. *Chepangs and Chiuri - The Use of Non-timber Forest Products in Nepal. Food Chain*. 26: pp 3–5
25. Rasmi, Sapna T. 2015. Phytochemical standardization of *Diploknema butyracea* (Roxb.) H.J. Lam. seeds by HPTLC technique. *Indian Journal of Natural Products and Resources*. 6 (4): 299–304.
26. Sofowora A. 1993. Recent trends in research into African medicinal plants. *Journal of Ethanopharmaclogy*. 38 (2–3): 209–214.
27. Trease GE, Evans WC. 1983. *Drugs of Biological Origin. Pharmacognosy*, 12th Edition. Balliere Tindall, United Kingdom. pp. 309–540.
28. Harborne JB. 1984. *Phytochemical Methods*. Chapman and Hall, New York. Vol. 2, No. 3: pp. 100–117.
29. Boham BA, Kocipal-Abyazan R. 1974. Flavonoids and condensed tannins from leaves of Hawaiian *Vaccinium vaticulatum* and *V. calycinum*. *Pacific Science*. 48: 458–463.
30. Obadoni BO, Ochuko PO. 2001. Phytochemical studies and comparative efficacy of crude extracts of some homeostatic plants in Edo and Delta States of Nigeria. *Global Journal of Pure and Applied Sciences*. 8: 203–208.
31. Sharma DK. 2006. Pharmacological properties of flavonoids including flavonolignans- Integration of petrocrops with the drug development from plants. *Journal of Scientific & Industrial Research*. 65: 477–484.

32. Winkel-Shirley B. 2002. Biosynthesis of flavonoids and effects of stress. *Current Opinion in Plant Biology*. 5 (3): 218–223.
33. Lu L, Liu SW, Jiang SB, Wu SG. 2004. Tannin inhibits HIV-1 entry by targeting gp41. *Acta Pharmacol Sin*. 25 (2): 213–218.
34. Akiyma H, Fujii K, Yamasaki O, Oono T, Iwattuski K. 2001. Antibacterial action of several tannins against *Staphylococcus aureus*. *Journal of Antimicrobial Chemotherapy*. 48: 487–491.
35. Kolodziej H, Kiderlen AF. 2005. Antileishmanial activity immune modulatory effects of tannins and related compounds on Leishmania parasitized RAW 264.7 cells. *Phytochemistry*. 66: 2056–2071.
36. Seyoum A, Asres K, El-Fiky FK. 2006. Structure-radical scavenging activity relationships of flavonoids. *Phytochemistry*. 67: 2058–2070.
37. Nautiyal TD, Kandpal BP. 2013. *Blog Butter Tree in India*. Department of Horticulture & Food Processing. Uttarakhand, India.
38. Tewari A, Dhar U. 1996. An investigation on seed germination on Indian butter tree-*Asiandra butyracea* (Roxb.) Baehni. *Seed Science and Technology*. 24: 211–218.
39. Tewari A. 1997. Clonal propagation of Indian Butter tree (*Diploknema butyracea*) through tissue culture. Ph. D. Thesis, Kumaon University, Nainital.
40. Medlicott HB, Blanford WT. 1879. *Manual of the Geology of India, Part 2*. Geological Survey of India, Calcutta.
41. Puri GS, Meher-Homji VM, Gupta RK, Puri S. 1983. Phytogeographical ecology. In: *Forest Ecology*. 2nd Edition. Oxford and IBH Publishers, New Delhi, India. pp. 115–210.

11 *Ficus auriculata* (Timla)

INTRODUCTION

Ficus auriculata Lour. (syn.; *Ficus roxburghii*) is a wild edible fruit tree belonging to the family Moraceae, reaching up to 20m in height. It can be deciduous during extended periods of cold temperatures, although it has been classified as an evergreen species. *F. auriculata* is widely distributed in tropical, subtropical, and temperate regions of about 1,800–2,600 MLS.[1] The common Indian names of the species are Gular, Timbal, Timal, Timla, Tirmal, Tremal, and Trimmal.[2] The plant contains an abundant amount of white latex in its parts.[3] Its bark is greyish brown with a rough texture. Its branchlets are reddish-brown, and the figs (also called fruits) are pear-shaped, depressed globose, or top-shaped, reddish-brown in color, and generally occur on leafless branchlets at the base of the trunk (Figure 11.1) and main branches.[4,5]

The figs of *F. auriculata* are key plant resources in tropical rainforests due to their rich and continuous production, serving as food for frugivores when the availability of other fruits is low.[6] The pollination process is specific to wasps and is an example of the mutual relationship between trees and their pollinators.[7] The species occur in the hills, especially in the conifer forests of Uttarakhand, some northeastern states of India, and from Pakistan to South China, up to an elevation of 1,700m from the foothills.[8] Its leaves are liked by cattle as fodder during the winter season.[9] Plates are made by stitching 3–4 leaves together for serving food during spiritual ceremonies and special occasions in villages of the hilly regions of India.[10] The regeneration of its trees is highly variable under natural conditions, and its poor regeneration in a forest is an indicator of the scarcity of seedlings and saplings. The regeneration of species, their survival, and the growth of seedlings depend on abiotic and biotic factors such as cattle browsing, human disturbance, and trampling by cattle. Poor regeneration in wild habitats is mainly due to heavy biotic pressure.[11] Its fruits are edible, eaten raw, and also used as a vegetable. For eating purposes, fruits are collected before maturation, resulting in low availability of seeds, a problematic situation, and threatening natural regeneration of *F. auriculata* in the region. The color change of fruits from green to red is an indicator of their maturity. Color changes have also been recommended as a ripeness indicator in several wild fruiting plants.[8] A decline in the moisture content of *F. auriculata* fruits is a good indicator of seed maturity.[8]

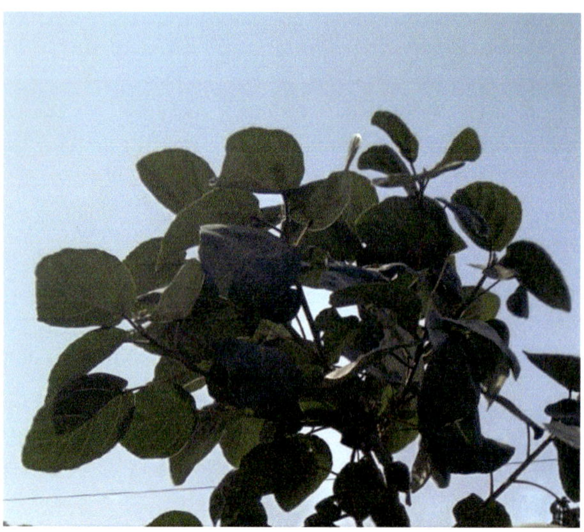

FIGURE 11.1 *F. auriculata* branch-bearing flower.

ETHNOPHARMACOLOGY

The traditional applications of *F. auriculata* in treating cholera, diarrhea, jaundice, cuts, wounds, mumps, dysentery, etc.[12] reveal its antimicrobial and antioxidant properties, although clinical studies have not been carried out for each activity. Fruits of *F. auriculata* are rich in polyphenolics and flavonoids and are very tasty. These are used in the treatment and prevention of stress-related diseases (such as hepatic and neurodegenerative ailments, stomachic, and astringents), as well as vermicides, carminatives, hypotensive, and anti-dysentery drugs. The paste of leaves is applied to the wounds for healing purposes.[13] The latex-like material within the vasculatures of the species grants protection and self-restoration from bodily assaults to the plant.[14]

The stem bark juice is effective in curing skin cuts, wounds, and diarrhea. Roasted figs are taken to treat diarrhea and dysentery. Latex of roots is used in diarrhea, cholera, mumps, and vomiting. The mixture of root powder of the species and the bark of *Oroxylum indicum* (Indian trumpet tree) is taken to treat jaundice.[15] Ethnic people in the Khagrachari hill district, Bangladesh, also use the species as food.[16]

Fresh juice of leaves with water (50–100mL) is used for about 10days to cure gastrointestinal problems.[17] Barks and roots are used to treat hypoglycemia and for their anthelmintic activity.[18,19] Fruit extracts are used for antitumor activity,[20] and the leaves are used for hypotensive activity.[21]

PHYTOPHARMACOLOGY

Phytochemical screening of *F. auriculata* fruits and leaves reveals the presence of tannins, phenols, resins, flavonoids, and glycosides, but alkaloids are absent.[22,23] On a dried weight basis, the total phenolic content in leaves of *F. auriculata* has been reported as 21.404mg GAE/mg, and the total flavonoid content is 50.83 ± 1.32 mg GAE/mg.[24] The stem bark extracts of *F. auriculata* have been reported to

DOI: 10.1201/9781003512868-13

present alkaloids, resins, carbohydrates, glycosides, saponins, amino acids, phenols, diterpenes, tannins, fatty oils, proteins, flavonoids, and phytosterols.[25]

Fatty acid profiling of *F. auriculata* fruits by GC-MS reveals the presence of stearic acid, oleic acid, linolenic acid, palmitic acid, vaccenic acid, and 3-hydroxy lauric acid. Unsaturated fatty acids, linoleic acid, and linolenic acid have health-protective and curative properties. Saturated fatty acids (palmitic acid, stearic acid, etc.) have industrial applications.[25] The nutritional components of fruits of *F. auriculata* vary as per geo-climatic regions, and fruits are a potent source of nutrients, including lipids, proteins, and carbohydrates.[16]

The reducing properties of *F. auriculata* fruits, leaves, and bark are important indicators of the antioxidant properties of the species associated with traditional and folk utilization.[24] The antioxidant potential of the species has been reported as dose-dependent, with fruit extracts showing more antioxidant potential compared to the leaves.[26] Alcoholic extracts of fruits and leaves of *F. auriculata* reveal the potential against human pathogenic bacteria (*Pseudomonas aeruginosa*, *Escherichia coli*, *Bacillus aureus*, *Bacillus subtilis*, and *Staphylococcus aureus*), but the inhibition zones were smaller compared to standard drugs. The leaves have been reported to have higher antibacterial activity compared to fruits.[26]

Studies conducted on the anti-cancerous activities of chloroform and methanol extracts of *F. auriculata* reveal that there is no significant cancer cell-killing activity.[23] The aqueous bark extract of *F. auriculata* has antidiabetic activity, with different concentrations (10–100 μg/mL) revealing that the plant possesses inhibitory activity on salivary amylase. The inhibition of *F. auriculata* aqueous extract has been reported to range from 4.5% to 31.3%.[27]

Rosalind et al. have reported that the methanol leaf extract of *F. auriculata* can improve the fatty acid impairment metabolism in diabetes. It elevates the secretion of insulin from β-cells of the pancreas and stimulates fatty acid biosynthesis.[28] The fruit extracts of *F. auriculata* made from different solvents (ethyl acetate, chloroform, petroleum ether, and ethanol with water) have been reported to have activity against three fungal strains (*Candida albicans*, *Aspergillus flavus*, and *Aspergillus parasiticus*) at different concentrations (10 and 50 mg/mL).[29]

The induced liver serum enzymes in animals with CCl_4 (such as serum glutamate pyruvate transaminase, serum alkaline phosphatase, and serum glutamate oxaloacetate transaminase) are reduced by the aqueous and methanolic extract of *F. auriculata*.[26,30]

The increase of reactive oxidative species (ROS) in the body is due to hypoxia (lack of oxygen supply in tissues), resulting in various hepatic diseases. The imbalance between antioxidants and ROS is known as the oxidative stress state. The damage due to ROS is prevented by antioxidants present in the body. Glutathione (GSH) is an endogenous antioxidant that can be used as a parameter of antioxidant content in the body. The *F. auriculata* leaf extract increases the GSH levels due to its enhanced antioxidant content.[31]

Anti-inflammatory activity evaluated on the rat hind paw edema model has revealed that increased concentrations of the *F. auriculata* extracts reduce inflammation in a dose-dependent manner. The alcoholic leaf extract (500 mg/kg) of *F. auriculata* has significant anti-inflammatory activity, and the presence of triterpenoids has been narrated to inhibit inflammation.[26]

There has been neither behavioral change nor mortality or toxicity reported after the administration of 1.00, 2.00, and 3.00 g/kg doses of methanolic leaf extract of *F. auriculata*. The LD_{50} of methanolic leaf extract of *F. auriculata* has been reported as 3.00 g/kg, and oral administration of the methanol leaf extract is associated with low toxicity.[28,32]

SCOPE AND OPPORTUNITY

The phytochemical constituents (flavonoids, glycosides, carbohydrates, tannins, alkaloids, and sterols) of *F. auriculata* are attributed to their biological properties. Additionally, the anti-diabetic, antioxidant, hepatoprotective, and other properties of the plant are currently used to treat diseases caused by pathogens. Antiproliferative activity has been traditionally attributed to the species, mainly activity against colon and liver cancer. This ability to induce apoptosis by DNA fragmentation deciphers it as a potent anticancer chemotherapeutic agent. These excellent properties of *F. auriculata*, based on the evidence from several research reports and review articles, make it a very helpful drug due to its curative properties, and it is easily available at a very low cost.

Detailed investigations on pharmacological activity with a preliminary phytochemical screening of the *F. auriculata* plant for antibacterial and antioxidant efficacy to select crude plant extracts may lead to new applications for a pivotal role.

The different extracts of *F. auriculata* are used for strengthening the antioxidant defense system to combat a wide range of degenerative diseases (e.g., atherosclerosis, cancer, coronary ailments, inflammation, liver injury, Alzheimer's, and Parkinson's) resulting from oxidative stress and free radicals.[33–35] The prime cause of oxidative stress is free radicals, namely, hydroxyl (OH^-), peroxyl (RO_2), nitric oxide (NO^-), superoxide ($O2\cdot^-$), peroxy-nitrite (ONO_2^-) radicals, along with non-free radical species such as nitrous acid (HNO_2), hydrogen peroxide ($H_2O_2\cdot$), and hypochlorous acid (HOCl).[36]

The use of synthetic antioxidants is associated with higher risks of side effects; therefore, the focus of consumers and doctors is on herbal antioxidants,[37] as natural antioxidants have hardly any harmful impacts. *F. auriculata* species has a huge number of antioxidants, and its use either alone or in synergistic combination can lead to new modern green medicine or food supplements with fewer or no side effects.

The phytopharmacological screening of *F. auriculata* for active compounds as promising sources of novel antibiotic prototypes is very important, as the antibacterial activities of its ingredients are associated with fewer side effects and have therapeutic potential to cure many infectious diseases.[38] The antibacterial compounds found in F. auriculata are promising. These may help in developing new herbal medicines to fight germs effectively while reducing the chances of developing resistance. This makes them a good option for treating infectious diseases naturally.[39] Further, phyto-ingredients are one of the potent alternatives to control these antibiotic-resistant human pathogens.[40] The purified and isolated antibacterial biomolecules would have an equivalent antibacterial activity to that of standard antibiotics. So, detailed investigations are necessary for maximum benefits from the *F. auriculata* plant. Further, clinical data may have a pivotal role in changing the traditional system of medicine into a scientific and standard medication system.

REFERENCES

1. Kala CP. 2007. Prioritization of cultivated and wild edibles by local people in the Uttaranchal hill of Indian Himalaya. *Indian Journal of Trading Knowledge*. 6: 239–244.
2. Shilpakar A, Gaire BP, Bahadur SC, Lamichhane R, Neupane S. 2009. Phytochemical screening and analysis of antibacterial and antioxidant activity of *Ficus auriculata* Lour. stem bark. Ph.D. Thesis, Pokhara University, Nepal.
3. Weiblen GD. 2000. Phylogenetic relationships of functionally dioecious *Ficus* (Moraceae) based on ribosomal DNA sequences and morphology. *American Journal of Botany*. 87: 1342–1357.
4. Wang HK, Hyde KD, Soytong K, Lin FC. 2008. Fungal diversity on fallen leaves of *Ficus* in northern Thailand. *Journal of Zhejiang University Science B*. 9: 835–841.
5. Schulz JB, Lindnau J, Seyfriend J, Dichgans J. 2000. Glutathione oxidative stress and neurodegeneration. *European Journal of Biochemistry*. 267: 4904–4911.
6. Pothasin P, Compton SG, Wangpakapattanawong P. 2014. Riparian *Ficus* tree communities: the distribution and abundance of Riparian Fig trees in Northen Thailand. *PLoS One*. 9(10) : e108945. doi: 10.1371/journal.pone.0108945
7. Machado CA, Jousselin E, Kjellberg F, Compton SG, Herre EA. 2001. Phylogenetic relationships, historical biogeography, and character evolution of Fig-pollinating wasps. *Proceedings of the Royal Society of London, Series B*. 268: 685–694.
8. Jyotsna TA, Shah S, Tamta KK, Singh N. 2020. Fruit maturation and germination in *Ficus auriculata* Lour. A lesser-known multipurpose tree species in Kumaun Himalayan region. *Ecology Environment & Conservation*. 26 (1): 142–147.
9. Roder W, Gyeltshen T. 2003. *Ficus auriculata*- its relative importance in Bhutan, farmer's preference, and fodder quality. *Agroforestry System*. 57 (1): 11–17.
10. Parmar C, Kushal MK. 1982. *Ficus auriculata*, Wild Fruits. Kalyani Publication, New Delhi, India. pp. 35–37.
11. Sundriyal M, Sundriyal RC. 2001. Seed germination and response of stem cuttings to hormonal treatment in six priority wild edible fruit species of Sikkim Himalaya. *Indian Forester*. 127 (6): 695–705.
12. Gairola Y, Biswas S. 2008. Bioprospecting in Garhwal Himalayas, Uttarakhand. *Current Science*. 94: 1139–1144.
13. Maxwell SR. 1995. Prospects for the use of antioxidant therapies. *Drugs*. 49: 345–361.
14. Schinor EC, Salvador MJ, Ito IY, Dias DA. 2007. Evaluation of the antimicrobial activity of crude extracts and isolated constituents from *Chresta scapigera*. *Brazilian Journal of Microbiology*. 38: 145–149.
15. Kunwar RM, Bussmann RW. 2006. Ficus (Fig) species in Nepal: a review of diversity and indigenous uses. *Lyon*. 11 (1): 85–97.
16. Khatun MJM, Rahman MM, Rahim MA, Jakariya M, Mirdah MH. 2016. Study on the ethnobotany and nutritional status of three edible *Ficus* species in hill district of Bangladesh. *International Journal of Minor Fruits, Medicinal and Aromatic Plants*. 2 (1): 35–40.
17. Rout SD, Panda T, Mishra N. 2009. Ethnomedicinal plants used to cure different diseases by Tribal's of Mayurbhanj district of North Orissa. *Ethno-Medicine*. 3 (1): 27–32.
18. Mazumder PM, Farswan M, Parcha V. 2009. Hypoglycaemic effect of *Ficus arnottiana* Miq. Bark extracts on streptozocin induced diabetes in rats. *Natural Product Researh*. 8 (5): 478–482.
19. Ghosh R, Sharathchandra K, Rita S, Thokchom IS. 2004. Hypoglycaemic activity of *Ficus hispida* (bark) in normal and diabetic albino rats. *Indian Journal of Pharmacology*. 36 (4): 222–225.
20. Aswar M, Aswar U, Watkar B, Vyas M, Wagh A, Gujar KN. 2008. Anthelmintic activity of Ficus bengalensis. *International Journal of Green Pharmacy*. 2 (3): 170–172.
21. Buniyamin A, Ayinde EI, Fabain O, Amaechina C. 2007. Pharmacognosy and hypotensive evaluation of *Ficus exasperata* Vahl (Moraceae) leaf. *Acta Poloniae Pharmaceutica*. 64 (116): 543–546.
22. Saklani S, Chandra S. 2012. In vitro antimicrobial activity, nutritional profile and phytochemical screening of wild edible fruit of Garhwal Himalaya (*Ficus auriculata*). *International Journal of Pharmaceutical Sciences Review and Research*. 12 (2): 61–64.
23. Kumari A, Verma R, Sharma M, Chauhan P, Kumar A. 2018. Evaluation of phytochemical, antioxidant, antibacterial and anti-cancerous activity of *Ficus auriculata* Lour. and *Osyris wightiana* Wall. ex Wight. *Bulletin of Environment, Pharmacology and Life Sciences*. 7 (8): 64–70.
24. Rosalind TH, Dutta BK, Paul SB. 2012. In vitro antioxidant capacity of estimation of total phenolic and flavonoid content of Ficus auriculata Lour. *International Journal of Pharmacy and Pharmaceutical Science*. 4 (4): 518–521.
25. Anjum N, Tripathi Y. 2019. In vitro alpha-amylase and alpha-glusidase inhibitory activities of fruits of *Ficus auriculata*. *International Journal of Pharma and Bio Sciences*. 10 (4): 134–141.
26. El-Fishawy A, Zayed R, Afifi S. 2011. Phytochemical and pharmacological studies of *Ficus auriculata* Lour. *Journal of Natural Products*. 4: 184–195.
27. Tiwari Y, Singh A, Kumar B, Kumar A. 2017. In vitro evaluation of alpha amylase activity of bark extracts of *Ficus Auriculata*. *International Journal of Innovative Science and Research Technology*. 12 (2): 2456–2165.
28. Rosalind T, Biman K, Satya B. 2013. Anti-hyperglycemic and antihyperlipidemic activity of *Ficus auriculata* lour. leaf extract in streptozotocin-induced diabetic mice. *World Journal of Pharmacy and Pharmaceutical Sciences*. 3 (1):412–427.

29. Jamil EF, Abdul Ghani R. 2017. *Ficus auriculata* (fig) extracts induced cell cycle profile changes and apoptosis through caspase independent pathway in human lung adenocarcinoma cell lineA549. *Journal of Medicinal Plants.* 3 (63): 57–67.
30. Kumar SS, Rekka R, Thankachan J, Santhosh T. 2018. Identification of aphrodisiac properties of *Ficus auriculata* Lour. fruit extract. *European Journal of Biomedicine.* 5 (2): 454–460.
31. Tamta G, Mehra N, Tandon S. 2021. Traditional uses, phytochemical and pharmacological properties of Ficus auriculata: A review *A review, Journal of Drug Delivery and Therapeutics*, 11(3): 163–169. http://dx.doi.org/10.22270/jddt.v11i3.4853 .
32. Doley BK, Kakoti BB. 2018. Hepatoprotective potential of *Ficus auriculata* and *Sarcochlamys pulcherrima*, two ethnomedicinal plants used by the mishing community of Assam. *World Journal of Pharmacy and Pharmaceutical Sciences.* 15 (7): 913–922.
33. Veerapur VP, Prabhakar KR, Parihar VK, Kandadi MR, Ramakrishana S, Mishra B, Rao S, Satish BS, Srinivasan KK, Priyadarsini KI, Unnikrishnan MK. 2009. *Ficus racemosa* stem bark extract: a potent antioxidant and a probable natural radioprotector. *eCAM.* 6: 317–324.
34. Lu JM, Lin PH, Yao Q, Chen C. 2010. Chemical and molecular mechanisms of antioxidants: experimental approaches and model systems. *Journal of Cellular and Molecular Medicine.* 14: 840–860.
35. Sanchez JC, Garcaia RF, Cors MM. 2010. 1,1-Diphenyl-2-picrylhydrazyl radical and superoxide anion scavenging activity of *Rhizophora mangle* (L.) bark. *Pharmacognosy Research.* 2: 279–284.
36. Mavi A, Terzi Z, Ozgen U, Yildirim A, Coskun M. 2004. Antioxidant properties of some medicinal plants: *Prangos ferulacea* (apiaceae), *Sedum sempervivoides* (crassulaceae) *Malva neglecta* (malvaceae), *Cruciata taurica* (rubiaceae), *Rosa pimpinellifolia* (rosaceae), *Galium verum subspecies verum* (rubiaceae), *Urtica dioica* (urticaceae). *Biological and Pharmaceutical Bulletin.* 27: 702–705.
37. Koduru S, Grierson DS, Afolayan AJ. 2006. Antimicrobial activity of *Solanum aculeastrum. Pharmaceutical Biology.* 44: 283–286.
38. Torres JA, Villegas MV, Quinn JP. 2007. Current concepts in antibiotic resistant Gram-negative bacteria. *Expert Review of Anti-infective Therapy.* 5: 833–843.
39. Usman H, Abdulrahman FI, Usman A. 2009. Qualitative phytochemical screening and in vitro antimicrobial effects of Methanol stem bark extract of *Ficus thonningii* (moraceae). *African Journal of Traditional, Complementary and Alternative Medicines.* 6:289–295.
40. Roopashree TS, Raman D, Rani SRH, Narendra C. 2008. Antibacterial activity of antipsoriatic herbs: *Cassia tora, Momordica charantia* and *Calendula officinalis. International Journal of Applied Research in Natural Products.* 1:20–28.

12 *Ficus palmata* (Bedu)

INTRODUCTION

Ficus palmata Forsk. (family: Moraceae) is a wild Himalayan plant, commonly known as Wild Himalayan Fig or Bedu.[1–3] It is highly variable and occurs in the northwest Himalayan hills of India (Uttarakhand, Punjab, and Kashmir), Nepal, the Arabian Peninsula, Afghanistan, Pakistan, Iran, Sudan, Ethiopia, Somalia, and southern Egypt, typically on dry-hot slopes with clay-loam soils.[1] Flowering (March-April) and fruiting (second fortnight of June to the first half of July) occur from spring to summer seasons.[4]

ETHNOPHARMACOLOGY

The whole fruit of *F. palmata,* along with its seeds, is edible. Its fruits are juicy and sweet, with some astringency due to the white latex just beneath the pericarp. Traditionally, the astringency is removed by immersing fruits in water for about 10–15 min before use.[4] Overall, the fruit quality is excellent. The young growth and unripe fruits are cooked and eaten as vegetables. Young growth or unripe fruits are boiled, water is removed by squeezing the biomass, and they are then fried.[4] The squeezed biomass is laxative, poultice, demulcent, and emollient. Fruits are used in the food diet to treat constipation and diseases of the bladder and lungs. The sap of *F. palmata* is used to treat warts.[4] The *F. palmata* leaves, fruits, bark, latex, and roots are traditionally used for anti-ulcer, antidiabetic, anti-tumor, hypoglycemic, antifungal, and lipid-lowering properties.[2,3] Traditionally, deeply lodged spines in the flesh are extracted by the application of stem latex.[1,2]

PHYTOCONSTITUENTS OF *F. PALMATA*

Joshi et al. have reported that fruits of *F. palmata* have 45.2% juice and 48.2% moisture content. Juice has dissolved solids, sugars, pectin content, and vitamins. Fruits are rich in minerals (Table 12.1).[4]

Anjum and Tripathi have studied the phytochemical composition of *F. palmata* fruit using different solvents such as n-BuOH, EtOAc, MeOH, and water and the standard protocols of analysis[6–8] to detect the presence of various phytochemicals such as alkaloids, phenols, coumarins, flavonoids, tannins, saponins, terpenoids, steroids, etc.[6] Either a change in color or precipitation with the specified detecting reagents of various fractions was observed and documented for the presence (+) or absence (–). Based on the observations, each test was replicated thrice for confirmation.[6–8] In another investigation, the *F. palmata* plant extracts have been reported for the presence of the same chemical classes.[9] The aerial parts of *F. palmata* have furanocoumarins (psoralen and bergapten), germanicol acetate, trans-psoralenoside, vanillic acid, and rutin.[10]

The comparative nutritional analysis deciphers that *F. palmata* fruits have higher levels of minerals, fiber, protein, and fat compared to cultivated mango fruits.[5] Additionally, 500 g of *F. palmata* fruits contain enough nutrients required per day by a person.[5]

PHARMACOLOGICAL PROPERTIES OF *F. PALMATA* PLANT

The presence of phytochemicals like glycosides, flavonoids, phenols, tannins, resin, etc. in the *F. palmata* plant supports its ethnopharmacological applications. The plant species has been reported to possess antioxidant,[11] antimicrobial,[12] anticancer, anti-inflammatory,[13] and antidiabetic[14] properties, along with mechanisms of action of some of its chemical constituents in the management of type 2 diabetes mellitus.[15]

The bark of *F. palmata* has been reported to have antibacterial and antioxidant properties,[9] whereas latex from stems has antibacterial properties.[16] As α-amylase and α-glucosidase retard the absorption of dietary carbohydrates and suppress postprandial hyperglycemia,[17,18] Anjum and Tripathi have studied the α-amylase and α-glucosidase inhibitory action of *F. palmata* fruits and reported their potent inhibitory action and utilization in the management of type 2 diabetes mellitus.[6] The results of the study have further validated the ethnomedicinal uses of *F. palmata* fruits to reduce elevated blood glucose levels.[6]

Saini et al. have studied the antioxidant activities of *F. palmata* fruits using ferric-reducing properties and free radical scavenging assays. The free radical scavenging assay was conducted with 2,2-diphenyl-1-picrylhydrazyl (DPPH) and 2,2′-azinobis-3-ethylbenzo thiazoline-6-sulphonic acid (ABTS). The DPPH scavenging activity was 104.9 mg catechin equivalents/100 g fruit weight in methanolic extract of fruits. In the acetone extract, it was 146.9 mg catechin equivalents/100 g. The ABTS cation scavenging activity of the methanolic extract of fruits was 557.09 mg butylated hydroxyl-anisole/100 g, while in acetone extract, it was 729.45 mg butylated hydroxyl-anisole/100 g fruit weight. The Fe^{+++} activity of the methanolic extract was 77.6 mg ascorbic acid/100 g fruit weight, while the acetone extract was 146.67 mg ascorbic acid/100 g fruit weight.[19]

The in vitro antibacterial and antifungal activities of *F. palmata* extract using ethyl acetate, methanolic, ethanolic, chloroform, petroleum ether, acetone, and water extracts reveal that ethanolic bark extract has significant

DOI: 10.1201/9781003512868-14

TABLE 12.1
Chemical Composition of *F. palmata* Plant Fruits[5]

Nutrients	Value	Nutrients	Value
Moisture (%)	48.20 ± 0.10	Insoluble ash (%)	9.46 ± 0.10
Total nitrogen (%)	0.73 ± 0.05	Mg (mg/100 g)	0.92 ± 0.15
Ash (%)	4.06 ± 0.15	Soluble ash (%)	7.54 ± 0.10
Total protein (%)	4.06 ± 0.08	K (mg/100 g)	1.58 ± 0.20
Crude fiber (%)	17.65 ± 0.14	Ca (mg/100 g)	1.54 ± 0.13
Crude fat (%)	4.71 ± 0.20	Na (mg/100 g)	0.75± 0.12
Organic matter (%)	95.90 ± 0.15	Fe (mg/100 g)	0.018 ± 0.02
Carbohydrate (%)	20.78 ± 0.10	P (mg/100 g)	1.88 ± 0.02

activity against *Staphylococcus aureus*.[20] The methanolic extract of the leaves of *F. palmata* possesses potent antimicrobial activity and supports its ethnopharmacological applications.[21]

The antiproliferative activity of *F. palmata* fruit extract has been reported on cervical cancer cell lines, namely C33A, HeLa, and normal peripheral blood mononuclear cells. Different concentrations of fruit extracts have demonstrated potent antiproliferative activity against C33A cells but do not have antiproliferative activity against HeLa cells. Acetone extract has been reported to have the highest anti-proliferative activity, and it was lowest in methanolic extract.[19]

Namola et al. have studied the in vitro effect of the aqueous extract of *F. palmata* leaves on growth and demineralization and concluded that the aqueous extract of *F. palmata* has dose-dependent anti-calcinogenic action in the demineralization of the calcium phosphate.[22] Studies on CCl_4-induced hepatic toxicity reveal that the use of *F. palmata* extract has a dose-dependent hepatoprotective action.[10] Alqasoumi et al. studied the anticoagulant effects of *F. palmata* herb extract in different solvents against the clotting time (CT) using warfarin as a standard and concluded that the petroleum ether and chloroform extracts had time-dependent and dose-dependent effects on clotting.[10]

SCOPE AND OPPORTUNITIES

The roots, bark, and fruits of *F. palmata* contain compounds like fixed oil, fats, alkaloids, flavonoids, steroids, tannins, carbohydrates, and proteins. The TLC results of the water, ethanol, and methanol extracts decipher six different constituents present in each extract of *F. palmata* bark.[5] More detailed investigations are to be done for isolation and characterization to know more about the pure ingredients.

The detailed literature survey revealed that the *F. palmata* plant has a wide therapeutic potential against various diseases and body disorders. The property of its fruits as potent α-amylase and α-glucosidase inhibitory activity has wide scope in the management of postprandial hyperglycemia in T2DM. Different fractions of the fruit extracts showed considerable enzyme inhibitory action in a dose-dependent manner, and the methanol fraction demonstrated the highest inhibitory efficacy compared to other fractions, which may be due to the presence of bioactive phytochemicals like phenolics, flavonoids, and terpenoids, as detected in the phytochemical screening in higher concentration. This therapeutic potentiality of the specific fraction of FPFE could be beneficially exploited in the treatment of Type2DM. The study further validates the ethnomedicinal uses of *F. palmata* fruits in the management of diabetes, though it directs further research on the isolation and characterization of specific ingredients responsible for the enzyme inhibitory activity of *F. palmata* fruits, as well as in vivo studies for further confirmation of the obtained results.

All species of *Ficus* plants possess antioxidant potential due to a higher concentration of phytochemical compounds. They have a valuable role in human nutrition and the treatment of body ailments due to a variety of bioactive therapeutic compounds. The main phytochemicals present in *Ficus* species are carotenoids, glycosides, phenolic acids, flavonoids, anthocyanins, some water-soluble vitamins, and polyphenols. The presence of these ingredients makes *Ficus* a medicinal plant with various biological properties, particularly antioxidant activity. On account of its high antioxidant potential, all parts of the *Ficus* plant are used for the treatment of various diseases and the management of oxidative stress.

REFERENCES

1. Parmar C, Kaushal MK. 1982. *Ficus palmata in Wild Fruits*. Kalyani Publishers, New Delhi, India. pp. 31–34.
2. Chopra RN, Nayar SL, Chopra IC. 1986. *Glossary of Indian Medicinal Plants (Including the Supplement)*. Council of Scientific and Industrial Research, New Delhi.
3. Khare CP. 2007. *Indian Medicinal Plants- An Illustrated Dictionary*. Springer. Berlin. pp. 267–268.
4. Joshi Y, Joshi A K, Prasad N, Juyal D. 2014. A review on *Ficus palmata* (Wild Himalayan Fig). *The Journal of* Phytopharmacology. 3 (5): 374–377.
5. Saklani S, Chandra S. 2012. Phytochemical screening of garhwal Himalaya wild edible fruit *Ficus palmata*. *International Journal of PharmTech Research*. 4 (3): 1185–1191.
6. Anjum N, Tripathi YC. 2019. Phytochemical screening and in-vitro evaluation of antidiabetic activity of *Ficus palmata* fruits. *European Journal of Pharmaceutical and Medical Research*. 6 (11): 251–258.

7. Raaman N. 2006. *Phytochemical Techniques*. New India Publishing Agency, New Delhi.
8. Evan WC, Evans T. 2003. *Pharmacognosy*, 5th Edition. Cambridge University Press, London. pp. 336–393.
9. Chauhan PK, Sharma S, Chandrika, Harsh, Manisha, Mansi. 2014. Evaluation of phytochemical and in-vitro antioxidant and antibacterial activities of wild plant species of *Bauhinia* and *Ficus* of HP. *World Journal of Pharmacy and Pharmaceutical Sciences*. 3 (4): 659–668.
10. Alqasoumi SI, Basudan OA, Al-Rehaily AJ, Abdel-Kader MS. 2014. Phytochemical and pharmacological study of *Ficus palmata* growing in Saudi Arabia. *Saudi Pharmaceutical Journal*. 22 (5): 460–471.
11. Sirisha N, Sreenivasulu M, Sangeeta K, Chetty CM. 2010. Antioxidant properties of *Ficus* species – a Review. *International Journal of PharmTech Research*. 2: 2174–2182.
12. Salem MZM, Salem AZM, Camacho LM, Ali HM. 2013. Antimicrobial activities and phytochemical composition of extracts of *Ficus* species: an overview. *African Journal of Microbiology Research*. 7: 4207–4219.
13. Lansky EP, Paavilainen HM, Pawlus AD, Newman RA. 2008. *Ficus* spp. (Fig): ethnobotany and potential as anticancer and anti-inflammatory agents. *Journal of E*thnopharmacology. 119: 195–213.
14. Khan KY, Khan MA, Ahmad M, Hussain I, Mazari P, Fazal H, Ali B, Khan IZ. 2011. Hypoglycemic potential of genus *Ficus* L.: a review of ten years of plant-based medicine used to cure diabetes (2000–2010). *Journal of Applied Pharmaceutical Science*. 1: 223–227.
15. Deepa P, Sowndhararajan K, Kim S, Park SJ. 2018. A role of *Ficus* species in the management of diabetes mellitus: a review. *Journal of Ethnopharmacology*. 215: 210–232.
16. Kumar A, Gularia R, Bhardwaj A. 2013. Antibacterial screening of *Ficus palmata* Forsk pure latex and its methanolic and ethanolic extracts. *Indian Journal Natural Product Resources*. 4: 271–274.
17. Subramanian R, Asmawi MZ, Sadikun A. 2008. *In-vitro* alpha-glucosidase and alpha-amylase enzyme inhibitory effects of *Andrographis paniculata* extract and andrographolide. *Acta Biochimica Polonica*. 55: 391–398.
18. Hossain SJ, Tsujiyama I, Takasugi MT, Islam MA, Biswas RS, Aoshima H. 2008. Total phenolic content, anti-oxidative, anti-amylase, anti-glucosidase and antihistamine release activities of Bangladeshi fruits. *Food Science and Technology Research*. 14: 261–268.
19. Saini R, Garg V, Dangwal K. 2012. Comparative study of three wild edible fruits of Uttarakhand for antioxidant, antiproliferative activities and polyphenolic composition. *International Journal of Pharma and Bio Sciences*. 3 (4): 158–167.
20. Saklani S, Chandra S. 2011. Antimicrobial activity, nutritional profile and quantitative study of different fractions of *Ficus palmata*. *International Research Journal of Plant Science*. 2 (11): 332–337.
21. Chandra S, Saklani S. 2017. Isolation and identification of *Ficus palmata* leaves and their antimicrobial activities. *Journal of Scientific Research*. 9 (2): 193–200.
22. Namola V, Agarwal K, Saini P. 2013. In vitro evaluation of leaves of *Ficus palmata* on calcium phosphate crystallization. *World Journal of Pharmaceutical Research*. 2 (4): 875–877.

13 *Garcinia cowa* (Kuji Thekera)

INTRODUCTION

Fruits of Kuji Thekera (*Garcinia cowa* Roxb. ex Choisy) (Figure 13.1a) are a dietary source of nutrition that play a vital role in folklore healing practices of Assam, India.[1] It is one of the important indigenous fruits of ancient Kamrup culture, currently known as the State of Assam, India. These fruits are highly perishable and concerned for retaining quality during long-distance transport. The sliced sun-dried fruits are used for garnishing curries and as folk medicine. Hydroxy citric acid (HCA) is the principal ingredient of the species, an anti-obesity compound. HCA inhibits fatty acid synthesis and accumulation of lipids in living organisms.[2] *G. cowa* is widely distributed throughout Thailand, Myanmar, and Malaysia. The young leaves and fruits have a sour taste and are edible. The bark of the species is dark brown with yellow latex (Figure 13.1b). Male flowers of the species are found along the branches as clusters and female flowers in yellow-orange color at the end of branches (Figure 13.1c). *G. cowa* has unisexual branches. The leaves are deep green, oblong, and glossy. The fruits are green when young (2.5–6.0 cm in size), and at maturity, they have a dull orange or yellow color with 5–8 shallow grooves and 6–8 large 3-angled seeds.[3]

Different parts of *G. cowa* are used in traditional medicinal purposes. Their bark, latex, and roots are used to treat fever,[4,5] and fruits and leaves are used to treat indigestion, improve blood circulation, and act as an expectorant.[5] The chemical composition and biological utilities of various parts of the *G. cowa* plant have been investigated at the molecular level. The derivatives of xanthones and phloroglucinols have been reported as the major ingredients; however, depsidones, flavonoids, terpenoids, and steroids are reported as minor ingredients.[6]

G. cowa in Bangladesh

In Bangladesh, *G. cowa* is described as an evergreen medium-sized tree with horizontal branches and an oval-shaped crown. Leaves are long, broadly elliptical lanceolate, and acuminate. Flowers are rather small and yellow; female flowers are located at the end of the branchlets. Male flowers are dense, located at the terminal clusters, and are smaller than female flowers. The bark is used in spasms and astringent. Fruits are used to treat headaches. Sliced, and subsequently, sun-dried fruits are used in dysentery. The gum resin may produce nausea and is drastic cathartic, even may cause vomit.[7]

G. cowa in China

Liu et al. have studied the interspecific associations and spatial patterns of plant species to understand the processes and mechanisms of coexistence, using point pattern analysis. For quantification (positive or negative associations), the 'torus-translation test' was used for topographic habitats. The results showed that (i) a total of 14–20 tree species were associated with one or two of the topographic variables indicating the spatial pattern of these species; (ii)

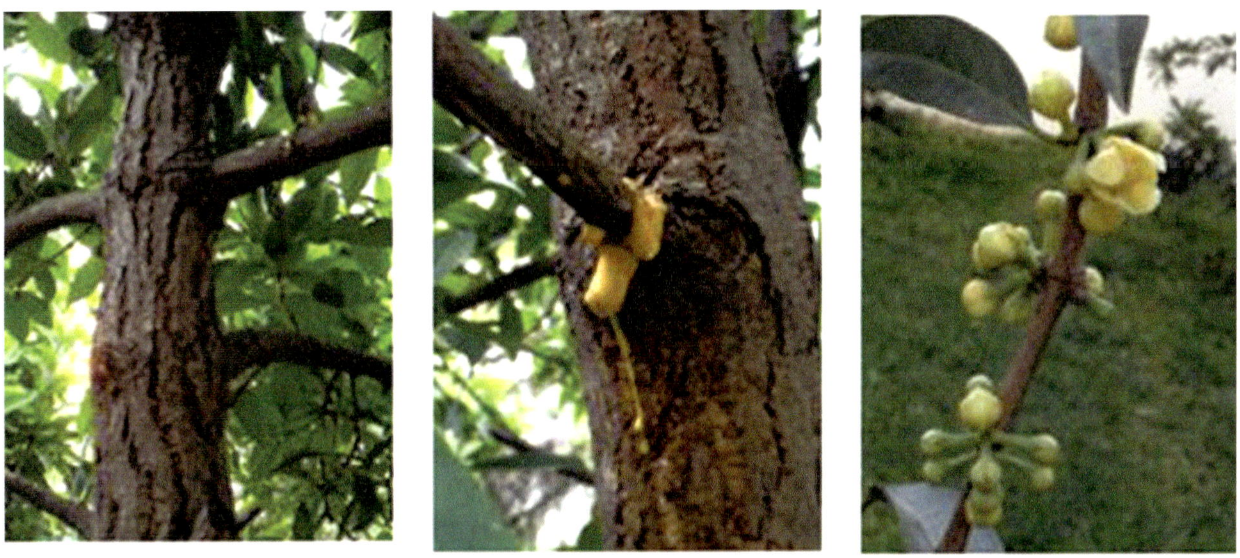

(a) (b) (c)

FIGURE.13.1 (a–c) *G. cowa* stem latex on trunk flowers as cluster.

DOI: 10.1201/9781003512868-15

most saplings of the *G. cowa* showed a clumped distribution at small scales (0–10 M) which was lost at a larger range (10–30 M); (iii) the degree of spatial clumping decreases from saplings to poles, to adults which indicates that density-dependent mortality of the offspring is ubiquitous in species; and (iv) a high number of positive small-scale interactions were found among the 20 species. For saplings, 38.4% were negative, while 42.6% of all combinations of species pairs showed positive associations at neighborhood scales up to five meters. The positive associations made up 45.5% and 29.5% for poles and adults, respectively. The study concluded with considerable evidence for the positive interactions among the tree species with *G. cowa* in the spatial patterns in Xishuangbanna, China.[8]

G. cowa in Thailand

G. cowa is commonly known as 'Kandis' or 'forest mangosteen' in Cha Muang and West Sumatra in Thailand.[6] The pericarp of the fruits (Figure 13.2) is used as kitchen jams and spices. Fresh fruits are used for pickles and different dishes in Western Sumatra. Seeds from the plant are used as supplementary feed for livestock. The fruits are considered safe and effective for good health.[9,10] *G. cowa* seeds have anti-nutrient compounds that inhibit the absorption of saponins and tannins.[11] Currently, antibiotics are banned in animal feed to prevent cases of antibiotic resistance in humans,[12] but phyto-probiotics are added in animal feed to increase livestock productivity. These phyto-probiotics are extracted from plant sources in different forms such as dry extract, oleoresin, or essential oil.[13] Flavonoids, the active ingredient in seeds of *G. cowa*, affect the metabolism, immunity, nervous system, and digestive conditions. The use of *G. cowa* fruits after removing seeds increases digestive enzymes due to increased digestive fluid production and, finally, regulates the microbial activity in the digestive tract.[14] The use of whole fruits without seeds for livestock food is supposed to have a healthy composition. Ouyang et al. have reported the use of *G. cowa* seeds in Thailand to increase carcass weight in broilers.[15] Further, research data have revealed that the use of *G. cowa* seed powder up to 1% dose in animal feed does not affect the appearance of broiler livestock production.[16]

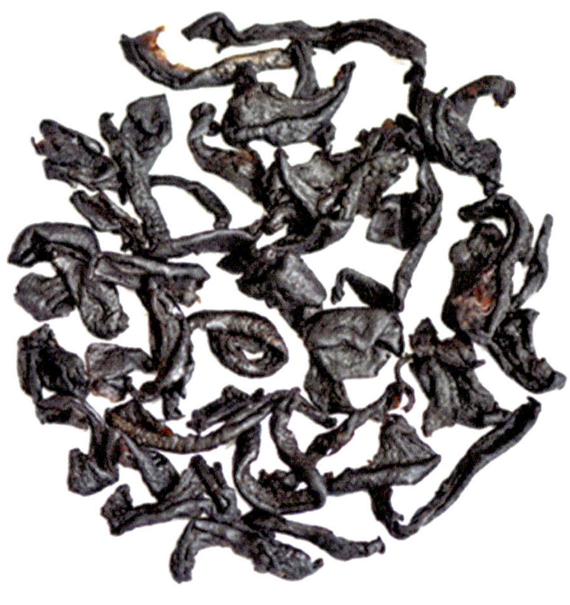

FIGURE 13.2 Sliced and sun-dried fruits.

G. cowa in Assam, India

Kuji Thekera (*G. cowa*) fruits are the source of carbohydrates, organic acids, minerals, proteins, and vitamins along with digestive enzymes. The use of *G. cowa* fruits in the diet stimulates appetite and helps in proper digestion. Neog has studied the floral biology, growth, and development of Kuji Thekera from Assam and reported that the flowering period of the species is from April to May. Anthesis time has been noted from 2 am to 4 am, dehiscence is completed within 3 to 4 h of anthesis, and pollen fertility is about 75%.[1] Baruah and Borthakur have reported the morphology and ethnobotany of the genus *Garcinia* including *G. cowa* and reported that the species is evergreen, and its flowering period is from March to April.[17]

Parthasarathy and Nandakishore have studied *G. cowa* from the Western Ghats, India, and reported that the species is evergreen and has an opposite decussate foliar arrangement. It has simple petiolate leaves. The petioles are so small and appear sessile. In the Western Ghats, the flowering season is different (December–March) from Northeast India where it starts in the summer (i.e., April–June).[18]

Neog and Mohan have studied the developmental physiology of the *G. cowa* fruit and reported the growth of *G. cowa* fruits in three distinct phases.[1,19] *G. cowa* (Kuji Thekera) fruits have 9.8% total soluble solids, 8.64 mg/100 g ascorbic acid, 4.7% acids, and 3.84% total sugar.[1]

PHYTOCHEMISTRY OF *G. COWA*

The traditional utility of *G. cowa* for healthcare has increased the attention of scientists for its phytochemical screening to identify medicinally active compounds. Further research is to develop value-added products, such as making derivatives of more therapeutic utility from the identified compounds. The following classes of compounds have been described by different researchers.

Depsidone: Depsidones are compounds comprised by the condensation of condensed ortho-positions through ester and ether linkages of benzoic acid and phenol skeletons. Depsidones are a well-known chemical class of natural products in the *Garcinia* spp.[20,21] The cowadepsidone is the first and only known depsidone from *G. cowa*. It has been isolated from the twig extract and has cytotoxicity against NCI-H187 and MFC-7 cancer cell lines.[22]

Flavonoids: A total of 12 flavonoids have been isolated from *G. cowa*.[23] The morelloflavone and morelloflavone-7″-O-glucoside have been reported as potent antioxidants.[5]

Phloroglucinols: Phloroglucinols are compounds having 1,3,5-benzenetriol core skeleton (phloroglucinol) or phloroglucin (1,3,5-cyclohexanetrione) tautomer. *G. cowa* has been reported for 15 phloroglucinols compounds. These are chamuangone, guttiferone K, garcicowins A, B, C, and D and nine others [namely cambogin, oblongifolins (B, C, A, and D), guttiferones (K, B and F), and 30-epicambogin.[6] A few of these have been reported for selective cytotoxicity against two cancer cell lines (HCT-116 and HT-29) and normal colon cells (CCD-18Co). Among all compounds, guttiferone K and 30-epicambogin have been identified for the highest efficacy against cancer cell line HT-29.[24] Further, chamuangone[5] exhibited antibacterial activity against *S. viridans* and *H. pylori* (minimum inhibitory concentration [MIC] = 15.6 µg/mL), *S. pyogenes* (MIC = 7.8 µg/mL), and *S. aureus*, *B. subtilis*.[25]

Terpenes and steroids: Terpenes and steroids are rare in *G. cowa*, and only four compounds, namely, friedelin, daucosterol, β-sitosterol, and stigmasterol, have been identified from the *G. cowa*[26]; but they have not been studied for biological activities although had been investigated from other plants after isolation.[27–30]

Xanthones: Xanthones are widely distributed in the plant kingdom, from higher plants to fungi, and lichens, and are known for their therapeutic properties. The basic chemical skeleton with two aromatic rings linked via ether and carbonyl linkages, xanthones, are the major ingredients of the *Garcinia* genus and commonly found in different parts of *G. cowa*, especially in the latex, fruit, and stem. Nineteen xanthones have been isolated from *G. cowa*. These have been named as cowagarcinone C, cowanol, cowanin, 1,3,6-trihydroxy-7-methoxy-2,5-bis-(3-methyl-2-butenyl)-xanthone, norcowanin, cowaxanthone, cowagarcinones A, B, E, and D from the latex,[4,31] cowaxanthones (B, C, D) and E from the fruit,[32] 7-O-methylgarcinone E, 4-(1,1-dimethyl-prop-2-enyl)-1,5,6-trihydroxy-3-methoxy-2-(3-methylbut-2-enyl) xanthen-9(9H)-one,1,5,6-trihydroxy-3-methoxy-4-(3-hydroxyl-3-methylbutyl)-xanthone, and 1,5-dihydroxy-3methoxy-6′,6′-dimethyl-2H-pyrano (2′,3′:6,7)-4-(3-methylbut-2-enyl) xanthone from the stem,[23,33] and cowaxanthone F.[5] Most of these xanthones have been reported for interesting biological activities.

Panthong et al. have reported that eight xanthones from the *G. cowa* fruits (cowaxanthones B, 7-O-methylgarcinone E, cowaxanthones C, α-mangostin, mangostanin, β-mangostin, cowanin, and cowanol) have antibacterial activity against *S. aureus* and MRSA (methicillin-resistant *Staphylococcus aureus*). α-Mangostin and mangostanin have been reported for significant potential activity against these bacteria. α-Mangostin had an MIC value of 8 µg/mL, against both *S. aureus* and MRSA, while mangostanin had an MIC value of 4 µg/mL against both bacteria.[32] Eight xanthones [α-mangostin, cowaxanthones (A, B, C, and D), mangostanin, cowanin, and cowanol] from *G. cowa* have been tested for their anti-inflammatory activity using the ethyl phenylpropiolate–induced ear edema assay. All xanthones except cowanol were more active than the standard drug, phenylbutazone.[5] Five xanthones isolated from the stem bark, namely 7-O-methylgarcinone E, α-mangostin, cowaxanthone, cowanol, and cowanin, had significant *in vitro* antimalarial activity against *Plasmodium falciparum* with IC_{50} values ranging between 1.5 and 3.0 µg/mL.[34] Six xanthones (cowaxanthone, cowanol, cowanin, norcowanin, 3,6-di-Omethyl-γ-mangostin, and dulxanthone A) isolated from twigs of *G. cowa* have been evaluated for their cytotoxicity against NCI-H187, KB, MFC-7, and/or HepG2 cell lines. Cowaxanthone, cowanin, norcowanin, and 3,6-di-O-methyl-γ-mangostin have exhibited significant cytotoxicity against the NCI-H187 cell line with IC_{50} values ranging between 3.87 and 8.58 µg/mL and moderately inhibited KB and MCF-7 cancer cell lines with IC_{50} values ranging between 6.43–15.43 and 10.59–21.38 µg/mL, respectively.[22] Dulxanthone A has been reported cytotoxic against the HepG2 cell line.[35]

Wahyuni et al. have reported ten miscellaneous classes of compounds (13% of the total isolated compounds) isolated from *G. cowa*,[36] but none of these has been tested for its biological activities.[6] The fruit, twig, and stem of *G. cowa* are the best source of secondary metabolites, and a few of these have interesting pharmacological activities such as α-mangostin, cowanin, and cowanol. These compounds are present in every part of the *G. cowa* plant and are used as chemotaxonomic markers of the plant species.

Different Extracts and Biological Activities

Chloroform and hexane extracts of the fruit rind and methanolic extract of leaves and twigs of *G. cowa* have been investigated for biological activities. They have been tested against four gram-positive bacteria (*Bacillus subtilis*, *B. coagulans*, *B. cereus*, and *S. aureus*) and one gram-negative bacterium (*Escherichia coli*)). Both extracts have potentially inhibited bacterial growth of the gram-positive bacteria (IC50s 15–30 µg/mL) but not gram-negative bacterium (i.e., *E. coli*) (IC_{50s} 250–500 µg/mL).[37]

Both these extracts have been reported to inhibit the growth of the common fungal food contaminant *Aspergillus flavus* ATCC 46283, which produces aflatoxin B1.[38]

The methanol extracts of the leaves and twigs of *G. cowa* have been reported rich in phenolic content.[39]

Chemical Composition of *G. cowa* Fruits

Dutta et al. collected the fruits of *G. cowa* from the Assam Agriculture University, Jorhat, Assam, India, and studied for chemical composition. The results have revealed the potential applications in healthcare practices and supported the traditional utilization. For stability study, after proper cleaning, fruits were subjected to various post-harvest treatments and coded as T1, T2, T3, and T4, but T5 was used as a control sample and not treated with any chemical. Fruit samples (T1–T4) were packed in perforated (0.2% ventilation) low-density polyethylene, 100 gauge bags, and stored at ambient conditions, with four replications to each, and analyzed for biochemical parameters at 3-day intervals for up to 9 days.[40] Ascorbic acid content was determined by visual titration method and expressed in mg 100/g.[41] Total sugars,[42] total phenols,[43] and HCA[44] content of Kuji Thekera fruits were quantified. The gross food energy of fruits was expressed in kcal/100 g on a dry basis.[45]

Ascorbic acid: A significant decrease of ascorbic acid content in Kuji Thekera fruits has been reported during the storage period. The cause of reduction was due to the presence of ascorbinase enzyme as it converts into dehydro-ascorbic acid.[46–48] Similarly, packaged fruits have been reported for more ascorbic acid content than the control, due to the reduced rate of respiration in the polyethylene bags that retards aging and depletion of acids.[49] It was also noted that ample oxygen gas (O_2) has increased enzymatic activities that lead to a biochemical breakdown of fruits' ingredients,[50] compared to the treated and packed fruits.[51]

Total sugar: The total sugar content in the fruits has been reported to decrease with the storage duration; despite the conversion of pectin and starch into simple sugar, there was an increase in the sugar content, but simultaneous decomposition of these sugars was also noticed.[40] Similar observations have been reported by Patel et al. in a study on custard apple.[52]

Total phenol: During storage, the non-protected/-treated fruits have been reported for the lowest level of total phenol content due to oxidation by polyphenol oxidase (PPO), which converts phenol to quinines.[53] The decreasing trend in the total phenol content was also observed by Kopjar et al.[54] The reduction in total phenol has been explained by the interconversion of free and bound phenolic substances.[55] In wax-coated fruits, the activity of PPO is reduced and resulted in the least deterioration of phenols during storage.[40]

Hydroxy citric acid: HCA is the main organic acid in the *Garcinia* species. HCA inhibits adenosine triphosphate citrate lyase and is hence used to treat obesity. Due to the inhibition of adenosine triphosphate citrate lyase, the starting material (oxaloacetate and acetyl-CoA) for fatty acid biosynthesis is blocked, and it affects lipid metabolism. At harvest time, fruits have been reported for 6.97 g/100 g HCA in pulp and 8.17 g/100 g in the peel portion.[40] Jena et al. reported 2.3% and 12.7% HCA in fruits and rinds, respectively, of *G. cowa*.[56]

Energy value: The energy values of fruits have been reported to decrease during storage in pulp and peel, due to a decrease in fat, protein, and carbohydrate contents.[40,57]

Scope for research: Wahyuni et al. have reported that tetra-prenyl-toluquinone (TPTQ) has cytotoxicity towards the H460 lung cancer cell line, which is isolated from the stem and bark of *G. cowa*, and TPTQ caused cell cycle arrest in G0/G1 phase. It was concluded that TPTQ may be a potential new chemotherapeutic agent for lung cancer,[58] and detailed studies along its validations are to be done.

The very-short shelf-life of *G. cowa* fruits and their wide applications are to be studied either for increasing the shelf-life of fruits or preparing its value-added products for the taste and feeling of fresh fruits of *G. cowa* around the year, globally. Currently, the freshness of *G. cowa* fruits is evaluated based on visual quality (color).[59] The shelf-life of the fruit depends on the presence of microorganisms and loss of organoleptic qualities such as loss of nutrient value, texture, taste, and color. Visual quality scoring has indicated that without treatment fruits have a shelf-life of two days only; even at room temperature fruits shrank in size, became unmarketable, and got fully spoiled. The wax-coated fruits had a maximum shelf-life of 6 days. Garg and Ram reported that wax emulsion combined with 0.5% Standard Operating Procedures and Policies (SOPP) can extend the shelf-life up to 6 days.[60]

G. cowa plant is a source of many antimicrobial compounds against several pathogenic microbes. These compounds may be of societal utility as there is a rapid rise in population; subsequently, there is a higher demand for the food supply to feed millions of people. Human dependence on the few major staple crops to meet the needs of the people has led to increases in starvation and poverty. Underutilized edible plants offer a more affordable and cheaper option and provide food security to the poor in the world. Current studies on *G. cowa* reveal the need to promote the species for cultivation to increase income through sustainable collection and marketing, prevent loss of the natural habitat caused by anthropogenic activities, and develop its value-added products to harness nutraceutical properties. This chapter describes the information on chemical constituents of the *G. cowa*, its biology, and physiology. Additional research, awareness about its uses as medicine, waste treatment, and biofuel are still needed for the beneficial purpose. *G. cowa* plant has a high potential to solve environmental problems and sustain human health and well-being from lifestyle-based health challenges.

REFERENCES

1. Neog M. 1990. Studies on the floral biology, growth and development of few minor species of Assam. M.Sc. (Agri) Thesis, Assam Agricultural University, Jorhat, India.
2. Lewis YS, Neelakantan S. 1965. Hydroxy citric acid the principal acid in the fruits of *Garcinia cambogia* desr. *Phytochemistry*. 4: 616–625.
3. Lim TK. 2012. *Edible Medicinal and Non-medicinal Plants. Volume 2, Fruits*. Springer Science and Business Media BV, London. pp. 29–34.
4. Mahabusarakam W, Chairerk P, Taylor WC. 2005. Xanthones from *Garcinia cowa* Roxb. Latex. *Phytochemistry*. 66: 1148–1153.
5. Panthong K, Hutadilok-Towatana N, Panthong A. 2009. Cowa xanthone F, a new tetra oxygenated xanthone, and other anti-inflammatory and antioxidant compounds from *Garcinia cowa*. *Canadian Journal of Chemistry*. 87: 1636–1640.
6. Ritthiwigrom T, Laphookhieo S, Pyne S G. 2013. Chemical constituents and biological activities of *Garcinia cowa* Roxb. *Maejo International Journal of Science and Technology*. 7 (2): 212–231.

7. Yusuf M, Chowdhury JU, Wahab MA, Begum J. 1994. *Medicinal Plants of Bangladesh*. Bangladesh Council of Scientific and Industrial Research, Dhaka, Bangladesh. pp. 17–66.
8. Liu B, Zhang X, Bussmann RW, Hart RH, Li P, Bai Y, Long C. 2017. Garcinia in Southern China: ethnobotany, management, and niche modelling. *Economic Botany*. 70 (4): 416–430.
9. Johanis Ly. 2016. Effect of fermented tamarind seeds (FTS) supplementation to sows during estrus to lactation period on sow reproduction performances and piglet mortality at weaning. *Journal of Agricultural Science and Technology* A. 7: 493–500.
10. Abreu AC, McBain AJ, Simoes M. 2012. Plants as sources of new antimicrobials and resistance-modifying agents. *Natural Product Reports*. 29: 1007–1021.
11. Pulaganthi M, Vadivel V, Gurumoorthi P, Janardhanan K. 2004. Comparative nutritional evaluation of little-known legumes, *Tamarindus indica*, *Erythrina indica* and *Sesbania bispinosa*. *Tropical and Subtropical Agro Ecosystems*. 4: 107–123.
12. Barton MD. 2000. Antibiotic use in animal feed and its impact on human health. *Nutrition Research* Reviews. 13 (2): 1–19.
13. Windisch W, Schedle K, Plitzner C, Kroismayr A. 2008. Use of phytogenic products as feed additives for swine and poultry. *Journal of Animal Science*. 86 (14): E140–E148.
14. Coates ME, Fuller R, Harrison GF, Lev M. 1963. A comparison of the growth of chicks in the Gustafsson germ-free apparatus and in a conventional environment, with and without dietary supplements of penicillin. *British Journal of Nutrition*. 17 (1): 141–150.
15. Ouyang KM, Jiang Xu Y, Wang W. 2016. Effects of alfalfa flavonoids on broiler performance, meat quality, and gene expression. *Journal of Animal Science*. 96: 332–341.
16. Kamboh AA, Zhu WY. 2013. Effect of increasing levels of bioflavonoids in broiler feed on plasma anti-oxidative potential, lipid metabolites, and fatty acid composition of meat. *Poultry Science*. 92: 454–461.
17. Baruah S, Borthakur SK. 2012. Studies on morphology and ethnobotany of six species of *Garcinia* L. (Clusiaceae) found in the Brahmaputra Valley, Assam, India. *Scholars Research Library*. 2 (3): 389–396.
18. Parthasarathy U, Nandakishore OP. 2014. Morphological characterization of some important Indian *Garcinia* species. *Dataset Papers in Science Volume*. Article ID 823705. https://doi.org/10.1155/2014/823705
19. Neog M, Mohan NK. 1992. Some aspects of development physiology of cowa (*Garcinia cowa* Roxb) fruit. *Horticultural Journal*. 5(1): 37–42.
20. Rukachaisirikul V, Naklue W, Phongpaichit S, Towatana NH, Maneenoon K. 2006. Phloroglucinols, depsidones and xanthones from the twigs of *Garcinia parvifolia*. *Tetrahedron*. 62: 8578–8585.
21. Ha LD, Hansen PE, Duus F, Pham HD, Nguyen LHD. 2012. liveridepsidones A-D, antioxidant depsidones from *Garcinia oliveri*. *Magnetic Resonance in Chemistry*. 50: 242–245.
22. Cheenpracha S, Phakhodee W, Ritthiwigrom T, Prawat U, Laphookhieo S. 2011. A new depsidone from the twigs of *Garcinia cowa*. *Heterocycles*. 83: 1139–1144.
23. Shen J, Tian Z, Yang JS. 2007. The constituents from the stems of *Garcinia cowa* Roxb. And their cytotoxic activities. *Pharmazie*. 62: 549–551.
24. Xu G, Kan W L T, Zhou Y, Song JZ, Han QB, Qiao CF, Cho CH, Rudd JA, Lin G, Xu HX. 2010. Cytotoxic acylphloroglucinol derivatives from the twigs of *Garcinia cowa*. *Journal of Natural Products*. 73: 104–108.
25. Sakunpak A, Panichayupakaranant P. 2012. Antibacterial activity of Thai edible plants against gastrointestinal pathogenic bacteria and isolation of a new broad spectrum antibacterial polyisoprenylated benzophenone, chamuangone. *Food Chemistry*. 130: 826–831.
26. Shen J, Yang J. 2007. Chemical constituents of branch of *Garcinia cowa* Roxb. *Zhongcaoyao*. 38: 993–994.
27. Mann A, Ibrahim K, Oyewale AO, Amupitan J O, Fatope MO, Okogun JI. 2011. Antimycobacterial friedelane-terpenoid from the root bark of *Terminalia avicennioides*. *American Journal of Chemistry*. 1: 52–55.
28. Viswanathan MB, Ananthi JDJ, Kumar PS. 2012. Antimicrobial activity of bioactive compounds and leaf extracts in *Jatropha tanjorensis*. *Fitoterapia*. 83: 1153–1159.
29. Lee JH, Lee JY, Park JH, Jung HS, Kim JS, Kang SS, Kim YS, Han Y. 2007. Immuno-regulatory activity by daucosterol, a β-sitosterol glycoside, induces protective Th1 immune response against disseminated Candidiasis in mice. *Vaccine*. 25: 3834–3840.
30. Ahamed BMK, Krishna V, Gowdru HB, Rajanaika H, Kumaraswamy HM, Rajshekarappa S, Dandin CJ, Mahadevan KM. 2007. Isolation of bactericidal constituents from the stem bark extract of *Grewia tiliaefolia* Vahl. *Research Journal of Medicinal* Plants. 1: 72–82.
31. Pattalung P, Thongtheeraparp W, Wiriyachitra P, Taylor WC. 1994. Xanthones of *Garcinia cowa*. *Planta Me*dica. 60: 365–368.
32. Panthong K, Pongcharoen W, Phongpaichit S, Taylor WC. 2006. Tetraoxygenated xanthones from the fruits of *Garcinia cowa*. *Phytochemistry*. 67: 999–1004.
33. Shen J, Yang JS. 2006. Two new xanthones from the stems of *Garcinia cowa*. *Chemical and Pharmaceutical Bulletin*. 54: 126–128.
34. Likhitwitayawuid K, Phadungcharoen T, Krungkrai J. 1998. Antimalarial xanthones from *Garcinia cowa*. *Planta Medica*. 64: 70–72.
35. Tian Z, Shen J, Moseman AP, Yang Q, Yang J, Xiao P, Wu E, Kohane IS. 2008. Dulxanthone A induces cell cycle arrest and apoptosis *via* up-regulation of p53 through mitochondrial pathway in HepG2 cells. *International Journal of Cancer*. 122: 31–38.
36. Wahyuni FS, Byrne LT, Dachriyanus NV, Dianita R, Jubahar J, Lajis NH, Sargent MV. 2004. A new ring-reduced tetra-prenyltoluquinone and a prenylated xanthone from *Garcinia cowa*. *Australian Journal of Chemistry*. 57: 223–226.
37. Negi PS, Jayaprakasha GK, Jena BS. 2008. Antibacterial activity of the extracts from the fruit rinds of *Garcinia cowa* and *Garcinia pedunculata* against food borne pathogens and spoilage bacteria. *LWT-Food Science and* Technology. 41: 1857–1861.
38. Joseph GS, Jayaprakasha GK, Selvi AT, Jena BS, Sakariah KK. 2005. Anti-aflatoxigenic and antioxidant activities of *Garcinia* extracts. *International Journal of Food Microbiology*. 101: 153–160.
39. Jantan I, Jumuddin FA, Saputri FC, Rahman K. 2011. Inhibitory effects of the extracts of *Garcinia* species on human low-density lipoprotein peroxidation and platelet aggregation in relation to their total phenolic contents. *Journal of Medicinal Plants Research*. 5: 2699–2709.

40. Dutta S, Neog M, Saikia A. 2017. Shelf-life enhancement of cowa (*Garcinia cowa* Roxb.). *International Journal of Processing and Post harvest Technology*. 8 (1): 50–55.
41. Ranganna S. 1986. *Handbook of Analysis and Quality Control for Fruit and Vegetable Products*, 2nd Edition. McGraw Hill Publishing Co., New Delhi. p. 122.
42. Sadasivam S, Manickam A. 1992. *Biochemical Methods for Agricultural Science*. New Delhi. pp. 6–7.
43. Malik E P, Singh MB. 1980. *Plant Enzymol. Hittoenzymol*. Kalyani Publishers, New Delhi. p. 286.
44. Benny A, Varghese W, Elias M. 1999. Spectrophotometric determination of hydroxy citric acid. *Indian Journal of Pharmaceutical Sciences*. 61: 316–317.
45. Osborn DR, Voogt P. 1978. *Calculation of Calorific Value in the Analysis of Nutrients in Foods*. Academic Press, New York. pp: 239–240.
46. Gohlani S, Bisen BP. 2012. Effect of different coating material on the storage behavior of custard apple (*Annona squamosa* L.). *The* Bioscan. 7: 637–640.
47. Piga A, Caro AD, Pinna I, Agabbio M. 2003. Changes in ascorbic acid, polyphenol content and antioxidant activity in minimally processed cactus pear fruits. *Lebensmittel-Wissenschaft und Technologie*. 36: 257–262.
48. Akhtar A, Abbasi NA, Hussain A, Bakhsh A. 2012. Preserving quality of loquat fruit during storage by modified atmosphere packaging. *Pakistan Journal of Agricultural Sciences*. 49: 419–423.
49. Azene M, Workneh TS, Woldetsadik K. 2014. Effect of packaging materials and storage environment on postharvest quality of papaya fruit. *Journal of Food Science and Technology*. 51: 1041–1055.
50. Yoshida O, Nakagawa H, Ogura N, Sato T. 1984. Effect of heat treatment on the development of poly galacturonase activity in tomato fruit during ripening. *Plant and Cell Physiology*. 25: 500–509.
51. Kader AA. 1985. Postharvest biology and technology: an overview. In: *Postharvest Technology in Horticultural Crops*. Academic Press, New York. pp: 39–47.
52. Patel N, Naik AG, Arbat Shakti S. 2011. Response of post-harvest chemical treatments on shelf-life and quality of custard apple cv. Balanagar. *Indian Journal of Horticulture*. 68: 547–550.
53. Li H, Guo A, Wang H. 2008. Mechanisms of oxidative browning of wine. *Food* Chemistry. 108: 1–13.
54. Kopjar M, Piližota V, Hribar J, Simcic M. 2009. Total phenol content and antioxidant activity of water solutions of plant extracts. *Croatian Journal of Food Science and Technology*. 1: 1–7.
55. Ferrante A, Maggiore T. 2007. Chlorophyll a fluorescence measurement to evaluate storage time and temperature of Valeriana leafy vegetables. *Postharvest Biology and Technology*. 45: 73–80.
56. Jena BS, Jayaprakasha GK, Sakariah KK. 2002. Organic acids from leaves, fruits and rinds of *Garcinia cowa*. *Journal of Agricultural and Food Chemistry*. 50: 3431–3434.
57. McEvily AJ, Inengar R, Otwell WS. 1992. Inhibition of enzymatic browning in foods and beverages. *Critical Reviews in Food Science*. 32: 253–273.
58. Wahyuni FS, Johnson S, Nordin HL, Dachriyanus. 2015. Cytotoxic studies of tetraprenyltoluquinone, a prenylated hydroquinone from the *Garcinia cowa* Roxb on H-460, MCF-7 and DU-145. *International Journal of Pharmacy and Pharmaceutical Sciences*. 7(2): 60–63.
59. Bhowmick SR, Pan JC. 1992. Shelf-life of mature green tomatoes started in controlled atmosphere and high humidity. *Journal of Food Science*. 4: 948–953.
60. Garg RC, Ram HB. 1972. Effect of different concentration of wax emulsion on the storage behaviour of litchi (*Litchi chinensis*). *Progressive Horticulture*. 3: 33–39.

14 *Garcinia pedunculata* (Bor Thekera)

INTRODUCTION

Garcinia pedunculata Roxb. ex Buch.-Ham. (Assamese; Bor Thekera, Ayurvedic; Amlavetasa)[1,2] is an evergreen tree (Figure 14.1) with short spreading branches and a fluted trunk. The leaf blade is oblong and oblong-lanceolate. Fruits are large, and yellow on ripping, oblate and concave on both ends on maturation.[3] Seeds, per fruit, are four to eight in number and fleshy or succulent aril inside. The mature fruits are eaten either raw or in a cooked form.[4] *G. pedunculata* is a tree common in dense forests of the Northeast region and Andaman Nicobar Islands of India. *G. pedunculata* is an exotic plant to the rest of the world, and people are looking to the Indian subcontinent for its potential biodefensive effects. The fruit rind is one of the important medicinal parts of the plant and is used as a condiment in the Indian kitchen. The dried rind of the mature fruit but not fully ripened has high medicinal value and is used in the diet of tribes of Assam, in particular, and the Northeast regions of India.[5] It is used in various ailments such as asthma, cough, fever, bronchitis, obesity, and rheumatoid arthritis and is used as a cardiotonic drug.[6] Old dried fruits are a good source of antioxidants and are used to cure dysentery.[6]

SALIENT FEATURES OF FRUITS OF *G. PEDUNCULATA*

Fruits of *G. pedunculata* are large, green in color (Figure 14.2), and become yellow on ripening. The weight of young mature fruit is about 50 g and has a shiny smooth appearance with a measurement of 7–8 × 25–29 cm in size. The fruit is covered by a thick skin; the inside aril is pulpy or succulent. Seeds are embedded in a fleshy pulp, and each fruit has 4–8 seeds, which are slimy and have medicinal value. The sun-dried longitudinally sliced fruit rind is flattened, flexible, and arcuate. The loss on drying is about 36.67% (w/w), the pH value of 10% aqueous solution is 1.75, and total ash 11.50% (w/w), water-soluble ash 0.37% (w/w), and acid-insoluble ash 0.75% (w/w) reveal the inorganic contents in the fruit rind. Fruits have 41.36% water, 12.40% ethanol, and 0.80% chloroform-soluble extractive values (w/w). Water, ethanol, and chloroform were used as a solvent for the qualitative phyto-screening of different ingredients of the fruit rind. The chemical screening reveals the presence of saponins, glycosides, phenols, carbohydrates, and carboxylic acids. The steroids, alkaloids, protein, tannin, anthocyanin, flavonoids, and phenols were absent in all the extracts tested.[7]

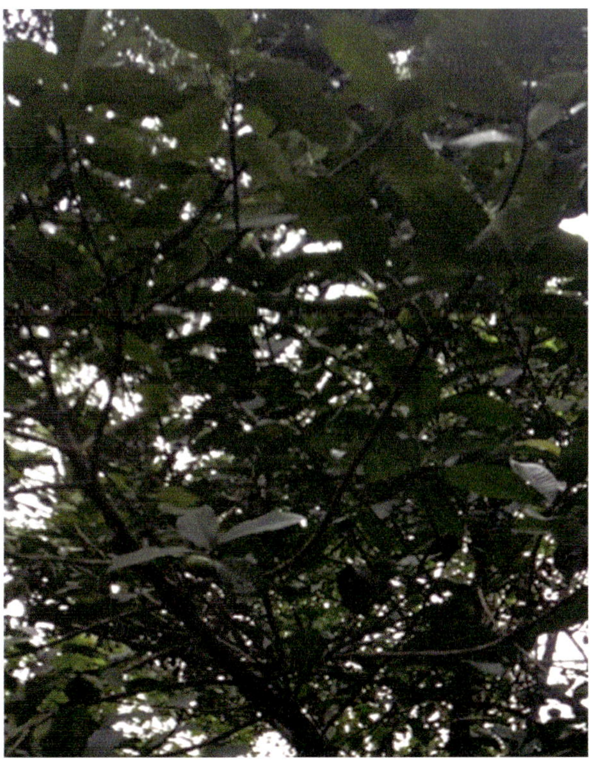

FIGURE 14.1 A branch of *G. pedunculata*.

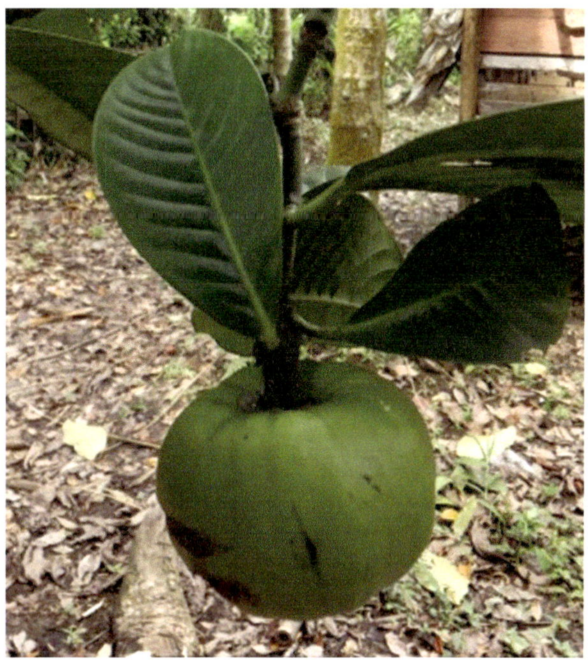

FIGURE 14.2 Immature fruit.

DOI: 10.1201/9781003512868-16

G. pedunculata in Assam, India

Studies on the folklore use of *G. pedunculata* fruits in Assam, India, revealed that most of the rural population utilize it as a medicine to cure different stomach-related diseases rather than allopathic drugs.[8] *G. pedunculata* fruit is used as both medicine and food. For medicinal uses, fruits are sliced into small pieces and dried under direct sunlight for about 10–15 days to remove water content. The seeds are separated from the sliced fruits and discarded, and the resulting product is known as 'Suthi' in Assamese. The healing potential of 'Suthi' depends on the duration of its preservation, as it is older, it is more effective. In folklore practices, a known quantity of dried pulp (Suthi) is mixed with water and prepared as a kind of juice to treat gastrointestinal problems. The juice is used as medicine for a person suffering from different stomach-related disorders. In rural Assam, most of the inhabitants suffer from gastrointestinal diseases due to floods, insanitation, lack of pure drinking water, drought, etc. As a result, rural people have been traditionally using herbals as medicine for recovery from these diseases, and the *G. pedunculata* fruit is highly preferred by the rural people in Assam to treat dysentery.[8] Sarma and Devi have reported that fresh fruits are not consumed as medicine or food as it causes blood dysentery.[8] The information was based on the response of questionnaires (i) the local name, (ii) the fruit part used, (iii) the method of preparation, (iv) the mode of application, (v) Bor Thekera fruits for other medicinal uses, (vi) dose and dosage forms (vii) whether they get relief by using it, and (viii) conservation status of the plant. During the whole study, it was observed that only dried fruits *G. pedunculata* are traditionally used as medicine by the people of Assam.[8]

The state of Assam, India, is divided into 33 administrative geographical units called district.[9] Assam is famous for beautiful rivers, floras, and faunas with unique biodiversity, and habitats of different ethnic groups. The fruits of *G. pedunculata* are used traditionally by all for the treatment of different kinds of diseases like cardiovascular, inflammation, diabetes, and stomach-related diseases without any scientific basis.[5,8] The species *Garcinia* play a significant role in healthcare practices including diabetes, Alzheimer's disease (AD), and normal aging.[10] It contains 2.3% garcinol[11] and is a rich source of lactones, xanthones, benzophenones, phenolic acids, and flavonoids with a wide range of biological and pharmacological applications.[6]

G. pedunculata in Ayurveda

The dried fruit rind of *G. pedunculata* is used in Ayurveda (Amlavetasa),[2] and dried pericarps of the fruits are extensively used in the diet by tribes across the Northeast States of India.[5] As per Ayurveda, *G. pedunculata* fruit is an excellent cardiotonic, rejuvenator, and laxative. It is used to treat cough, asthma, obesity, and arthritis.[6] It has (-) hydroxycitric acid, benzophenones, garcinol, etc.[12] and screened for different activities such as anti-inflammatory, hepatoprotective, cardioprotective, and in vitro antioxidant activities.[13–15] Mundugaru et al. studied an aqueous extract of *G. pedunculata* fruits to treat acetic acid–induced ulcerative colitis in Swiss albino mice and confirmed the traditional healing applications. They reported that the fruit possesses potent antioxidant and anti-inflammatory properties to treat the acetic acid–induced colonic damage.[16]

G. pedunculata in Arunachal Pradesh, India

G. pedunculata is known as Mibia/Meba by the Nyishi tribe of Arunachal Pradesh and uses only the fruits and leaves of the species to treat indigestion, dysentery, fever, diarrhea, and jaundice of which dysentery and diarrhea are most common ailments for which *G. pedunculata is* utilized. Though the species is wildly growing, it has been domesticated and grown in the backyards of most of the villages for fruits as medicine and food. Most people use only the fruit parts, and a few use the leaves for curing various body ailments. Tender leaves are consumed raw and used as vegetables. Its fruits are edible and used as 'chutney'.[17]

G. pedunculata in Bangladesh

G. pedunculata is known as Taikor in Bangladesh. Islam et al. have reported the Taikor as a new potential natural source of nutrients, as it is rich in phenolic compounds and is a good source of antioxidants. The edible portion of the fruit was analyzed for vitamins (thiamine and riboflavin, ascorbic acid), proteins, total soluble solids, minerals, heavy metals, and moisture. The study concluded with remarks that Taikor is a rich source of fiber, natural antioxidants, and phenols, with a high number of ascorbic acids, so there is scope to develop value-added products or medicine from it for industrial adoptions. As a raw material, fruits have good stability for ascorbic acid content and their antioxidant capacity during cold storage, with little loss in these properties.[18]

In Vietnam, fruits of *G. pedunculata* are used to treat constipation and digestive problems.[19]

PHYTOCHEMICAL SCREENING

G. pedunculata is a potential source of unique health-promoting compounds. Gogoi et al. have conducted a study to examine the total phenols, ascorbic acid, carotenoids, and total antioxidant activity of the *Garcinia* species (*G. cowa, G. lanceifolia, G. pedunculata,* and *G. xanthochymus*) collected from Assam, India. Ascorbic acid content was reported highest in *G. pedunculata* (88.92 mg/100 g) and least in *G. xanthochymus* (35.37 mg/100 g).[20] Pedunxanthons A–C were obtained from the bark of the tree.[21]

The mature but not fully ripe fruit's dried rind of *G. pedunculata* has high medicinal value and is used in the diet of tribes of Assam and the North-Eastern region of India.[5] The mature but not fully ripened fruits have pedunculol, garcinol, and (-)-hydroxycitric acid.[22] Chloroform and hexane extracts of mature but not fully ripened fruits have free radical scavenging properties, antioxidant activity, and strong anti-mutagenicity, while hexane extract is more active than chloroform.[12] The chloroform and hexane extract of mature but not fully ripened fruits showed minimum inhibitory concentration on the growth of *Aspergillus flavus* at 3,000 and 4,000 ppm, respectively.[6] The mature but not fully ripe fruits are reported to have antibacterial,[23] hepatoprotectives,[14] antiinflammatories,[24] and cardioprotective activities.[15]

Islam et al. reported *G. pedunculata* fruits having total polyphenol 19.45±1.0 (mg GAE/100g), total flavonoids 18.33±1.12 (mg RE/g), and antioxidant activity 16.20±0.04 [ABTS (μM TE/g fruit)], and 1,813.88±12.62 [DPPH (μM TE/g fruit)].[18] Two xanthones [1,3,5,7- and 1,3,6,7-tetrahydroxyxanthone], two bioflavonoids [GB-1a and Talbotaflavone], and four benzophenones [pedunculol, cambogin, garcinol, and 2,4,6,30,50-penta-hydroxy-benzophenone] have been isolated from the species.[12,25] Hau et al. extracted three new xanthones, pedunxanthones A–C (1–3), together with five known compounds, namely, 1,5-dihydroxy-3-methoxy-4-(3-methylbut-2-enyl) xanthone, dulxanthone A, 1,5-dihydroxy-3-methoxy-60,60-dimethyl-2H-pyrano-(20,30:6,7)-4-(3-methylbut-2-nyl)xanthone, oleanolic acid, and garbogiol, from a petroleum ether extract of the bark of *G. pedunculata* collected from Vietnam.[21]

PHYTOPHARMACOLOGY OF FRUITS

G. pedunculata, a medicinal plant available particularly in West Bengal, Arunachal Pradesh, and Assam in India, has been utilized to cure several ailments such as cough, asthma, bronchitis, chronic catarrh, and fever, and is used as a cardiotonic in folk.[5] A few studies to establish the molecular mechanism were conducted by different researchers and are summarized below.

Hepatoprotective Activity

The liver, a vital organ of the body, supports almost every organ and is important for survival because of its multidimensional functions. Though it is prone to many diseases, the most common diseases are fatty liver, cancer, hepatitis, cirrhosis, alcohol damage, and drug-induced liver damage.[26] The liver has a unique property to regenerate and has a large reserve capacity. Mostly, the liver only produces toxic symptoms after its extensive damage. Paracetamol, when taken at recommended doses for a limited duration and under medical supervision, serves as an antipyretic and is effective in treating mild to moderate pain. However, an overdose can lead to severe hepatic damage.[4,27] Mundugaru et al. have reported the hepatic healing properties of the aqueous extract of fruits of *G. pedunculata* in paracetamol-induced liver toxicity in rats.[24,28]

Neuroprotective Activity

AD is a type of dementia accompanied by memory impairment and neuronal loss. Environmental neurotoxins like $AlCl_3$ interact with enzymes and biomarkers related to AD.[5] Occupational exposure to aluminum can be through food during processing and storage in aluminum vessels, foil, cans, medicines such as antacids, cosmetic agents, drinking water, vaccines, etc. The average dietary intake of aluminum ranges from 3 to 12 mg/day, and the population routinely exposed to the product may have higher chances of neurotoxicity.[6,12] Repeated exposure to aluminum has been experimentally documented to be able to cross the blood–brain barrier and implicate pathological changes in the brain, resulting in neurodegenerative disorders. The chronic exposure of $AlCl_3$ studied on rats has been reported for neurodegeneration in the forebrain, midbrain, hippocampus, and changes in the cerebellum in a few rats.[24]

Several herbal products such as quercetin, naringin, catechins, and curcumin have potential neuro-protective activities against $AlCl_3$-induced neurotoxicity.[29,30] The phytochemicals from the fruit rinds of *G. pedunculata* are major contributors to the antioxidant activity of the fruit.[31] In a study *G. pedunculata* fruits were collected from Assam (April 2015) authenticated, shade dried, and powdered. A total of 500 g powder was soaked in 2.0 L of cold distilled water for 24 h, filtered, and concentrated by evaporation in a water bath until free from water. Acute oral toxicity study of *G. pedunculata* fruit's aqueous extract has no mortality in doses up to 2,000 mg/kg, and it was revealed that LD_{50} is much more than 2,000 mg/kg. The 1/10th (200 mg/kg) and 1/5th (400 mg/kg) doses were selected by the research team for the neuroprotective study.[7]

Chronic administration of $AlCl_3$ in experimental animals has triggered lipid peroxidation, and Acetylcholinesterase (AChE) activity developed behavioral deficits and reduced levels of glutathione peroxidase, catalase, and histological aberrations. Co-administration of aqueous extract of *G. pedunculata* has attenuated the $AlCl_3$-induced alteration biological system. The study has concluded that the aqueous extract of fruits of *G. pedunculata* has significant neuroprotection against $AlCl_3$-induced neurotoxicity in mice.[24]

Nephroprotective Effect

Mundugaru et al. have studied the fruits of *G. pedunculata* for nephroprotective activity in cisplatin-induced nephrotoxicity animal models.[7] Cisplatin, a cytotoxic agent used in the treatment of cervical, head, neck, and testicular cancer, and used for chemotherapy in different solid tumors. It has a severe side-effect on normal tissues (such as the neuronal system, liver, and kidney) limiting its utilization.[32] The water extract of fruits of *G. pedunculata* is effective against cisplatin-induced nephrotoxicity and reveals that *G. pedunculata* is a potential source to prevent the nephrotoxicity induced by cisplatin.[33–35]

The comparative histopathological studies of kidneys from cisplatin control and treated models support the generalized cytoprotective effect of aqueous extract of the fruits of *G. pedunculata*. The results of the study can be used for developing new drugs for nephroprotection.[24]

TREATMENT OF Β-THALASSEMIA

Amlavetasa (Ayurvedic name of *G. pedunculata*)[2] is used as an excellent laxative, digestive, and cardiac stimulant in Ayurveda since 1500 BC. Its classical uses are in the treatment of bronchitis, asthma, heart diseases, cough, piles, constipation, abdominal pain due to digestion imbalance and bloating, anemia, anorexia, intestinal worms, splenomegaly, and indigestion, and for the treatment of epilepsy, toxic conditions, dysuria, ascites, malabsorption syndrome, etc. The plant is commonly found and harvested in the Northeast States of India like Manipur, Assam, and Shillong (Meghalaya).[36] Primary studies on the fruit of *G. pedunculata* reveal the potential to provide a better quality of life and to reduce complications related to blood transfusion on its use as per Ayurvedic procedure.

Thalassemia as per Ayurvedic parlance is a blood-related disease ('Beeja Dushti Janya Vikara').[2,37] The Ayurvedic books (Samhitas) indirectly decipher it as disease caused by the abnormal composition of blood ('Beeja Dosha Janya Sahaja Vyadhi').[38]As per modern molecular science, β-thalassemia is caused by point mutations or, more rarely, deletions in the beta-globin gene on chromosome 11, resulting in reduced (beta+) or absent (beta) synthesis of the beta chains of hemoglobin.[39] Hemoglobin E (Hb E) disease is an inherited blood disorder characterized by an abnormal form of hemoglobin. Patients with this condition may have very mild anemia, but the condition typically does not cause any symptoms. It is inherited in an autosomal recessive manner and is caused by a mutation in the HBB gene.[40] Most people with Hb E disease do not need any treatment.[41]

A case study by Ray et al.[2] has described a patient who has reported a major complaint of recurrent fever, jaundice, anemia, and generalized weakness, for the last few months. Further, she has revealed that she was a known case of Hb E-beta thalassemia by birth with repeated blood transfusions. The patient was given Amlavetasa fruit pulp in the dose of 10 g once daily to be taken in the early morning on an empty stomach for regular use for 8 months. The *G. pedunculata* fruits were soaked in water, and a paste was made from the wet pulp, which was used as the medicine. During the scheduled treatment, the patient was not advised to follow any specific diet-related instructions (Pathya–Apathya).

The treatment was based on the hypothesis that Amlavetasa (*G. pedunculata*) fruit has the potential of iron-chelating activity and can contribute to a reduction of S. ferritin (i.e., iron deficiency symptoms). After 6 months of uninterrupted treatment, patient's serum iron level decreased up to 168.71 μg/dL, but no relevant changes in hemoglobin and bilirubin parameters were noticed. Her body weight increased from 17 kg to 20.71 kg. After treatment, her spleen measured 2.5 cm, which was initially up to 4 cm in the abdomen initially. It was reported that there was reduction in the symptoms associated with *G. pedunculata*, such as weakness, fever, nausea, and whole-body ache.[2]

It was a successful treatment using *G. pedunculata* fruits without any adverse effects and concluded that *G. pedunculata* fruits have an iron-chelating agent. The fruit pulp is helpful to normalize iron metabolism, decrease iron overload in the body, prolong the red blood cells' life span, relieve signs and symptoms of the disease, and increase blood transfusion interval. The use of *G. pedunculata* fruits increases the expectancy and improves the quality of life of a thalassemic patient.[2]

SCOPE FOR BIOTECH INTERVENTION

G. pedunculata is used for various ailments such as jaundice, urinary troubles, fever, and stomach diseases. Traditional practitioners prescribe a precise *G. pedunculata* dose to the patients depending on the degree and duration of the ailment, based on age and health status. This therapeutic knowledge of *G. pedunculata* needs to be conserved for exploration in pharmaceutical industries after molecular studies as a clue for a mode of drug delivery. A cross-culture study on the ethnic utilization pattern of the species may be helpful in the exploration of ethnobotanical utilities among different communities of the region.

Propagation of the Species

Bhuyan et al. carried out studies on seeds of *G. pedunculata* collected from Dulung Forest Reserve, Assam, India, to find out the most effective treatments for germination. Different treatments were applied to coated and de-coated seeds of the species, and it was reported that Gibberellin (GA) 250 ppm was the most effective treatment in de-coated seeds with 100% seed germination with the highest seedling vigor index (21.23).[42]

Value-Added Products

Chemical information of plants (i.e., phenolic compounds, glycosides, alkaloids, amino acids, carbohydrates, saponin, fixed oils, fats, proteins, etc.) is important to utilize as a medicine. The curative properties of medicinal plants are due to the presence of various secondary metabolites such as alkaloids, flavonoids, glycosides, terpenoids, phenolics, and saponins. Plant materials contain alkaloids and flavonoids, which have potent antioxidant, anti-inflammatory, and pain-relieving properties. Phenolic compounds like tannins are potent inhibitors of many hydrolytic enzymes, and saponins act as an antibacterial chemical class used in hypercholesterolemia, hyperglycemia, antioxidant, anticancer, anti-inflammatory, and weight loss.[43–45] These different chemical classes are present in *G. pedunculata*, a significant indication for innovative scope for biotech interventions. The presence of these secondary metabolites in the methanolic extract of fruits of *G. pedunculata* has higher affirmative results than the leaves and barks.[43] The chemical composition of various parts of *G. pedunculata* indicates that fruits of *G. pedunculata* have higher medicinal values for curing various ailments.

- Though *G. pedunculata* fruits have higher HCA content and enormous health benefits, the fruits are underutilized due to their seasonal availability and short shelf life. It is necessary to prepare value-added products to processing techniques blending with traditional knowledge to reduce losses due to rot/damage of ripe fruits. *G. pedunculata* fruits can play a major role in the village economy as they are consumed as an added source of diet. Sometimes these are sold in local markets, and local village people dwelling in the forests could generate additional income also. It has higher dietary importance even cooked or raw. Usually, the ripe or raw fruits are sliced, sun-dried, preserved, and prepared for the sour fish curry. In Assam, there are several traditional uses of *G. pedunculata* fruit products. One of the most popular traditional preparations is 'tenga diya masor jol' (fish curries with *G. pedunculata* sun-dried fruit) prepared from sun-dried sliced fruits of *G. pedunculatat*.[43] These slices of *G. pedunculata* enhance the flavor of the fermenting bamboo shoots. The fermenting bamboo shoots are locally known as "Khorisa". Water extract from dry slices is used as a cooling drink taken in warm weather. It is reported as antiscorbutic, astringent, cardiotonic, and emollient. *G. pedunculata* has dietary importance and is widely utilized in the preparation of fish curries by the people of Assam. It has several medicinal properties and is used as an antiscorbutic and astringent. Due to its high HCA content, it is believed to be useful as a natural anti-obese agent. Despite such enormous health benefits, the fruits are underutilized due to their seasonal availability and very short shelf life. As the fruit is seasonal, maturing and ripening in the summer season, the value-added fruit products with superior nutritive and shelf stability may have a good seasonal market, which will help to develop the rural economy.

Because of the folklore utilities of the fruits of *G. pedunculata*, the rural population of Assam still cultivates the plant traditionally. Given its therapeutic properties, there is scope for more value-added products from seeds, fruits, tender leaves, and stems, so commercial cultivation with the conservation of the plant is equally important. Due to different social and environmental adversities, the plant population is under threat. So, it needs a specific strategy to increase the cultivation/plantation of valuable species on a priority basis.

REFERENCES

1. Biswas SC, Hazarika P, Dutta NB, Sarmah H. 2017. Few novel value added products prepared from fruits of *Garcinia pedunculata* Roxb. ex Buch.-Ham. *Research Journal of Chemical* Sciences. 7 (3): 23–29.
2. Ray C, Mitra A, Ravte RK, Hazra J. 2018. Role of Amlavetasa (*Garcinia pedunculata* Roxb. ex Buch.-Ham.), an Ayurvedic drug in E-ß Thalassaemia: a case study. *Indian Journal of Traditional Knowledge*. 17 (3): 598–601.
3. Baruah S, Borthakur SK. 2012. Studies on morphology and ethnobotany of six species of *Garcinia*L. (Clusiaceae) found in the Brahmaputra Valley, Assam, India. *Journal of Natural Product and Plant Resources*. 2 (3): 389–396.
4. Patiri B, Borah A. 2007. Wild edible plants of Assam. In: *Studies in Medical Anthropology*, 1st Edition. Sengupta S (Ed.) N L Publications, Dibrugarh, Assam. pp. 258–264.
5. Kagyung R, Gajurel PR, Rethy P, Singh B. 2010. Ethnomedicinal plants used for gastrointestinal diseases by Adi tribes of Dehang-Debang Biosphere Reserve in Arunachal Pradesh. *Indian Journal of Traditional Knowledge*. 9: 496–501.
6. Jayaprakasha GK, Negi PS, Jena BS. 2006. Antioxidative and antimutagenic activities of the extracts from the rinds of *Garcinia pedunculata*. *Innovative Food Science & Emerging* Technologies. 7 (3): 246–250.
7. Mundugaru R, Sivanesan SK, Udaykumar P, Joy F, Narayana SKK, Rajakrishnan L, AlFarhan AH, Jacob T, Rajagopal R, Hisham SM. 2017. Quality standardization and nephroprotective effect of *Garcinia pedunculata* Roxb. fruit rind. *Indian Journal of Pharmaceutical Education and Research*. 51 (4): 713–721.
8. Sarma R, Devi R. 2015. Ethnopharmacological survey of *Garcinia pedunculata* Roxb. fruit in six different districts of Assam, India. *International Journal of Pharmaceutical Science Invention*. 4 (1): 20–28.
9. Anonymous. 2019. The Office of Registrar General and Census Commissioner of India. https://en.wikipedia.org/wiki/List_of_districts_of_Assam#cite_ref-4, as on 24th April 2021.
10. Yamaguchi F, Ariga T, Yoshimura Y, Nakazawa H. 2000. Antioxidative and anti-glycation activity of garcinol from *Garcinia indica* fruit rind. *Journal of Agricultural and Food Chemistry*. 48: 180–185.
11. Krishnamurthy N, Lewis YS, Ravindranath B. 1981.On the structures of garcinol, isogarcinol and camboginol. *Tetrahedron Letters*. 22: 793–796.
12. Sahu A, Das B, Chatterjee A. 1989. Polyisoprenylated benzophenones from Garcinia pedunculata. *Phytochemistry*. 28: 1233–1235.
13. Ravi M, Febin J, Shrinidhi R, Lipika D, Sudhakara B, Ravishankar B. 2014. Anti-inflammatory activity of aqueous extract of fruits of *Garcinia pedunculata* in experimental animals. *American Journal of PharmTech Research*. 4: 3–6.
14. Ravi M, Madhan C, Ravishankar B. 2014. Hepatoprotective activity of fruits extract of *Garcinia pedunculata*. *Bangladesh Journal of Pharmacology*. 9: 4–8.
15. Ravi M, Senthilkumar S, Padmaja UK, Sudhakara B. 2016. Cardio protective activity of fruits extract of *Garcinia pedunculata*. *Bangladesh Journal of Pharmacology*. 11: 5–9.
16. Mundugaru R, Udaykumar P, Kumar KNS, Nayak S, Jacob T, Ah A, Rajakrishnan R. 2019. Protective effect of *Garcinia penduncculata* fruit rind in acetic acid induced ulcerative colitis. Farmacia. 67: 160–166.

17. Srivastava RC, *Nyishi* Community. 2010. Traditional knowledge of *Nyishi* (Daffla) tribe of Arunachal Pradesh. *Indian Journal of Traditional Knowledge*. 9 (1): 26–37.
18. Islam MZ, Hoque MM, Asif-UI-Alam SM, Monalisha K. 2015. Chemical composition, Antioxidant capacities and storage stability of *Citrus macroptera* and *Garcinia pedunculata* fruits. *Emirates Journal of Food and Agriculture*. 27 (3): 275–282.
19. Pham HH, 2006. *Vietnamese Medicinal Plants*. Youth Publishing House, Ho Chi Minh City. pp. 91.
20. Gogoi B, Das R P, Barua U. 2016. Antioxidant activity of *Garcinia* species of Assam. *International Journal of Agriculture Science*. 8 (29): 1611–1612.
21. Hau V, Nguyen NT, Mass G, Werz U, Pham HD, Nguyen LH. 2012. Xanthones from the bark of Garcinia pedunculata. *Phytochemistry Letters*. 5 (4): 766–769.
22. Jayaprakasha GK, Jena BS, Sakariah KK. 2003. Improved liquid chromatographic method for determination of organic acids in leaves, pulp, fruits, and rinds of *Garcinia*. *Journal of AOAC International*. 86 (5): 1063–1068.
23. Negi PS, Jayaprakasha GK, Jena BS. 2008. Antibacterial activity of the extracts from the fruit rinds of *Garcinia cowa* and *Garcinia pedunculata* against food borne pathogens and spoilage bacteria. *LWT-Food Science and Technology*. 41 (10): 1857–1861.
24. Mundugaru R, Joy F, Shrinidhi R, Das L, Sudhakara RB. 2014. Anti-inflammatory activity of aqueous extract of fruits of *Garcinia pedunculata* in experimental animals. *American Journal of PharmTech Research*. 4 (3): 278–283.
25. Rao AVR, Sarma MR, Venkataraman K, Yemul SS.1974. A benzophenone and xanthone with unusual hydroxylation patterns from the heartwood of Garcinia pedunculata. *Phytochemistry*. 13: 1241–1244.
26. Graham GG, Davies MJ, Day RO, Mohamudally A, Scott KF. 2013. The modern pharmacology of paracetamol: therapeutic actions, mechanism of action, metabolism, toxicity and recent pharmacological findings. Inflammopharmacology. 21: 201–232.
27. Larson AM, Polson J, Fontana RJ. 2005. Acetaminophen-induced acute liver failure: results of a United States multicenter, prospective study. *Hepatology*. 42: 1364–1372.
28. Bradly DW, Maynard JE, Emery G, Webster H. 1972. Transaminase activities in serum of long-term hemodialysis patients. *Clinical Chemistry*. 18: 1442.
29. Bancroft JD, Gamble M. 2002. *Theory and Practice of Histological Techniques*, 5th Edition. Churchill Livingstone, Edinburgh.
30. Sinha AK. 1972. Colorimetric assay of catalase. *Analytical Biochemistry*. 47 (2): 389–394.
31. Rotruck JT, Pope AL, Ganther HE, Swanson AB, Hafeman DG, Hoekstra W. 1973. Selenium: biochemical role as a component of glutathione peroxidase. *Science*. 179 (4073): 588–590.
32. Kuhad A, Tirkey N, Pilkhwal S, Chopra K. 2006. Renoprotective effect of *Spirulina fusiformis* on cisplatin-induced oxidative stress and renal dysfunction in rats. *Renal Failure*. 28 (3): 247–254.
33. Ramesh G, Reeves WB. 2003. TNFR2-mediated apoptosis and necrosis in cisplatin-induced acute renal failure. *American Journal of Physiology-Renal Physiology*. 285 (4): F610–618.
34. Ramesh G, Reeves WB. 2004. Inflammatory cytokines in acute renal failure. *Kidney International*. 66: S56–61.
35. Tsuruya K, Ninomiya T, Tokumoto M, Hirakawa M, Masutani K, Taniguchi M, Fukuda K, Kanai H, Kishihara K, Hirakata H, Iida M. 2003.Direct involvement of the receptor-mediated apoptotic pathways in cisplatin-induced renal tubular cell death. *Kidney International*. 63 (1):72–82.
36. Sharma PV. 2012. *Dravyaguna-Vijnana*. Chaukhamba Bharati Academy, Varanasi. Vol II. pp. 338.
37. Panigrahi HK, Kushawa H, Sharma SS. 1997. Treatment of sickle cell disorders by ayurvedic medicine. *Ancient Science of Life*. 17 (1): 15–22.
38. Gameti R, Kori VK, Patel KS, Rajagopala S. 2017. Ayurvedic management of Thalassemia Major (*Beeja Dushtijanya Pandu*): as an adjuvant therapy. *International Ayurvedic Medical Journal*. 5 (3): 998–1004.
39. Hazza AM, Al-Jamal G. 2006. Dental development in subjects with Thalassemia Major. Journal of Contemporary Dental Practice. 4 (7): 063–070.
40. Bachir D, Galacteros F. 2004. Haemoglobin E. Orphanet Encyclopedia. November.
41. Evan N, Braunstein M. 2017. Haemoglobin E Disease. Merck Manual. January.
42. Bhuyan L, Sharma CL, Singh B, Sharma M, Bharali P. 2017. Regeneration of two medicinally important *Garcinia* species of Assam, NE India. *International Journal of Recent Scientific Research*. 8 (8): 19372–19377.
43. Gogoi G, Das AK. 2016. Ethnomedicobotany and phytochemical screening of *Garcinia pedunculata* Roxb. ex Buch.–Ham from Arunachal Pradesh, India. *Journal of Bioresources*. 3 (1): 16–23.
44. Mandal P, Sinha Babu SP, Mandal NC. 2005. Antimicrobial activity of saponins from *Acacia auriculiformis*. *Fitoterapia*. 76 (5): 462–465.
45. Manjunatha BK. 2006. Antibacterial activity of *Pterocarpus santalinus*. *Indian Journal of Pharmaceutical Sciences*. 68 (1): 115–116.

15 *Juglans regia* (Walnut/Akhrot)

INTRODUCTION

Juglans regia Linn. (family: Juglandaceae) occurs natively and is cultivated commercially in Asia, Europe, and the southeastern parts of the United States for the quality timber and edible kernels.[1,2] Wild trees of *J. regia* (Eng.: walnut) have been reported in the temperate and semi-arid mountain areas of Central and Southeast Asia, the Middle East, and the Caucasus region.[3–5] The walnut tree species is native to the western Himalayas[6] and was cultivated in Europe as early as 1000 BC. Currently, walnuts are cultivated commercially in northern Africa, eastern Asia, southern Europe, the USA, and western South America. China is the leading world producer, followed by the USA, Iran, Turkey, Ukraine, Romania, France, and India, but its production in Argentina and Chile has been increasing rapidly.[7]

According to the International Union for Conservation of Nature, it is a red list of threatened species and is globally assessed as a 'least concerned' species.[8] The plant is a light-demanding species and has strong positive phototropism at every stage of life.[9] Propagation of walnut is more difficult compared to other fruit species.[10] Forests with wild walnut plants are characterized by an extraordinary physiological and morphological diversity[11] and are home to numerous wild relatives of cultivated species.[12] The natural walnut forests suffer from forest degradation and deforestation, a major threat to the species.[13]

J. regia L. is commonly known as 'Akhrot' in India,[14] and most of the walnut products are from trees of seedling origin grown in a semi-wild state (Figures 15.1 and 15.2). There are genetically diverse seedling trees of walnuts in India, and the major production of walnuts is from farmers' backyards and wild habitats.[14] In Himachal Pradesh and the Uttarakhand hills of India, trees are growing naturally in wild habitats on rocky soils along streams, with some scattered populations in farmers' backyards and on hillocks. Nuts are collected by hill people during winter for self-consumption and sold in nearby markets. The chemical profile of walnuts, compared to the other common nuts, such as almonds, peanuts, and hazelnuts, contains the highest spectrum of antioxidants and fiber.[15] The walnut fruit consists of the innermost edible kernel, the kernel's skin, a surrounding hard shell, and the outermost green husk. The nut is collected for its edible kernel, and a high amount of the husk is discarded. Recently, walnut green husk has been identified as a source of different natural bioactive compounds with potent antimicrobial and antioxidant properties.[16]

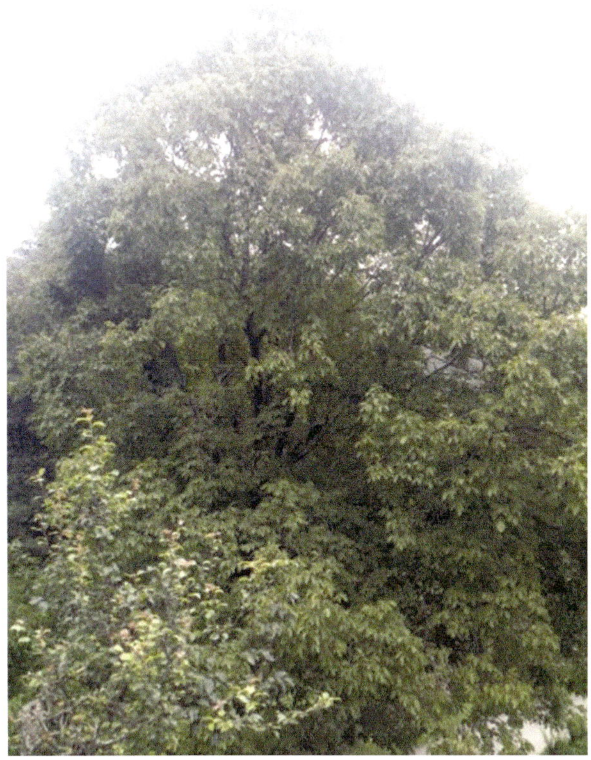

FIGURE 15.1 *J.regia* tree.

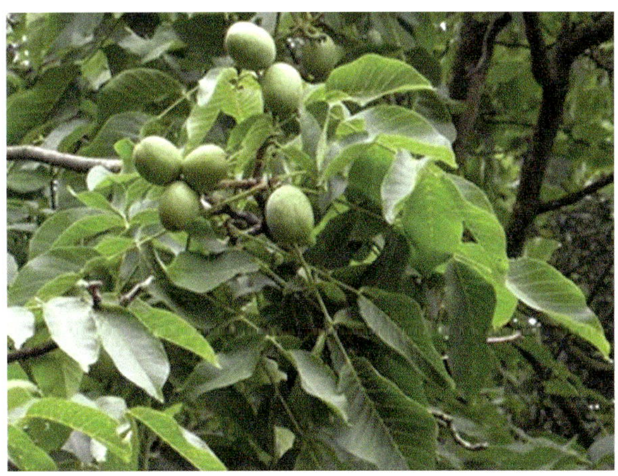

FIGURE 15.2 *J. regia* fruit-bearing branch.

ETHNOPHARMACOLOGY

The walnut tree has socio-economic importance globally. Though it is cultivated in the temperate zones of the world, the trade covers the whole world because of its quality timber and edible seeds. The seed oil is rich in tocopherols, phytosterols, and unsaturated fatty acids.[17–20] Walnuts are

DOI: 10.1201/9781003512868-17

consumed traditionally to cure many health ailments, and many more traditional uses have been proved in pharmacological investigations also.[21,22] Walnuts have been listed in the FAO list of priority plants and described as a strategic plan for human nutrition.[10] Nearly all the parts of walnuts – like green husk, bark, flowers, leaves, kernels, oil, and septum – have folk medicinal applications.[23]

The walnut plant has economic, nutritional, and medicinal value.[24] The trade of walnut fruits is the backbone of the economy of the region of its cultivation and is directly connected to the economic prosperity of the people living in remote areas. Hassan et al. (2013) have reported that walnuts from Kashmir, India, are exported to more than 49 countries, and their annual production is 3,73,474 M tones. The annual earnings of revenue have been reported as more than 543 crores.[25] It has been reported that walnut in Jammu and Kashmir, India, is used to treat 17 different types of diseases, and their leaves are used as a mosquito repellent, additionally. Further, it is narrated that some plant parts are used to treat more than one disease; likewise, more than one plant part is used to treat a particular disease. Fruits have been reported to treat nine different diseases, followed by leaves.[25]

Walnuts are widely used in traditional medicines around the globe. Its kernels have been documented for anti-atherogenic, lipid-lowering, anti-inflammatory, anti-mutagenic, and antioxidant properties.[21] Walnuts do not affect antioxidant status in the fasted state after chronic feeding but increase antioxidant capacity postprandially, and their inclusion in the diet improves endothelial function.[26] Leaves of walnut trees are used as antiseptic, chemo-preventive, antibacterial, depurative, and anthelmintic, for the treatment of skin inflammation and for astringent purposes.[27] Walnut kernels are supposed to nourish brain cells and are used to improve human memory. In Nepal, the bark paste of walnuts is used to treat skin diseases, toothache, and arthritis and to promote hair growth. The seed coat of the plant is used for wound healing,[28] and bark is utilized to treat cancer.[29] Walnuts are used to cure toothaches in the Himalayan regions.[30] In India, fruit shells and bark have been described for cleaning teeth and treating cuts, pyorrhea, and wounds.[31] In Nepal, bark is used as an anthelminthic and treatment for tuberculosis.[32] In Ladakh, Kashmir, and Jammu, it is used as an anthelmintic, to treat gum problems, constipation, liver ailments, skin diseases, toothache, sore throat, alopecia, joint pain, frostbite, anemia, and skin eruptions.[33]

The roots of the plant are used as a demulcent and an anti-diarrheal.[34] Fruits and barks are used as an antiseptic, tonic, and for dental health.[35] Dried fruit is mixed with honey and coconut, and the mixture is used as a tonic. The decoction of leaves is used against intestinal worms and eczema.[36,37] The whole plant is known to be useful to treat weakness in the legs, constipation, and cough.[38] In Iran, the bark tincture is used to cure hemorrhoids, the decoction of fruits is used to treat high arterial pressure and cardiac diseases, and it is used as a mouthwash for gingivitis. The fruit bark juice is used for external ulcers, eczema, and itchy dermatosis. Batsatsashvili et al. reported that the leaf infusion is orally used to cure skin diseases and treat gastrointestinal problems, diabetes, tuberculosis, and venereal diseases.[39] In Gilgit-Baltistan, walnut fruits are used as a brain tonic and for cardiac problems.[40]

In Turkish folk medicine, the juice of fresh leaves of walnut is applied on the naked skin to reduce fever and headache, and even on the swelled joints to alleviate rheumatic pain.[41,42] The kernel is used to treat inflammatory bowel disease in Iranian traditional medicine.[43] In Palestinian folklore, walnut is used to treat diabetes and asthma[44,45] and to cure prostate and vascular disturbance.[46] The plant is used as a topical remedy for dermal inflammation and excessive perspiration of the hands and feet. Leaves of walnuts are used topically to treat scalp itching and dandruff, sunburn, superficial burns, and skin disorders.[47] Walnut has high anti-atherogenic potential and remarkable osteoblastic activity, so it is recommended in the diet for cardio-protection and prevention of bone loss.[48] The bark, branches, and exocarp of the immature green fruit of the walnut plant have been used to treat gastric, liver, and lung cancer in Chinese folklore.[49] It is used by traditional healers in the northeastern region of Mexico to protect the liver from damage.[50] The shells of walnut fruits are used in Calabrian folk medicine to heal malaria.[51]

PHYTOPHARMACOLOGY

The kernel of walnut is a rich source of phenolics, which have high antioxidant activity.[16] Kernels are eaten raw or used in ice cream, cakes, confections, and other items. The walnut husk, a residue after walnut farming and processing, is also a source of phenolics.[52] The kernel of the fruit is covered by a thin, light brown layer, known as the skin. Walnut skin contains high amounts of antioxidant compounds,[53,54] which protect the kernel against the deleterious effects of extreme UV radiation, including bacterial, viral, and fungal infection/contamination.[55] Kernels contain amino acids (aspartic acid, glutamic acid, valine, threonine, serine, proline, glycine, methionine, leucine, tyrosine, phenylalanine, lysine, and arginine),[56] phenolic compounds (phenolic acids and tannins), vitamins (A, B, and C), and stepophyllarin.[57] Kernels are rich in linoleic acid (58%) and linolenic acid (12%); both these essential fatty acids are required for a sustainable, healthy body. It has about 14.5%–24% of protein and rises to 61%–66% in the dry, defatted cake. The protein is of good quality and is therefore easy to digest.[58]

Antimicrobial Activities

Walnut husk has naphthoquinones and derivatives. Maleita et al. have studied the effects of pure naphthoquinones, including juglone, plumbagin, and 1,4-naphthoquinone, on the root-knot nematode and reported that 1,4-naphthoquinone is the most active compound.[52] Additionally, it was reported that the dried husk extract has repellent properties and reduces the penetration of the nematode into the root, but it did not affect reproduction. Maleita et al. have recommended using walnut husk as a bio-nematicide against *Meloidogyne* spp.[52]

Anti-Platelet Activities

Plant-derived polyphenolic compounds have protective effects on human health, particularly affecting platelet function during hemostasis. The green husk of walnut fruits has anti-platelet activity and antioxidant properties due to polyphenolic compounds. Meshkini and Tahmasbi have suggested using the walnut husk for thrombotic disorder treatment.[59]

Cytotoxic Activities

Juglanones A and B, isolated from *J. regia* and investigated with seven different human cancer cell lines (BEL-7402, A549, HeLa, MCF-7, COLO205, SKOV3, and BGC-823) for cytotoxic effects, have been reported for IC_{50} values in the range of 0.26–1.67 μM.[60]

SCOPE AND OPPORTUNITIES FOR BIOTECH INTERVENTIONS

Currently, plant-based materials have gained more attention and interest for new drug discovery,[61–63] due to the richness of valuable compounds that have fewer side effects, if any.[64–66] Walnuts are mainly cultivated for kernels, but other parts of the fruit such as the shell and husk, are by-products during fruit harvesting and processing.[7,55] It has been well documented that these by-products can be employed in different industries as low-cost materials.[16]

Dilute acid hydrolysis of walnut husk produces glucose, revealing that walnut husk is a source of sugar.[60] The study has concluded that walnut green husk could be a source of raw material for producing bioethanol.[67]

Walnut fruit by-products: The hard shell and green husk of the walnut fruit are the by-products that are generated in walnut harvesting. The walnut's hard shell and husk are traditionally used to generate heat.[68] The green husk of the walnut fruit is a traditional therapeutic herb.[68,69] The walnut shell has lignin (50.3%), ash (3.4%), cellulose (23.9%), and hemicellulose (22.4%). The lesser quantities of hygroscopic components and higher quantities of hydrophobic components in walnut shells are significant for their application in outdoor products, which makes them suitable for high environmental resistance in flooring and fencing.[67,70–73]

The thick outer green layer of the walnut fruit, the husk, is an abundant by-product of fruit harvesting.[55] It is a valuable source of phenolic compounds and antioxidants. It is used in the traditional treatment of skin ailments and reduction of pain.[74] The walnut husk is used as a natural dyeing source, such as juglone (5-hydroxy-1,4-naphthoquinone),[75] a brown pigment of walnut trees from different parts, such as the bark, leaf, root, and husk.[76] The green husk has scarce utilization in agriculture, and its application as a source of natural manure, rich in antimicrobials and antioxidants, can be useful in agriculture-related areas.[75,77]

The extracts of walnut husk have high antioxidant activity and are rich in total flavonoid content, total phenolic content, and total condensed tannin content, resulting in a higher bioactive potential item.[78]

The available research reports on different applications of walnut husk in the pharmaceutical, food, and cosmetic industries. The trapping and removal of hazardous materials, including synthetic heavy metal ions and dyes from industrial effluents, is the main use of walnut husk finally divided into powder form. Proper characterization and specification for walnut husk is a need of the hour to use in medicine and food items. It can be used in green medicine as an excellent antioxidant, antimicrobial, antifungal, and anticancer ingredient.[75,77,78]

Recently, the husk of the walnut fruit has been used to remove hazardous materials generated because of industrial activities such as BR 46 dye from an aqueous solution.[79,80] The environmental toxicity of heavy metals and the threat to life are matters of current concern.[81,82] Wang et al. have reported the removal of Cr^{4+} ions from water by the walnut husk. Wang et al. have reported a maximum removal (97.3%) at pH = 1.[83] Walnut husk is an affordable and effective low-cost water treatment material.[84] The adsorption of Cd^{2+} ions by walnut green husk from polluted water has been reported as pH-dependent, and it is maximum at pH = 7.[85]

Walnut green husk is a cost-effective, health-friendly, valuable, and safe ingredient for antimicrobial and cosmetic dyeing applications. Its uses as a natural hair color agent, fastness of induced color, antimicrobial behavior of coloring material, coloring properties, and skin irritation tests have been reported as safe. Its combination with $FeSO_4$ (as a mordant), ascorbic acid (as a developer), and *Aloe vera* extract (as a secondary mordant) develops dark brown-colored hair, which has good daylight fastness, excellent appearance for a hair surface, and adequate color strength. Natural mordants such as lactic acid, oxalic acid, etc., are used to avoid any side effects.[75]

Studies have revealed the use of green walnut husk extract at 100 mg/kg concentration could well slow the oxidation process, and it is comparable with tert-butyl hydroquinone at 200 mg/kg. Results from the study reveal that green walnut husk has high antioxidant value, and its low price could be a source to replace synthetic antioxidants.[86]

The walnut green husk is used as a functional additive in the meat processing industry to reduce weight loss in cooked sausages during storage and to maintain the color during the storage of meat. Furthermore, the addition of green husk of the walnut extract is used to improve sensory acceptance and check the growth of microorganisms during the storage of cooked sausages.[87]

The immature walnut fruits, just before the hardening of the endocarp, are picked, sliced, and left to steep in food-grade ethanol alcohol for a delicious beverage, the walnut liqueur. 'Nocino', an Italian name for a walnut drink, is prepared by a similar method as the aforementioned young green walnut fruits.[88] In folk medicine, the traditional drink from fresh green walnut fruits has extensive applications as it is rich in phenolic compounds and vitamins.[89] The fresh green walnut fruits are used to prepare jam.[78,90] Walnut liqueur, a dark brown, bitter, and tasty drink, is used as an aperitif and to treat stomachaches. The unique astringency and bitterness of the beverage are due to the phenolics.[91] The traditional walnut liqueur is considered a cocktail of phenolics.[89] Its quality depends on the selection of cultivar and phenolic content in the fruits at the time of picking for liqueur preparation,[91] but the concentration of individual phenolics in liqueur may be relatively low compared to the green husk.[89] A higher quantity of ethanol in walnut liqueur increases the content of total phenolics and certain individual phenolic compounds (e.g., 1,4-naphthoquinone, p-coumaric acids, sinapic, and protocatechuic).[92] Phenolic compounds (syringic acid, chlorogenic acid, vanillic acid, caffeic acid, protocatechuic acid, ferulic acid, sinapic acid, epicatechin, gallic acid, ellagic acid, catechin, myricetin, juglone, and 1,4-naphthoquinone) have been identified as a marker in the walnut liqueur.[89] The antioxidant activity and antioxidant potential of walnut liqueur did not change even after many years of storage; however, the temperature and duration of soaking of fruits in ethanol are significant for the phenolic composition and efficacy of the liqueur.[88]

The young green walnuts, which fall due to hell storms, may be used as per traditional practices for making a walnut liqueur. The chemical composition of walnut husk deciphers the presence of naphthoquinones, α-tetralones, and triterpenoids. These compounds have potent anticancer properties. These ingredients alone could be studied as novel drugs after purification and characterization for developing new anticancer agents.

Ethno-botanical knowledge is a very important clue as it deciphers the practices and problems solved by the indigenous communities through their long experience and provides valuable baseline information for the commercial exploitation of natural resources. The folklore clue could be useful for physicians, pharmacologists, phytochemists, botanists, and others alike interested in the development of herbal therapies as a safe and more reliable option.

REFERENCES

1. McGranahan G, Leslie C. 1991. Walnuts (*Juglans*). In *Genetic Resources of Temperate Fruit and Nut Crops*. International Society for Horticultural Science, Moore JN, Ballington Jr. JR (Eds.) Leuven, Belgium. pp. 907–974.
2. Bernard A, Lheureux F, Dirlewanger E. 2018. Walnut: past and future of genetic improvement. *Tree Genetics & Genomes*. 14: 1–28. https://doi.org/10.1007/s11295-017-1214-0
3. Malhotra SP. 2008. *World Edible Nuts Economy*. Concept, New Delhi.
4. Shah UN, Mir JI, Ahmed N, Zaid A, Jan S, Fazili KM, Wani SH. 2017. Bio-techniques for improvement of qualitative and quantitative traits in walnut (*Juglans regia*). *Advances in Horticultural Science*. 32: 113–135. https://doi.org/10.13128/AHS-21330
5. Molnar TJ, Zaurov DE, Capik JM, Eisenman SW, Ford T, Nikolyi LV, Funk R. 2011. Persian walnuts (*Juglans regia* L.) in Central Asia. *Annual Report of the Northern Nutrition Growers Association*:56–69.
6. Fernandez-Lopez J, Aleta N, Alıas R. 2000. *Forest Genetic Resources Conservation of Juglans regia* L. IPGRI Publishers, Rome.
7. Martinez ML, Labuckas DO, Lamarque AL, Maestri DM .2010. Walnut (*Juglans regia* L.): genetic resources, chemistry, by-products. *Journal of the Science of Food and Agriculture*. 90: 1959–1967.
8. Rivers MC, Allen DJ. 2017. *Juglans regia*. The IUCN Red List of Threatened Species: e.T63495A 61526700. 2017. https://doi.org/10.2305/IUCN.UK.2017-3.RLTS.T63495A61526700.en
9. Mohni C, Pelleri F, Hemery GE. 2009. The modern silviculture of *Juglans regia* L.: a literature review. *Die. Bodenkultur*. 60: 19–32.
10. Gandev S. 2007. Budding and grafting of the walnut (*Juglans regia* L.) and their effectiveness in Bulgaria. *Bulgarian Journal of Agricultural Science*. 13: 683–689.
11. Feng X, Zhou H, Zulfiqar S, Luo X, Hu Y, Feng L, Malvolti ME, Woeste K, Zhao P. 2018. The phytogeographic history of common walnut in China. *Frontiers in Plant Science*. 9: 1399. https://doi.org/10.3389/fpls.2018.01399
12. Fisher B, Christopher T. 2007. Poverty and biodiversity: measuring the overlap of human poverty and the biodiversity hotspots. Ecological Economy. 62(1): 93–101.
13. Wilson B, Mills M, Kulikov M, Clubbe C. 2019. The future of walnut-fruit forests in Kyrgyzstan and the status of the iconic endangered apple Malus niedzwetzkayana. *Oryx*. 53(3): 415–423. https://doi.org/10.1017/S0030605318001230
14. Luo X, Zhou H, Cao D, Yan F, Chen P, Wang J, et al. 2022. Domestication and selection footprints in Persian walnuts (Juglans regia). PLoS Genet 18(12): e1010513. https://doi.org/10.1371/journal.pgen.1010513.
15. Pandey G, Shukla SK. 2007. The walnut industry in India-Current status and prospects. *International Journal of Fruit Science*. 6 (4): 67–75. https://doi.org/10.1300/J492v06n04_07
16. Jahanban-Esfahlan A, Ostadrahimi I A, Tabibiazar M, Amarowicz R. 2019. A comprehensive review on the chemical constituents and functional uses of walnut (*Juglans* spp.) Husk. *International Journal of Molecular Sciences*. 20: 3920. https://doi.org/10.3390/ijms20163920
17. Amaral JS, Casal S, Pereira JA, Seabra RM, Oliveira BP. 2003. Determination of sterol and fatty acid compositions, oxidative stability, and nutritional value of six walnut (*Juglans regia* L.) cultivars grown in Portugal. *Journal of Agricultural and Food Chemistry*. 51: 7698–7702.
18. Amaral JS, Seabra RM, Andrade PB, Valentao P, Pereira JA, Ferreres F. 2004. Phenolic profile in the quality control of walnut (*Juglans regia* L.) leaves. *Food Chemistry*. 88:373–379.
19. Amaral JS, Alves MR, Seabra RM, Oliveira BP. 2005. Vitamin E composition of walnuts (*Juglans regia* L.): a 3-year comparative study of different cultivars. *Journal of Agricultural and Food Chemistry*. 53: 5467–5472.
20. Amaral JS, Valentão P, Andrade PB, Martins RC, Seabra RM. 2008. Do cultivar, geographical location and crop season influence phenolic profile of walnut leaves? *Molecules*. 13: 1321–1332.

21. Anderson KJ, Teuber SS, Gobeille A, Cremin P, Waterhouse AL, Steinberg FM. 2001. Walnut polyphenolics inhibit in vitro human plasma and LDL oxidation. *Journal of Nutrition*. 131: 2837–2842.
22. Fukuda T, Ito H, Yoshida T. 2004. Effect of the walnut polyphenol fraction on oxidative stress in type 2 diabetes mice. *Biofactors*. 21:251–253.
23. Gupta A, Behl T, Panichayupakaranan P. 2019. A review of phytochemistry and pharmacology profile of *Juglans regia*. *Obesity Medicine*. 16: 100142. https://doi.org/10.1016/j.obmed.2019.100142
24. Khan SA, Bhatia S, Tripathi N. 2013. Entomological Studies of *Chaetoproctaodata*, An Important Pest on Walnut Trees (*Juglans regia* L.) in Kashmir Valley. *Journal of Academia and Industrial Research*. 2 (6): 378–381.
25. Hassan GA, Bilal T, Ahmad BT, Sameena W, Irshad N. 2013. Economic and ethno-medicinal uses of *Juglans regia* L. in Kashmir Himalaya. *UJAHM*. 1 (3): 64–67.
26. Stonehouse W. 2011. The effects of walnuts (*Juglans regia*) on the characteristics of the metabolic syndrome. In: *Nuts and Seeds in Health and Disease Prevention*. Elsevier, Amsterdam. pp. 1141–1148.
27. Eidi A, Moghadam JZ, Mortazavi P, Rezazadeh S, Olamafar S. 2013. Hepatoprotective effects of *Juglans regia* extract against CCl_4-induced oxidative damage in rats. *Pharmaceutical Biology*. 51: 558–565.
28. Kunwar RM, Adhikari N. 2005. Ethnomedicine of Dolpa district, Nepal: the plants, their vernacular names and uses. *Lyonia*. 8: 43–49.
29. Palit D, Banerjee A. 2016. Traditional uses and conservative lifestyle of Lepcha tribe through sustainable bioresource utilization – case studies from Darjeeling and North Sikkim, India. *International Journal of Conservaton Science*. 7(3): 735–752.
30. Bhat J, Malik ZA, Ballabha R, Bussmann RW, Bhatt AB. 2015. Ethnomedicinal plants traditionally used in health care practices by inhabitants of Western Himalaya. *Journal of* Ethnopharmacology. 172: 133–144.
31. Singh A, Nautiyal MC, Kunwar RM, Bussmann RW. 2017. Ethnomedicinal plants used by local inhabitants of Jakholi block, Rudraprayag district, Western Himalaya, India. *Journal of Ethnobiology and* Ethnomedicine. 13: 49. https://doi.org/10.1186/s13002-017-0178-3
32. Kunwar RM, Nepal BK, Kshetri HB, Rai SK, Bussmann RW. 2006. Ethnomedicine in Himalaya: a case study from Dolpa, Humla, Jumla and mustang districts of Nepal. *Journal of Ethnobiology and* Ethnomedicine. 2 (1): 27. https://doi.org/10.1186/1746-4269-2-27
33. Gairola S, Sharma J, Singh Bedi Y. 2014. A cross-cultural analysis of Jammu, Kashmir and Ladakh (India) medicinal plant use. *Journal of Ethnopharmacology*. 155: 925–986.
34. Shah GM, Khan MA. 2006. Checklist of medicinal plants of Siran Valley, Mansehra, Pakistan. *Ethnobotanical Leaflets*. 10: 63–71.
35. Yousufzai SA, Khan N, Wahab M, Ajaib M. 2010. Ethnomedicinal study of Marghazar Valley, Pakistan. *International Journal of Biology and Biotechnology*. 7: 409–416.
36. Akhtar N, Rashid A, Murad W, Bergmeier E. 2013. Diversity and use of ethno-medicinal plants in the region of swat, North Pakistan. *Journal of Ethnobiology and* Ethnomedicine. 9 (1): 25. https://doi.org/10.1186/1746-4269-9-25
37. Ahmad KS, Habib S. 2014. Indigenous knowledge of some medicinal plants of Himalaya region, Dawarian village, Neelum valley, Azad Jammu and Kashmir, Pakistan. *Universal Journal of Plant Science*. 2(2): 40–67.
38. Abbasi AM, Khan MA, Khan N, Shah MH. 2013. Ethnobotanical survey of medicinally important wild edible fruits species used by tribal communities of lesser Himalayas-Pakistan. *Journal of Ethnopharmacology*. 148 (2): 528–536.
39. Batsatsashvili K, Mehdiyeva N, Fayvush G, Kikvidze Z, Khutsishvili M, Maisaia I, Sikharulidze S, Tchelidze D, Alizade V, Aleksanyan A, Paniagua Zambrana NY, Bussmann RW. 2017. *Juglans regia* L. In: *Ethnobotany of the Caucasus*. Bussmann RW (Ed.) Springer International Publishing, Cham. https://doi.org/10.1007/978-3-319-49412-8_22
40. Wali R, Rahman K, Raja NI, Qureshi R, Bussmann RW, Mashwani ZUR. 2019. A quantitative medico botanical expedition of Fairy Meadows National Park, Diamir, Gilgit Baltistan, Pakistan. *Ethnobotany Research and Applications*. 18 (35): 1–30. https://doi.org/10.32859/era.18.35.1-30
41. Fujita T, Sezik E, Tabata M, Yesilada E, Honda G, Takeda Y, Tanaka T, Takaishi Y. 1995. Traditional medicine in Turkey VII. Folk medicine in Middle and West Black Sea regions. *Economic Botany*. 49: 406–422.
42. Yesilada E. 2002. Biodiversity in Turkish folk medicine. In: *Biodiversity: Biomolecular Aspects of Biodiversity and Innovative Utilization*. Sener B (Ed.) Kluwer Academic/Plenum Publishers, London. pp. 119–135.
43. Kim HG, Cho JH, Jeong EY, Lim JH, Lee SH, Lee HS. 2006. Growth inhibiting activity of active component isolated from *Terminalia chebula* fruits against intestinal bacteria. *Journal of Food Protection*. 69: 2205–2209.
44. Jaradat NA. 2005. Medical plants utilized in Palestinian folk medicine for treatment of diabetes mellitus and cardiac diseases. *Journal of al-Aqsa University*, 19: 1–28.
45. Kaileh Mb, Berghea WV, Boonec E, Essawib T, Haegemana G. 2007. Screening of indigenous Palestinian medicinal plants for potential anti-inflammatory and cytotoxic activity. *Journal of Ethnopharmacology*. 113: 510–516.
46. Spaccarotella KJ, Kris-Etherton PM, Stone WL, Bagshaw DM, Fishell VK, West SG, Lawrence FR, Hartman TJ. 2008. The effect of walnut intake on factors related to prostate and vascular health in older men. *Nutrition Journal*. 7: 13. https://doi.org/10.1186/1475-2891-7-13
47. Gruenwald J, Brendler T, Jaenjke C. 2001. *PDR for Herbal Medicines*. Montvale, N.J.: Medicinal Economic.
48. Papoutsi Z, Kassi E, Chinou I, Halabalaki M, Skaltsounis LA, Moutsatsou P. 2008. Walnut extract (*Juglans regia* L.) and its component ellagic acid exhibit anti-inflammatory activity in human aorta endothelial cells and osteoblastic activity in the cell line KS483. *British Journal of Nutrition*. 99: 715–722.
49. Liu L, Li W, Koike K, Zhang S, Nikaido T. 2004. Newalphatetralonylglucosides from the fruit of *Juglans mandshurica*. *Chemical and Pharmaceutical Bulletin. Tokyo*. 52: 566–569.
50. Torres-Gonzalez. 2011. Protective effect of four Mexican plants against CCl_4-induced damage in the hyh7 human hepatoma cell. *Annals Hematology*. 10:73–79.
51. Tagarelli G, Tagarelli A, Piro A. 2010. Folk medicine used to heal malaria in Calabria (southern Italy). *Journal of Ethnobiology and Ethnomedicine*. 6: 27. https://doi.org/10.1186/1746-4269-6-27

52. Maleita C, Esteves I, Chim R, Fonseca L, Braga MEM, Abrantes I, de Sousa HC. 2017. Naphthoquinones from walnut husk residues show strong nematicidal activities against the root-knot nematode Meloidogyne hispanica. *ACS Sustainable Chemistry & Engineering*. 5: 3390–3398.
53. Labuckas DO, Maestri DM, Perelló M, Martínez ML, Lamarque AL. 2008. Phenolics from walnut (*Juglans regia* L.) kernels: antioxidant activity and interactions with proteins. *Food Chemistry*, 107: 607–612.
54. Trandafir I, Cosmulescu S, Botu M, Nour V. 2016. Antioxidant activity, and phenolic and mineral contents of the walnut kernel (*Juglans regia* L.) as a function of the pellicle colour. *Fruits*. 71: 173–184.
55. Jahanban-Esfahlan A, Amarowicz R. 2018. Walnut (*Juglans regia* L.) shell pyroligneous acid: chemical constituents and functional applications. *RSC* Ad*vances*. 8: 22376–22391.
56. Savage GP. 2001. Chemical composition of walnuts (*Juglans regia* L.) grown in New Zealand. *Plant Foods for Human Nutrition*. 56: 75–82.
57. Fukuda T, Ito H, Yoshida T. 2003. Antioxidative polyphenols from walnuts (*Juglans regia* L.). *Phytochemistry*. 63: 795–801
58. Milind P, Deepa K. 2011. Walnut: not a hard nut to crack. *International Research Journal of Pharmacy*. 2: 8–17.
59. Meshkini A, Tahmasbi M. 2017. Anti-platelet aggregation activity of walnut hull extract via suppression of ROS generation and caspase activation. *Journal of Acupuncture and Meridian Studies*. 10: 193–203.
60. Arasteh Nodeh A, Ardjmand M, Fanaei MA, Safekordi AA. 2013. Neural network for modeling of chemical reaction systems: kinetics of concentrated acid hydrolysis of walnut green skin. *Asian Journal of Chemistry*. 25: 1793–1799.
61. Chang SK, Alasalvar C, Bolling BW, Shahidi F. 2016. Nuts and their co-products: the impact of processing (roasting) on phenolics, bioavailability, and health benefits – a comprehensive review. *Journal of Functional Foods*. 26: 88–122.
62. Mourtzinos I, Goula A. 2019. Polyphenols in agricultural by-products and food waste. In: *Polyphenols in Plants*, Ronald Ross Watson (Ed.) 2nd Edition. Academic Press, Cambridge, MA. pp. 23–44.
63. Ignat I, Volf I, Popa VI. 2011. A critical review of methods for characterisation of polyphenolic compounds in fruits and vegetables. *Food Chemistry*. 126: 1821–1835.
64. Balasundram N, Sundram K, Samman S. 2006. Phenolic compounds in plants and agri-industrial by-products: antioxidant activity, occurrence, and potential uses. *Food Chemistry*. 99: 191–203.
65. Atanasov AG, Waltenberger B, Pferschy-Wenzig E, Linder T, Wawrosch C, Uhrin P, Temml V, Wang L, Schwaiger S, Heiss EH, Rollinger JM. 2015. Discovery and resupply of pharmacologically active plant-derived natural products: a review. *Biotechnology Advances*. 33: 1582–1614.
66. Haminiuk CWI, Maciel GM, Plata-Oviedo MSV, Peralta RM. 2012. Phenolic compounds in fruits-An overview. *International Journal of Food Science and Technology*. 47: 2023–2044.
67. Güngör A, Akbay I, Özdemir T. 2019. Waste walnut shell as an alternative bio-based filler for the EPDM: mechanical, thermal, and kinetic studies. *Journal of Material Cycles and Waste Management*. 21: 145–155.
68. Demirbas A. 2006. Effect of temperature on pyrolysis products from four nut shells. *Journal of Analytical and Applied Pyrolysis*. 76: 285–289.
69. Srinivasan A, Viraraghavan T. 2008. Removal of oil by walnut shell media. *Bioresources Technology*. 99: 8217–8220.
70. Ayrilmis N, Kaymakci A, Ozdemir F. 2013. Physical, mechanical, and thermal properties of polypropylene composites filled with walnut shell flour. *Journal of Industrial & Engineering Chemistry*. 19: 908–914.
71. Montava-Jorda S, Quiles-Carrillo L, Richart N, Torres-Giner S, Montanes N. 2019. Enhanced interfacial adhesion of polylactide/poly (ε-caprolactone)/walnut shell flour composites by reactive extrusion with maleinized linseed oil. *Polymers*. 11: 758. https://doi.org/10.3390/polym11050758
72. Barczewski M, Sałasińska K, Szulc J. 2019. Application of sunflower husk, hazelnut shell and walnut shell as waste agricultural fillers for epoxy-based composites: a study into mechanical behavior related to structural and rheological properties. *Polymer Testing*. 75: 1–11.
73. Salasinska K, Barczewski M, Górny R, Kloziński A. 2018. Evaluation of highly filled epoxy composites modified with walnut shell waste filler. *Polymer Bulletin*. 75: 2511–2528.
74. Oliveira I, Sousa A, Ferreira ICFR, Bento A, Estevinho L, Pereira JA. 2008. Total phenols, antioxidant potential and antimicrobial activity of walnut (*Juglans regia* L.) green husks. *Food and Chemical Toxicology*. 46: 2326–2331.
75. Beiki T, Najafpour GD, Hosseini M. 2018. Evaluation of antimicrobial and dyeing properties of walnut (*Juglans regia* L.) green husk extract for cosmetics. *Color Technology*. 134: 71–81.
76. Jahanban-Esfahlan A, Davaran S, Moosavi-Movahedi A, Dastmalchi S. 2017. Investigating the interaction of juglone (5-hydroxy-1, 4-naphthoquinone) with serum albumins using spectroscopic and in silico methods. *Journal of the Iranian Chemical Society*. 7: 1527–1540.
77. Fernandez-Agullo A, Pereira E, Freire MS, Valentao P, Andrade PB, González-Álvarez J, Pereira JA. 2013. Influence of solvent on the antioxidant and antimicrobial properties of walnut (*Juglans regia* L.) green husk extracts. *Industrial Crops and Products*. 42: 126–132.
78. Cosmulescu S, Trandafir I, Nour V, Ionica M, Tutulescu F. 2014. Phenolics content, antioxidant activity and color of green walnut extracts for preparing walnut liquor. *Notulae Botanicae Horti Agrobotanici*. 42: 551–555.
79. Yagub MT, Sen TK, Afroze S, Ang H. 2014. Dye and its removal from aqueous solution by adsorption: a review. *Advances in Colloid and Interface Science*. 209: 172–184.
80. Çelekli A, Bozkurt H, Geyik F. 2016. Artificial neural network and genetic algorithms for modeling of removal of an azo dye on walnut husk. *Desalination Water Treatment*. 57: 15580–15591.
81. Harrison RM. 2001. *Pollution: Causes, Effects and Control*. Royal Society of Chemistry, Cambrige, UK.
82. Köhler SJ, Cubillas P, Rodríguez-Blanco JD, Bauer C, Prieto M. 2007. Removal of cadmium from waste waters by aragonite shells and the influence of other divalent cations. *Environmental Science and Technology*. 41: 112–118.
83. Wang XS, Li ZZ, Tao SR. 2009. Removal of chromium (VI) from aqueous solution using walnut hull. *Journal of Environmental Management*. 90: 721–729.
84. Zafarani HR, Bahrololoom ME, Noubactep C, Tashkhourian J. 2015. Green walnut shell as a new material for removal of Cr (VI) ions from aqueous solutions. *Desalination Water Treatment*. 55: 431–439.
85. Dalali N, Hagghi, A. 2015. Removal of cadmium from aqueous solutions by walnut green husk as a low-cost biosorbent. *Desalination Water Treatment*. 57: 13782–13794.

86. Noshirvani N, Fasihi H, Moradipayam A. 2015. Study on the antioxidant effects of extract and powder of green walnut hulls on the oxidation of sunflower oil. *Iranian Journal of Nutrition Sciences & Food Technology.* 10: 79–90.
87. Salejda AM, Janiewicz U, Korzeniowska M, Kolniak-Ostek J, Krasnowska G. 2016. Effect of walnut green husk addition on some quality properties of cooked sausages. *LWT-Food Science and Technology.* 65: 751–757.
88. Alamprese C, Pompei C. 2005. Influence of processing variables on some characteristics of nocino liqueur. *Food Chemistry.* 92: 203–209.
89. Stampar F, Solar A, Hudina M, Veberic R, Colaric M. 2006. Traditional walnut liqueur–cocktail of phenolics. *Food Chemistry.* 95: 627–631.
90. Stampar F, Solar A, Hudina M, Veberic R, Colaric M, Fabcic J. 2007. Phenolics in walnut liqueur. *Acta Horticulturae.* 744: 451–454.
91. Jakopic J, Colaric M, Veberic R, Hudina M, Solar A, Stampar F. 2007. How much do cultivar and preparation time influence on phenolics content in walnut liqueur? *Food Chemistry.* 104: 100–105.

16 *Morus alba* (Mulberry)

INTRODUCTION

Mulberry is globally distributed under different climatic conditions, from temperate to tropical.[1,2] It belongs to the genus *Morus* (family: Moraceae) and has 24 species. *Morus alba* Linn. (Eng.: Mulberry, Hindi: 'Tut') is a dominant species among all.[3,4] It is 3–6 m high, a moderate-sized tree, and is cultivated throughout the world for rearing silkworms. Mulberry leaves are rich in flavones A, B, and C, morin, mulberrin, quercetin, and β-sitosterol. Mulberry is native to India, Nepal, Myanmar, Indochina, China, and Japan. It is extensively cultivated throughout the plains of India and in the Himalayan hills up to 3,300 MSL elevation.[5,6] India has the second-largest mulberry cultivation area, 280,000 ha, after China, which is above 626,000 ha.[7] The fruit of *M. alba* has a yield of more than 10 kg/tree from some cultivars in one fruiting season[8] and is commonly used as a fruit juice or jam, eaten either dried or fresh, and processed into wine. It has a low-calorie content, high nutrient content, pleasing color, and delicious taste.[9–11]

ETHNOPHARMACOLOGY

Mulberry fruits in Japan, Korea, and China are used in folk medicine to treat sore throats, lower blood pressure, improve eyesight, protect the liver and kidneys, and reduce fever.[12,13] Traditionally, *M. alba* is used to cure kidney and liver diseases, revive joint damage, and as an anti-aging food.[14]

The mulberry plant has been used in folklore for ailments such as bronchitis, insomnia, asthma, wound healing, cough, edema, diabetes, influenza, nosebleeds, and eye infections.[15] Traditionally, mulberry fruits are used as a medicinal agent to treat weakness, benefit the kidneys, nourish the blood, fatigue, premature graying of hair, and anemia. In elderly patients, it is also used to treat dizziness, urinary incontinence, constipation, and tinnitus.[16] All the parts of the white mulberry plant are used in Chinese medicine.[17] It has been used in the Indian indigenous system of medicine as a diuretic, purgative, anthelmintic, brain tonic, antibacterial, hepatopathy laxative, acrid, and for cooling purposes. Ayurveda recommends white mulberry to treat burning sensation symptoms.[18]

Dried mulberry fruits are powdered and stored. 10 g of dried fruit are reported for 100 mg of anthocyanins.[19] Due to the presence of resveratrol, mulberry fruits have an antimutagen effect and inhibit the mutation of healthy and normal cells. In folk medicine, it is believed that mulberry fruits inhibit cancer, heart disease, and chronic inflammation. Powder from dried fruits is used for maintaining a normal level of cholesterol and carbohydrates and has an anti-aging effect on the human body.[20]

Mulberry leaves are globally used as feed for the silkworm, while fruits are location-dependent and consumed fresh, as juice, or as jam. Mulberry fruits are used to treat liver, kidney, and urinary infections; tinnitus; dizziness; and constipation in the elderly, while in general they are used to cure anemia, sore throat, fever, and depression.[21] Young leaves and petioles are used as delicious vegetables. Leaves are used as a tea for therapeutic applications.[22]

The wine from mulberry fruits is sweet and sour and is used for the purification of blood. There is a common belief that one glass of mulberry wine per day improves health by pursuing fecal residues from the gastrointestinal tract.[23,24]

During the Middle Ages, mulberry was used as an ingredient in a mixture used for anesthesia. Hugh of Lucca, a surgeon of his period (the 13th century), prepared a sleeping sponge using the juice of the unripe mulberry with many more herbs.[25] The Jewish community of medieval times also used mulberry (during the 11th–14th centuries), which is mentioned.[26]

The overripened sour fruits of mulberry are converted into a wine with a sweet and sour taste and are used for the improvement of general vitality. In Armenia, Georgia, and Azerbaijan, the wine is consumed to increase potency and is a very popular liqueur. In Azerbaijan, it is believed that a small dose of mulberry wine protects the stomach and heart from diseases. In Greece, mulberry fruit is used to produce traditional, aromatic drinks called 'mouro distillate'.[27] In Europe, mulberry fruit wine is popular among ladies. As mulberry fruits are rich in anthocyanins,[27] the coloring compounds, and these anthocyanins are used in the food industry, specifically cyanin, a red pigment that imparts the red to purple color to fruits.[27]

Peng et al. have improved the bread quality by adding catechin- and epicatechin-rich grape seed extract.[28] Using the aforementioned concept, Kobus-Cisowska et al. have studied the effect of mulberry leaf-enriched bread and concluded that white mulberry leaf extract (WMLA)-enriched bread extends the shelf life of bread while maintaining high sensory, microbial quality, and functional properties. In mulberry-enriched bread, protocatechuic acid and chlorogenic acid contents were higher compared to the control sample by 50% and 160%, respectively.[29]

It was also observed that samples enriched with WMLA are more stable compared to the control sample. Further, it has been revealed that the addition of mulberry increases the phenolic acids and flavonols in the bread and stabilizes the presence of other polyphenolic substances.[30] Finally, it was concluded that the bread can be an attractive matrix as a carrier of mulberry bioactive ingredients.[30] Mulberry leaf extract and mulberry fruit extract in the production of bread do not alter the microbiological quality at all, even during freezing storage of the bread, and they can be an interesting alternative in the diet.[30]

DOI: 10.1201/9781003512868-18

PHYTO-CONSTITUENTS

The health-promoting effect of *M. alba* is due to the presence of polyphenolic compounds (astragalin, iso-quercetin, kaempferol, quercetin, rutin, and myricetin derivatives), other glucosides, and minerals.[31] Mulberry fruits and leaves are rich in phenolic acids (chlorogenic acid, caffeic acid, hydroxybenzoic or ferulic acid).[32]

MULBERRY FRUIT CHEMISTRY

M. alba fruits are a healthy food option for consumers as they have abundant lipids, protein, fiber, carbohydrates, vitamins, and minerals but are low in calories. 100 g of fresh mulberry fruits can produce 1.44 g of protein. From a total of 18 amino acids, all nine essential amino acids required by the human body are present in mulberry fruits.[33] The mature and fully ripened mulberry fruits have a mouth-watering taste with a pleasing aroma and flavor. These fruits are edible and used for making value-added products. Mulberry fruits have high nutritional significance[34] and several nutrient elements essential for a healthy metabolic process.[35] *M. alba* fruits are a good source of carbohydrates, lipids, protein, vitamins, minerals, and fibers. The quantity of protein in fresh *M. alba* fruits is higher than that of raspberries[36] and strawberries[37] and comparable to blackberries,[38] whereas the anthocyanin content is higher than blackberries, blueberries, blackcurrants, and redcurrants.[39] *M. alba* fruits contain both essential and nonessential amino acids. The essential amino acid vs total amino acid ratio is 42%, which is almost equal to the fish and milk combination.[40] Each species of genus *Morus* contains a significant amount of vitamin C. Ascorbic acid is 15.81 mg/100 g of the fresh fruit weight in *M. alba*.[41] Mulberries have some important alkaloids that activate macrophages by stimulating the immune system and are regarded as safeguarding the human body against health threats.[42] 1-deoxynojirimycin (DNJ), 1,4-dideoxy-1,4-imino-D-ribitol, and 1,4-dideoxy-1,4-imino-D-arabinitol are the main alkaloids isolated from mulberry leaves.[43] Fructose and glucose are the primary sugars present in mulberry fruits, which increase with ripening.[41] *M. alba* has a total fat of 1.10%. Oleic acid, palmitic acid, and linolenic acid are the major fatty acids in fruits.[3] The organic acids present in mulberry fruits are citric acid, fumaric acid, malic acid, succinic acid, and tartaric acid; however, malic acid is the most common acid found in all the species.[41]. Mulberry is an excellent source of minerals, particularly calcium, magnesium, sodium, phosphorus, and potassium.[35]

M. alba fruits have been recorded in the Chinese pharmacopoeia.[44] and support traditional applications.[45–47]Various studies have concluded that mulberry fruit extracts are potent neuroprotective antioxidants and anti-obesity effects and have cardioprotective, immunomodulatory, and antitumor effects.[3,40,48]

M. alba is a cosmopolitan species and experiences a great degree of environmental variability that influences its morphology and physiology, including the chemical characteristics and quality profiles of bioactive compounds such as carotenoids, flavonoids, and anthocyanins.[3,49]

M. ALBA LEAVES

The leaves of *M. alba* have nutritional applications, so they are used in several types of preparations. Its leaves have a high content of proteins (13.4%–19.4%) and are used with wheat flour to increase the nutritional value of the bread and improve the stability duration.[50] The phenolic fraction of leaves of *M. alba* has antioxidant activity. The main compounds identified for the antioxidant activity are catechin, chlorogenic acid, and rutin.[51]

A high concentration of sugar-mimicking alkaloids (1,4-dideoxy-1,4-imino-D-arabinitol, DNJ, and 1,4-dideoxy-1,4-imino-D-ribitol), which are also known for hypoglycemic properties, are present in the leaves of *M. alba*.[52] These compounds inhibit either all or a few intestinal disaccharidases and pancreatic amylases by regulating the uptake of monosaccharides, so they are used in the oral treatment of type 2 diabetes mellitus.[44] Mulberry leaf extract reduces insulin resistance by modulating gene and protein expression used in glucose homeostasis in the liver. The extract of leaves has a dose-dependent effect on gluconeogenic enzymes, specifically phosphoenolpyruvate carboxykinase, and glucose-6-phosphatase, while suppressing the activities of glycolytic enzymes, including glucokinase, phosphofructokinase, and pyruvate kinase.The extract of leaves has a dose-dependent impact on gluconeogenic enzymes phosphoenolpyruvate carboxykinase and glucose-6-phosphatase to suppress, and activities of glycolytic enzymes glucokinase, phosphofructokinase, and pyruvate kinase for stimulation. It also activates the different signaling pathways by elevating the translocation of the glucose transporter (GLUT-4) in adipose tissues and skeletal muscles.[45]

PHARMACOLOGICAL PROPERTIES

Antidiabetic Activity

Ethanolic extract of root barks *of M. alba* reduces the amount of glucose and increases insulin production, protects pancreatic β cells from degeneration, diminishes lipid peroxidation, inhibits low-density lipoprotein atherogenic modification and lipid peroxide formation, and increases the expression of adipogenic marker proteins (such as GLUT4, peroxisome proliferator-activated receptors γ, and adipocyte-specific fatty acid-binding protein 4).[53–55] Methanolic extract of *M. alba* has in vitro acetylcholine esterase inhibitory activity. Different doses of mulberry leaf extract administered to animal models for 35 days reveal reduced blood glucose levels through regeneration of β cells.[56]

Adaptogen Property

The ethyl acetate-soluble fraction from methanol extract of *M. alba* roots has adaptogen properties tested against a rat model of chronic stress, revealing its possible clinical applications as an anti-stress agent.[57]

Anthelmintic Activity

Leaf extracts of *M. alba* were studied for anthelmintic activity at different concentrations using albendazole as the standard. All extracts (petroleum ether, chloroform, and methanol) had dose-dependent effects and were comparable to the standard drug.[58]

Neuroprotective Activity

To reduce reactive oxygen species-induced damage, Kang et al. (2006) investigated mulberry fruit extract (MFE) and concluded that dietary MFE supplementation has a positive effect on neuron density and enhanced anti-oxidase activity.[59]

Hepatoprotection

The hepatoprotective action of mulberry water extract in mice has been revealed to effectively prevent liver injury, mainly via decreasing antioxidative stress and inhibiting lipogenesis and inflammation. It increases fatty acid transport and the rate of oxidation.[60]

ROLE OF *MORUS* IN FOOD INDUSTRIES

Mulberry fruits are well known throughout the world for their mouth-watering taste, making them a choice for consumption either fresh or as an ingredient in value-added products. Mulberry fruits are low-calorie edible fruits having a mood-refreshing taste that has led to increased demand in the food processing industries. Ripened mulberry fruits are harvested by slightly shaking trees.[8] Various investigations and results have concluded that *M. alba* can be effectively used in the food and beverage industries. *M. alba* fruits are a valuable source of antioxidants with a strong nutritional profile.[8]

SCOPE AND OPPORTUNITIES

The genus *Morus* is a rich source of phenolics[61] and is traditionally used for the prevention of kidney and liver diseases, the repair of joint damage, and anti-aging purposes. The therapeutic potential is due to the antioxidant properties of phenolics.[14] It has a hypoglycemic effect, so it is an ally in the treatment of type 2 diabetes mellitus.[50] Further, there is a need to develop the best cultivation techniques for mulberry leaves for the rearing of silkworms in a reasonably inexpensive manner, which is also another opportunity. Different synergistic formulations are possible from mulberry for use in pharmacy and as food. Its health properties are known from ancient times in the folklore of different civilizations, ranging from the treatment of depression to obesity. The pleasant taste and smell of its fruit extract as fresh food, and its value-added products as a sweet or alcoholic beverage, have been served on numerous occasions and offer has high health benefits. These products are localized and not available commercially. In modern medicine, its use is predominantly limited as an additive in syrups and as natural colors.

Mulberry fruit may be used to develop novel functional foods or potential drugs because the increased demand for healthy foods is on the rise. There is scope for various mulberry value-added products with specifications after their safety evaluation. Chang et al. have reported that mulberry fruits are non-carcinogenic and pose no health risks to consumers.[62] Therefore, the consumption of mulberry fruit is safe.[63]

Mulberry fruits have abundant nutrients and bioactive compounds and are known as potential disease-fighting food. Fruits are used for the prevention and cure of chronic illness, but there is still a knowledge gap between the phytochemicals and the mechanism of biological activities. The therapeutic ingredients of mulberries and their contents vary with varieties, cultivars, biotic and abiotic factors, and stages of harvest. Though the chemical composition of mulberry fruits has been extensively studied, there may still be a few unknown compounds that contribute to their biological activities. Therefore, detailed investigations, including synergistic behaviors with other fruits, may be conducted to explore the therapeutic mechanism.

REFERENCES

1. Pel P, Chae HS, Nhoek P, Kim YM, Chin YW. 2017. Chemical constituents with proprotein convertase subtilisin/kexin type 9 mRNA expression inhibitory activity from dried immature *Morus alba* fruits. *Journal of Agricultural and Food Chemistry*. 65: 5316–5321.
2. Yuan QX, Xie YF, Wang W, Yan YH, Ye H, Jabbar S, Zeng XX. 2015. Extraction optimization, characterization, and antioxidant activity in vitro of polysaccharides from mulberry (*Morus alba* L.) leaves. *Carbohydrate Polymers*. 128: 52–62.
3. Ercisli S, Orhan E. 2007. Chemical composition of white (*Morus alba*), red (*Morus rubra*), and black (*Morus nigra*) mulberry fruits. *Food Chemistry*. 103: 1380–1384.
4. Butt MS, Nazir A, Sultan MT, Schroën K. 2008. *Morus alba* L. nature's functional tonic. *Trends in Food Science and Technology*. 19: 505–512.
5. Bhat KKP. 1995. Medicinal plant information databases. In: *Non-Wood Forest Products. Medicinal Plants for Conservation and Health Care*. Food and Agriculture Organization, Rome.
6. Evans WC, Trease GE. 2002. *Trease and Evans Pharmacognosy*, 6th Edition. WB Saunders, China.
7. Sanchez MD. 2000. World distribution and utilization of mulberry, potential for animal feeding. FAO Animal Production and Health Paper. pp. 1–11.
8. Singhal BK, Khan MA, Dhar A, Baqual FM, Bindroo BB. 2010. Approaches to industrial exploitation of mulberry (*Mulberry* sp.) fruits. *Journal of Fruit and Ornamental Plant Research*. 18: 83–99.
9. Jelled A, Hassine R B, Thouri A, Flamini G, Chahdoura H, Arem A E, Lamine J B, Kacem A, Haouas Z, Cheikh H B. 2017. Immature mulberry fruits richness of promising constituents in contrast with mature ones: a comparative study among three Tunisian species. *Industrial Crops and Products*. 95: 434–443.

10. Pawlowska AM, Oleszek W, Braca A. 2008. Quali-quantitative analyses of flavonoids of *Morus nigra* L. and *Morus alba* L. (Moraceae) fruits. *Journal of Agricultural and Food Chemistry*. 56: 3377–3380.
11. Huang LX, Zhou YB, Meng LW, Wu D, He Y. 2017. Comparison of different CCD detectors and chemometrics for predicting total anthocyanin content and antioxidant activity of mulberry fruit using visible and near infrared hyperspectral imaging technique. *Food Chemistry*. 224: 1–10.
12. Zhou M, Chen QQ, Bi JF, Wang YX, Wu XY. 2017. Degradation kinetics of cyanidin 3-O-glucoside and cyanidin 3-Orutinoside during hot air and vacuum drying in mulberry (*Morus alba* L.) fruit: a comparative study based on solid food system. *Food Chemistry*. 229: 574–579.
13. Chen C, Zhang B, Fu X, You L J, Abbasi AM, Liu RH. 2016. The digestibility of mulberry fruit polysaccharides and its impact on lipolysis under simulated saliva, gastric and intestinal conditions. *Food Hydrocolloids*. 58: 171–178.
14. Mena P, Sanchez-Salcedo EM, Tassoti M, Martínez JJ, Hernandez F, Del Rio D. 2016. Phytochemical evaluation of eight white (*Morus alba* L.) and black (*Morus nigra* L.) mulberry clones grown in Spain based on UHPLC-ESI-MSn metabolomic profiles. *Food Research International*. 89: 1116–1122.
15. Anonymous. 1952. *The Wealth of India, A Dictionary of Indian Raw materials*. Council of Scientific and Industrial Research, New Delhi. Vol. 7. pp. 429–437.
16. Nadkarni AK. 1976. *Indian Materia Medica*. Popular Prakashan, Mumbai. Vol. 1. pp. 1292–1294.
17. Mhaskar KS, Latter EB, Caius JS, Kirtikar, Basu. 2000. *Indian Medicinal Plants*. Sri Satguru Publications. New Delhi, India. Vol. 3. pp. 3185.
18. Arya VS. 1997. *Indian Medicinal Plant*. Orient Longman Limited, Chennai. Vol. 14. pp. 65–67.
19. Singhal BK, Dhar A, Khan MA, Bindroo BB, Fotedar RK. 2009. Potential economic additions by mulberry fruits in sericulture industry. *Plant Horticultural Technology*. 9 (1): 47–51.
20. Liu LK, Chou FP, Chen YC, Chyn HH, Wang J. 2009. Effects of mulberry (*Morus alba* L.) extracts on lipid homeostasis *in- vitro* and *in- vivo*. *Journal of Agricultural and Food Chemistry*. 57 (16): 7605–7611.
21. Darias-Martin J, Lobo-Rodrigo G, Henrnandez-Cordero J, Diaz E, Diaz-Romero C. 2003. Alcoholic beverages obtained from black mulberry. *Food Technology and Biotechnology*. 41 (2): 173–176.
22. Masilimani S, Qadri SMH, Dandin SB. 2008. Mulberry fruits: a potential value-addition enterprise. *Indian Silk*. 46 (11): 12–13.
23. Elmaci Y, Altug T. 2002. Flavour evaluation of three black mulberry (*Morus nigra* L.) cultivars using GC/MS, chemical and sensory data. *Journal of the Science of Food and Agriculture*. 82 (6): 632–635.
24. Zhang W, He J, Pan Q, Han F, Duan C. 2011. Separation and character analysis of anthocyanins from mulberry (*Morus alba* L.) pomace. *Czech Journal of Food Sciences*. 29 (3): 268–276.
25. Robinson V. 1946. *Victory over Pain; A History of Anesthesia*. Henry Schuman, New York.
26. Lev E. 2007. Drugs held and sold by pharmacists of the Jewish community of medieval (11th-14th centuries) Cairo according to lists of Materia Medica found at the Taylor-Schechter Genizah collection. Cambridge. *Journal of Ethnopharmacology*. 110 (2): 275–293.
27. Giusti MM, Wrolstad RE. 2001. Characterization and measurement of anthocyanins by UV-visible spectroscopy. *Current Protocols in Food Analytical Chemistry*. F1.2.1–F1.2.13. https://doi.org/10.1002/0471142913.faf0102s00
28. Peng X, Ma J, Cheng KW, Jiang Y, Chen F, Wang M. 2010. The effects of grape seed extract fortification on the antioxidant activity and quality attributes of bread. *Food Chemistry*. 119: 49–53.
29. Kobus-Cisowska J, Szulc P, Szczepaniak O, Dziedzinski M, Szymanowska D, Szymandera-Buszka K, Goryńska-Goldmann E, Gazdecki M, Telichowska A, Ligaj M. 2020. Variability of *Hordeum vulgare* L. cultivars in yield, antioxidant potential, and cholinesterase inhibitory activity. *Sustainability*. 12: 1938. https://doi.org/10.3390/su12051938
30. Kobus-Cisowska J, Dziedzinski M, Szymanowska D, Szczepaniak O, Byczkiewicz S, Telichowska A, Szulc P. 2020. The effects of *Morus alba* L. fortification on the quality, functional properties and sensory attributes of bread stored under refrigerated conditions. *Sustainability*. 12: 6691. https://doi.org/10.3390/su12166691
31. Piechocka J, Szulc P, Dziedziński M, Kobus-Cisowska J, Szczepaniak O, Szymanowska-Powałowska D. 2020. Antioxidant potential of various solvent extract from *Morus alba* fruits and its major polyphenols composition. *Ciência Rural*. 50 (1). https://doi.org/10.1590/0103-8478cr20190371
32. Kobus-Cisowska J, Gramza-Michalowska A, Kmiecik D, Flaczyk E, Korczak J. 2013. Mulberry fruit as an antioxidant component in muesli. *Agricultural Science*. 4: 130–135.
33. Yuan Q, Zhao LJ. 2017. The mulberry (*Morus alba* L.) fruit- A review of characteristic components and health benefits. *Journal of Agricultural and Food Chemistry*. 65: 10383–10394.
34. Sengül M, Fatih Ertugay M, Sengül M. 2005. Rheological, physical, and chemical characteristics of mulberry pekmez. Food Control. https://doi.org/ 10.1016/j.foodcont.2003.11.010
35. Akbulut M, Özcan MM. 2009. Comparison of mineral contents of mulberry (*Morus* spp.) fruits and their pekmez (boiled mulberry juice) samples. *International Journal of Food Sciences and Nutrition*. https://doi.org/10.1080/09637480701695609
36. Rao AV, Snyder DM. 2010. Raspberries and human health: a review. *Journal of Agricultural and Food Chemistry*. https://doi.org/10.1021/jf903484g
37. Giampieri F, Tulipani S, Alvarez-Suarez JM, Quiles JL, Mezzetti B, Battino M. 2012. The strawberry: composition, nutritional quality, and impact on human health. *Nutrition*. https://doi.org/10.1016/j.nut.2011.08.009.
38. Kaume L, Howard LR, Devareddy L. 2012. The blackberry fruit: a review on its composition and chemistry, metabolism and bioavailability, and health benefits. *Journal of Agricultural and Food Chemistry*. https://doi.org/10.1021/jf203318p
39. Veberic R, Slatnar A, Bizjak J, Stampar F, Mikulic-Petkovsek M. 2015. Anthocyanin composition of different wild and cultivated berry species. *LWT - Food Science and Technology*. https://doi.org/10.1016/j.lwt.2014.08.033
40. Jiang Y, Nie WJ. 2015. Chemical properties in fruits of mulberry species from the Xinjiang province of China. *Food* Chemistry. 174: 460–466.
41. Eyduran SP, Ercisli S, Akin M, Beyhan O, Gecer MK, Eyduran E, Erturk YE. 2015. Organic acids, sugars, vitamin C, antioxidant capacity, and phenolic compounds in

fruits of white (*Morus alba* L.) and black (*Morus nigra* L.) mulberry genotypes. *Journal of Applied Botany and Food Quality*. https://doi.org/10.5073/JABFQ.2015.088.019
42. Kim SB, Chang BY, Jo YH, Lee SH, Han SB, Hwang BY, Kim SY, Lee MK. 2013. Macrophage activating activity of pyrrole alkaloids from *Morus alba* fruits. *Journal of Ethnopharmacology*. https://doi.org/10.1016/j.jep.2012.11.007
43. Sharma SB, Gupta S, Ac R, Singh UR, Rajpoot R, Shukla SK. 2010. Antidiabetogenic action of *Morus rubra* L. leaf extract in streptozotocin-induced diabetic rats. *Journal of Pharmacy and Pharmacology*. doi: 10.1211.jpp/62.02.0013.
44. Asano N. 2009. Sugar-mimicking glycosidase inhibitors: bioactivity and application. *Cellular and Molecular Life Sciences*. 66: 1479–1492.
45. Liu HY, Wang J, Ma J, Zhang YQ. 2016. Interference effect of oral administration of mulberry branch bark powder on the incidence of type II diabetes in mice induced by streptozotocin. *Journal of Food & Nutrition Research*. 60. https://doi.org/10.3402/fnr.v60.31606
46. Choi KH, Lee HA, Park MH, Han JS. 2016. Mulberry (*Morus alba* L.) Fruit extract containing anthocyanins improves glycemic control and insulin sensitivity via activation of AMP-activated protein kinase in diabetic C57BL/Ksj-db/db mice. *Journal of Medicinal* Food. 19: 1–9.
47. Ahn E, Lee J, Jeon YH, Choi SW, Kim E. 2017. Anti-diabetic effects of mulberry (*Morus alba* L.) branches and oxy-resveratrol in streptozotocin-induced diabetic mice. *Food Science and Biotechnology*. 26: 1693–1702.
48. Imran M, Khan H, Shah M, Khan R, Khan F. 2010. Chemical composition and antioxidant activity of certain Morus species. *Journal of Zhejiang University Science B*. 11: 973–980.
49. Jiao Y, Wang X, Jiang X, Kong F, Wang S, Yan C. 2017. Antidiabetic effects of *Morus alba* fruit polysaccharides on high-fat diet and streptozotocin-induced type 2 diabetes in rats. *Journal of Ethnopharmacology*. 199: 119–127.
50. Sanchez-Salcedo EM, Amorós A, Hernández F, Martínez JJ. 2017. Physicochemical properties of white (*Morus alba*) and Black (*Morus nigra*) mulberry leaves, a new food supplement. *Journal of Food & Nutrition Research*. 5: 253–261.
51. Zhang Y, Du W, Zhang X, Zhao H, Wang Y. 2017. Antioxidant activity and the potential for cholesterol-lowering of phenolic extract of *Morus alba*, *Morus multicaulis*, and *Morus laevigata* leaves from Yunnan (China). *Journal of Food Biochemistry*. 41: 1–8.
52. Konno K, Ono H, Nakamura M, Tateishi K, Hirayama C, Tamura Y, Hattori M, Koyama A, Kohno K. 2006. Mulberry latex rich in antidiabetic sugar-mimic alkaloids forces dieting on caterpillars. *Proceedings of the National Academy of Sciences of the United States of America*. 103: 1337–1341.
53. El-Beshbishy HA, Singab ANB, Sinkkonen J, Pihlaja K. 2006. Hypolipidemic and antioxidant effects of *Morus alba* L. (Egyptian mulberry) root bark fractions supplementation in cholesterol-fed rats. *Life Sciences*. 78: 2724–2733.
54. Oh TS, Choi DK, Yun JW. 2011. *Morus alba* L. root bark stimulates adipocyte differentiation in 3T3-L1 cells. *Biotechnology and Bioprocess* Engineering. 16: 978–986.
55. Singab ANB, El-Beshbishy HA, Yonekawa M, Nomura T, Fukai T. 2005. Hypoglycemic effect of Egyptian *Morus alba* root bark extract: effect on diabetes and lipid peroxidation of streptozotocin-induced diabetic rats. *Journal of* Ethnopharmacology. 100: 333–338.
56. Jamshid M, Prakash RN. 2012. The histopathologic effects of *Morus alba* leaf extract on the pancreas of diabetic rats. *Turkish Journal of Biology*. 36: 211–216.
57. Vandana SN, Laxman AK, Rashmi AN, Adhikrao VY. 2009. Adaptogenic effect of *Morus alba* on chronic foot shock-induced stress in rats. *Indian Journal of Pharmacology*. 41 (6): 246–251.
58. Aditya RSJ, Ramesh CK, Riaz M, Prabhakar BT. 2012. Anthelmintic and antimicrobial activities in some species of mulberry. *International Journal of Pharmacy and Pharmaceutical Science*. 4 (5): 335–338.
59. Kang TH, Hur JY, Kim HB, Ryu JH, Kim SY. 2006. Neuroprotective effects of the cyanidin-3-O-β-D-glucopyr anoside isolated from mulberry fruit against cerebral ischemia. *Neuroscience Letters*. 391: 122–126.
60. Tang CC, Huang HP, Lee YJ, Tang YH, Wang CJ. 2013. Hepatoprotective effect of mulberry water extracts on ethanol-induced liver injury via anti-inflammation and inhibition of lipogenesis in C57BL/6J mice. *Food and Chemical Toxicology*. 62: 786–796.
61. Kumar V, Chauhan S. 2008. Mulberry: life enhancer. *Journal of Medicinal Plants Research*. 2: 271–278.
62. Chang BY, Kim SB, Lee MK, Park H, Kim SY. 2016. Nonclinical safety assessment of *Morus alba* L. fruits: study of 90-d toxicity in sprague dawley rats and genotoxicity in salmonella. *Journal of Food Science*. 81: T1328–T1335.
63. Mehmood Abbasi A, Shah MH, Guo X, Khan N. 2016. Comparison of nutritional value, antioxidant potential, and risk assessment of the mulberry (*Morus*) fruits. *International Journal of Fruit Science*. 16:113–134.

17 *Myrica esculenta* (Kaphal)

INTRODUCTION

Myrica esculenta Buch.-Ham. ex. D. Don. (fam.: Myricaceae) Syn., *Myrica nagi* Hook., an Ayurvedic medicinal plant is known as Kaphal or Katphala in the Indian subcontinent.[1] The genus *Myrica* consists of about 97 species and is distributed in both subtropical and temperate regions globally.[2] Species *Myrica australiasica* F. Muell is confined only to Australia,[3] while *M. cerifera* L. (Southern wax myrtle/wax myrtle) and *M. pensylvanica* Mirb. (Northern bayberry)[4] are reported as official drugs of North America[5] and have been cited for similar medicinal properties as *M. esculenta* in the Indian systems of medicine.[6] Another species of the genus *Myrica*, namely *M. rubra* (Chinese bayberry), is common in China and Japan.[7–9] *M. esculenta* (Kathphala, Kaiphal, and Boxberry) has been reported to be the only species found in India (Figure 17.1).[10] It is an economical medicinal plant with multipurpose applications[11] and is an actinorhizal species, useful in the regeneration of nitrogen-depleted soils.[2] The plant is a source of the tastiest wild fruits of the sub-Himalayan region[12] and has been recognized for its therapeutic and nutritional potential.[13] Fruits of the plant are also used to prepare refreshing drinks, syrups, pickles, and jams.[14] It is a rich source of polyphenolic compounds (flavonols, flavonoids, phenols, and tannins) and vitamin C.[15]

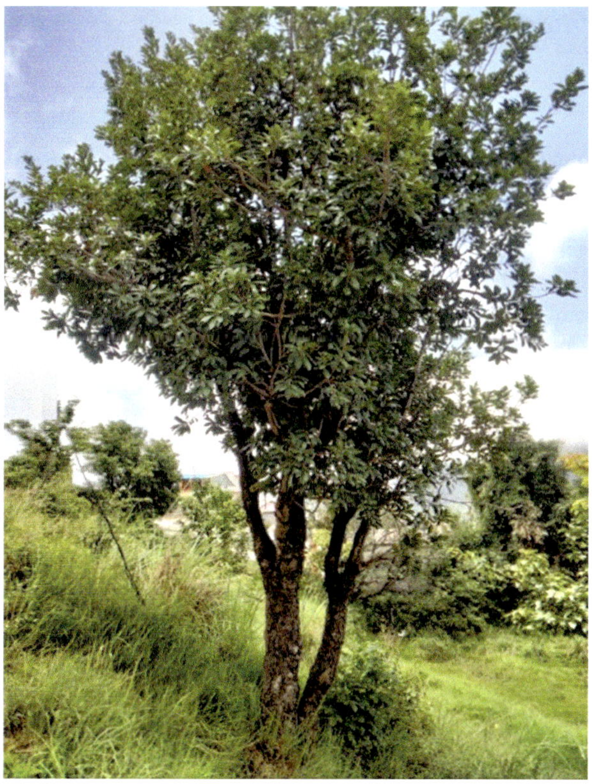

FIGURE 17.1 *M. esculenta* tree.

Local tribes utilize trees as fodder, timber, fuel, and wood,[16] as well as for tanning and yellow dye.[17,18] *M. esculenta* fruits have a unique taste and are a seasonal source of potential income generation for the local people of the sub-Himalayan region.[14,19] All the parts of the *M. esculenta* plant have huge therapeutic and nutritional importance. Fruits are used for syrups, jams, pickles, and preparation for refreshing drinks.[14] Traditionally, its roots, leaves, and bark are used for the treatment of various body ailments and disorders.[8,20,21] The bark of *M. esculenta* is used for making ropes, paper,[22] Ayurvedic medicines (Table 17.1),[23,24] and folk practices (Table 17.2).[25–29]

AYURVEDIC FORMULATIONS

M. esculenta fruits and roots are used to prepare Ayurvedic medicines such as Chyawanaprash and Brahmarasayan, which are used to enhance physical strength, memory, digestion, concentration, and intelligence.[30] The bark of *M. esculenta* is used as an ingredient of Vishweshwara rasa, a common Ayurvedic medicine to treat fever of kapha and pitta origin.[31] The bark or fruits of *M. esculenta* are used in Ayurvedic formulations, namely, Katphala taila, Katphaladi churna, Katphala kvatha, Kaas-har churna, Maha vatagajankush rasa, Khadiradi gutika, Brihat Phala ghrita, Pusyanuga churna, Bala taila, Arimedadi taila, and Mahavishagarbha taila, for the treatment of various ailments such as menstrual disorders, diarrhea, dysentery, menorrhagia, headache, and rheumatoid arthritis.[32,33]

M. esculenta is a multipurpose medicinal tree, but its cultivation is very limited. The traditional and commercial uses of the plant are dependent exclusively on wild-collection sources.[34] The increased urbanization, subsequent over-harvesting, negligence of sustainable utilization, and overexploitation of forests have affected the natural population of the *M. esculenta* plant.[35,36] The present text is an attempt to better harness the ethnomedical knowledge, phytochemistry, and therapeutic potential of *M. esculenta* as per modern molecular knowledge, along with its prospects for conservation, cultivation, and sustainable utilization.

ETHNOBOTANY

The plant is used in a wide range of ailments, specifying decoctions of fruits and stones, and its barks are claimed to be beneficial in cardiac debility, edema, and hemoptysis. A wax covering on the fruit is extracted by scalding the fruit with boiling water and used as an application for ulcer healing.[18,35] A large part of the population living in rural areas of Uttarakhand uses stem bark to cure

DOI: 10.1201/9781003512868-19

TABLE 17.1
Applications of *M. esculenta* in Different Ayurvedic Formulations[23,24]

S. No	Ayurvedic Formulation	Application
1	Arimedadi Taila	Helps to relieve tooth decay and breath problem
2	Bala Taila	Treatment of vata disorders, respiratory infections, and weakness
3	Brihat Phala Ghrita	Treatment of infertility
4	Chyawanprash	Improve immunity, digestion, and enhanced energy
5	Katphaladi Churna	Treatment of fever, throat infection, respiratory disorders, and abdominal pain
6	Khadiradi Gutika	Treatment of dental, oral, throat, and tonsillar infections
7	Pushyanug Churna	Treatment for bleeding disorders and candidiasis
8	Katphala Taila	Treatment of joint pain
9	Maha Visagarbha Taila	Used for neuromuscular conditions and vata imbalance.
10	Maha Vatagajankusha Rasa	Rheumatoid arthritis, asthma, migraine, cold, cough, and paralysis.

TABLE 17.2
Traditional Uses of Different Parts of *M. esculenta* Plant[25–29]

Plant Part	Traditional Applications
Bark	The bark oil of *M. esculenta* is used to treat earache[32] and acts as a fish poison.[29] Bark decoction with *Quercus lanata* bark is used to cure dysentery and applied as a poultice to cure sprains.[26]
	Bark powder with ginger paste is used as a rubefacient and to treat cholera. Its juice is externally applied to heal wounds and cuts, while internally it is used to cure headaches and catarrh.[26]
Flowers	Oil from flowers of *M. esculenta* is useful in earache, diarrhea, paralysis, and inflammation.[12,32,38]
Fruits	Fruits are claimed to act as an antiulcer, carminative, sedative, and stomachic agents,[26,48] and are used to treat abdominal tumors, irregular bowel function, asthma, piles, fever, anemia, nausea, oral disorders, dyspnea, and cough.[32] Fruits are useful for retaining placenta and bone fractures.[49] The juice of the unripe fruit is used as an anthelmintic.[26] Fruit oil or wax is used to cure toothache, menstrual disorders, bleeding piles, and menorrhagia.[49]
	Fruits have been reported to be used as antirheumatic, antiseptic, astringent, carminative, and stimulant.[49]
	Fruits are used to treat chronic bronchitis, abdominal tumors, fever, piles, asthma, ulcers, anemia, dysentery, indigestion, nausea, oral disorders, diarrhea, cough, dyspnea, anorexia, and ENT (ear, nose, and throat) disorders.[32,48,49]
Roots	Roots are used to treat asthma, bronchitis, cholera, and cough.[50]

ulcers, asthma, and chronic cough,[37] and powdered bark is inhaled to cure headaches.[38] The decoction of the bark is used to cure toothache and as a mouth freshener in the sub-Himalayan region.[39] The paste of barks is applied to joint pains, wounds, and paralysis, and is also used to cure colds and headaches.[40,41] Fruit juice is used to treat bacterial dysentery by tribals of Meghalaya, India, and fruits are eaten raw or used to prepare refreshing drinks.[42–44] Its bark is used for washing putrid sores and is chewed to relieve toothache.[45] Leaves paste is applied externally by the local tribe of Uttarakhand, India, to cure headaches.[46] *M. esculenta* has been a well-recognized medicinal plant (Table 17.2)[25–29] since the era of Ayurveda and Unani systems of medicine.[47–49]

Kabra et al. have described the ethnomedicinal uses of the *M. esculenta* plant for making jam, squash, and syrup. The bark of *M. esculenta* is used by the Khasi tribe of Meghalaya for fish poison, and its tannin is used as a tanning and dyeing agent. In Arunachal Pradesh, local people use the *M. esculenta* tree for fuel and timber.[51]

PHYTOCHEMISTRY OF THE *M. ESCULENTA*

Molecular knowledge has an impact on the utilization pattern of the *M. esculenta* plant. Different bioactive compounds, such as tannins, volatile oils, glycosides, saponins, terpenoids, alkaloids, and flavonoids, have been reported to have pharmacological effects.[51] A light-yellow crystalline compound, myricetin is extracted from members of the family Myricaceae[52] and is a key ingredient in many foods, used as a food additive due to its known antioxidant activity and ability to protect lipids from oxidation.[53] Myricetin was first isolated from the bark of *Myrica nagi* (currently known as *M. esculenta*) harvested in India, and it is used as an ingredient in various foods and beverages. Myricetin has potent antidiabetic, anti-inflammatory, anticancer, and antioxidant effects and has been reported to protect a wide variety of cells from in vitro and in vivo lesions.[54,55] Myricetin has been reported as neuroprotective and used to treat Parkinson's disease and Alzheimer's disease. It extends the shelf life of foods rich in oils and fats, and its ability is associated with protecting lipids against oxidation.[51]

Though myricetin occurs throughout the plant kingdom, plants from the families Myricaceae, Anacardiaceae, Polygonaceae, Pinaceae, and Primulaceae have a higher concentration of myricetin.[51] Myricetin, a phenolic compound, is common in vegetables, berries, and beverages (i.e., teas, wines, etc.) produced from various plants, in both the free and its glycoside forms. It is poorly soluble in water but dissolves rapidly in alkaline aqueous media. It has solubility with dimethylformamide, dimethylacetamide, tetrahydrofuran, and acetone.[56] It is most stable at pH = 2, but its degradation is pH- and temperature-dependent. It was first isolated from the bark of a plant harvested in India.[54] Its melting point is 357°C, and it is used in various derivatives such as ethyl, methyl, potassium, and bromo compounds.[57]

Myricetin is structurally related to quercetin, morin, kaempferol, and fisetin, the well-known phenolic compounds. The compound is sometimes referred to as hydroxyl-quercetin. The nutraceutical and antioxidant properties of myricetin are based on scientific evidence and claims for pharmacological activities such as analgesic, anti-inflammatory, antitumor, antidiabetic, and hepatoprotective applications.[58]

Myricetin has activity against several RNA polymerases, DNA polymerases, reverse transcriptases, telomerases, kinases, and helicases. Myricetin acts through additive or synergistic interactions in combination with other bioactive compounds.[59] It has a peripheral analgesic effect, and folk application of the *M. esculenta* plant is supported to cure pain and inflammation.[60] There is scope to develop an anti-inflammatory and analgesic drug based on the results from various in vivo studies of myricetin. Myricetin has been reported to decompose DNA, carbohydrates, and other non-lipid compounds present in food.[61] Hakkinen et al. have reported stability concerns at high temperatures and sensitivity to pH.[62] Intraperitoneal administration of myricetin at a dose of 1,000 mg/kg b.w. to mice did not reveal any fatalities or toxic effects.[63] Myricetin had no toxicity at doses above 100 mg/kg (LD_{50} value) in zebrafish larvae induced by UVB-generated ROS.[64] As it is nontoxic, it can be used to protect stored food grains.[65]

NUTRITIONAL VALUE OF FRUITS

M. esculenta fruits have been reported as a rich source of crude fiber, crude protein, crude fat, crude carbohydrates, and minerals (Ca, Fe, Mg, Na, Zn, Mn, K, Cu) (Table 17.3).[66,67]

TABLE 17.3
Chemical Composition of Fruits of *M. esculenta*[66,67]

Parameters	Value
Ash (%)	2.18 ± 0.02
Moisture content (%)	72.33 ± 0.23
Crude fat (%)	4.93 ± 0.06
Crude fiber (%)	5.22 ± 0.08
Crude protein (%)	9.62 ± 0.03
Carbohydrates (%)	78.03 ± 0.14
Energy (kcal/g)	395.04 ± 0.54
Minerals (mg/g):	
Calcium	4.63 ± 0.06
Magnesium	8.4 ± 0.20
Potassium	7.75 ± 0.11
Phosphorus	0.24 ± 0.25
Sodium	0.81 ± 0.013
Manganese	0.032 ± 0.0001
Zinc	0.216 ± 0.0016
Iron	0.404 ± 0.0021
Copper	0.004 ± 0.0002

PHARMACOLOGY

Various phytochemical investigations have been carried out on the bark, leaves, and fruits of *M. esculenta*, revealing the presence of different chemical classes as bioactives, including alkaloids, glycosides, steroids, saponins, triterpenoids, and volatile compounds. The traditional uses of *M. esculenta* have inspired researchers to investigate and verify its utility through pharmacological screening. Different extracts from various parts of the plant and purified bioactive compounds have been investigated for different biological activities, including analgesic, anti-asthmatic, anticancer, anti-inflammatory, antioxidant, antidiabetic, antiulcer, hepatoprotective, anxiolytic, chemopreventive, wound-healing, and hypotensive effects, by several in vitro and in vivo animal models for authentication of the traditional utilities of *M. esculenta* scientifically.

Pant et al. have reported the analgesic properties of methanol extract of *M. esculenta* fruits on oral feeding.[68] The ethyl acetate soluble fraction of the methanolic extract of leaves has a significant analgesic effect,[69] while the methanol extract of leaves has 54.56% inhibition at a dose of 200 mg/kg.[70]

The phytoconstituents of *M. esculenta* have a wide range of pharmacological effects. Kabra et al. have developed the HPTLC fingerprints of different extracts from several parts of the *M. esculenta* plant.[34,51] Extracts of stem, bark, and fine branches using n-hexane [mobile phase; toluene:ethyl acetate (5:5 v/v)], ethyl acetate [mobile phase; toluene:ethyl acetate (7:3 v/v)], and ethanol [mobile phase; toluene:ethyl acetate:formic acid (5:5:0.5 v/v)] were analyzed using HPTLC,[34] while for ethyl acetate, methanol, and water extracts of leaves, the mobile phase was toluene:ethyl acetate (7:3 v/v).[71]

M. esculenta bark has gallic acid, epigallocatechin-(4β→8)-epigallocatechin3-O-gallate, epigallocatechin-3-O-gallate, 3-O-galloyl-epigallocatechin-(4β→8)-epigalloc-atechin3-O-gallate, and castalagin. Reversed-phase high-performance liquid chromatography analysis of fruit extract deciphers the presence of chlorogenic acid, ρ-coumaric acids, catechin, and gallic acid. Leaves of *M. esculenta* are reported to contain 3-hydroxy-benzaldehyde, ethyl-β-D-glucopyranoside, isovanillin, 4-(hydroxymethyl)-phenol, and 4-methoxy benzoic acid. LC-MS analysis of fruit extract reveals the presence of other bioactive compounds, such as ferulic acids and gallic acid.[34]

Monoterpenoids from the leaves and triterpenoids in barks and leaves of *M. esculenta* have been reported.[34] The volatile compounds identified in the leaves are nerolidol, β-caryophyllene, α-pinene, β-selinen, α-selinene, α-cadinol, α-caryophyllene, and linalool. The bark contains volatile compounds such as eudesmol acetate, n-hexadecanol, and n-octadecanol.In the bark, the volatile compounds are eudesmol acetate, n-hexadecanol, and n-octadecanol.[35] *M. esculenta* barks have pro-anthocyanidins (proanthocyanidin methyl ether, proanthocyanidin acetate, and prodelphinidin).[35] *M. esculenta* roots, leaves, and bark have myricanone and myricanol.[35] β-sitosterol-β-D-glucopyranoside and β-rosasterol have been reported in leaves, whereas stigmasterol and taraxerol are present in bark. Both leaves and bark of *M. esculenta* have been reported to contain β-sitosterol.[35]

Phenolic compounds prevent oxidative losses and have adaptogen, cytoprotective, and anti-inflammatory properties. Herbals rich in phenolic compounds have a promising potential to treat degenerative ailments due to the ability to eliminate hydroxyl radicals,[72] superoxide anion radicals,[73] lipid peroxyl radicals,[74] and even chelate metals. Phenolic compounds have a vital role in the strong defense mechanisms of biological systems and the stability of food products. Extracts from *M. esculenta* are rich in phenolic compounds.

Different investigations have revealed that methanolic extract of *M. esculenta* leaves is not lethal at a 300 mg/kg dose on oral administration for 2 weeks. In Wistar rats, a dose of methanol extract at 2000 mg/kg has been noted for a lethal impact.[75] Extracts of *M. esculenta* bark in ethyl acetate and water have an LD_{50} dose of 1,000 mg/kg in mice.[76]

CURRENT STATUS AND SCOPE FOR BIOTECH INTERVENTION

Due to extreme overuse of the *M. esculenta* plant, its limited geographic dominance and seed germination are under threat.[37] Currently, the demolition of the plant is hundreds of times faster compared to the natural rate of elimination.[77] *M. esculenta* is most often used in traditional medication, and its use in domestic applications has led to an exceptional decline in population.[78] Although many studies have investigated its chemical constituents and pharmacological activity, the mechanisms of action and the metabolites responsible for these activities require study in more detail.

Myricetin, a principal ingredient of *M. esculenta* fruits, requires more study for diabetes and neuro-diseases. A detailed search of the existing literature reveals that it is an important molecule, and in the era of COVID-19, there is a need to focus studies related to its structure–activity relationships and mechanisms of action in various biological processes. *M. esculenta* is beneficial in diseased conditions as well as maintaining proper health, and it has an endangered stigma, so prompt attention is needed to protect the species from extinction.

REFERENCES

1. Prashar Y, Patel N J. 2018. A review on Myrica nagi: Approach in recognizing the overall potential of the plant.. *Research Journal of Life Science, Bioinformatics, and Chemical Science..* 4(6): 217. doi:10.26479/2018.0406.16.
2. Yanthan M, Misra AK. 2013. Molecular approach to the classification of medicinally important actinorhizal genus Myrica. *Indian Journal of* Biotechnology. 12: 133–136.
3. Lutzow-Felling C, Gardner DE, Markin GP, Smith CW. 1995. *Myrica faya: Review of the Biology, Ecology, Distribution, and Control, Including an Annotated Bibliography.* Cooperative National Park Resources Studies Unit, University of Hawaii, Honolulu, Hawaii.
4. https://www.gardenia.net/plant/morella-cerifera.
5. Gathercoal EN, Wirth EH. 1943. *Pharmacognosy*, 2nd Edition. Lea & Febiger, Philadelphia.
6. Singh J, Lan VK, Trivedi VP. 1986. Pharmacognostic evaluation of Katphala (The bark of *Myrica esculenta* Buch–Ham). *Ancient Science of Life*. 6: 85–87.
7. Kumar A, Rana AC. 2013. Pharmacognostic and pharmacological profile of traditional medicinal plant: *Myrica nagi*. *International Research Journal of Pharmacy*. 3: 32–37.
8. Sun C, Huang H, Xu C, Li X, Chen K. 2013. Biological activities of extracts from Chinese bayberry (*Myrica rubra* Sieb. et Zucc.): a review. *Plant Foods for Human Nutrition*. 68: 97–106.
9. Silva BJC, Seca AML, Barreto CMD, Pinto DCGA. 2015. Recent breakthroughs in the antioxidant and anti-Inflammatory effects of *Morella* and *Myrica* species. *International Journal of Molecular Science* 16: 17160–1780.
10. Haridasan K, Rao RR. 1987. *Forest Flora of Meghalaya. Caprifoliaceae to Salicaceae.* Bishen Singh Mahendra Pal Singh, Dehradun (India).
11. Maikhuri RK, Semwal RL, Singh A, Nautiyal MC. 1994. Wild fruits as a contribution to sustainable rural development: a case study from the Garhwal Himalaya. *International Journal of Sustainable Development & World Ecology*. 1: 56–68.
12. Parmar C, Kaushal MK. 1982. *Myrica nagi*. In: *Wild Fruits of the Sub-Himalayan Region*. Parmar C., Kaushal M. K., (Eds.) Kalyani Publishers, New Delhi. pp. 49–53.
13. Dhani A. 2013. Major wild edible fruits used by locals of Garhwal Himalaya. *International Journal of Advancement in Life Sciences*. 6: 145–149.
14. Ksanbok M, Lynser MB, Pala KHM. 2014. Marketing of indigenous fruits: a source of income among Khasi women of Meghalaya, Northeast India. *Journal of Agricultural Science*. 4 (5): 1–9.
15. Panthari P, Kharkwal H, Kharkwal H, Joshi DD. 2012. *Myrica nagi*: a review on active constituents, biological and therapeutic effects. *International Journal of Pharmacy and Pharmaceutical Science*. 4:38–42.
16. Dollo M, Samal PK, Sundriyal RC, Kumar K. 2009. Environmentally sustainable traditional natural resource management and conservation in Ziro valley, Arunachal Himalaya, India. *Journal of American* Science. 5: 41–52.

17. Kumar JK, Sinha AK. 2004. Resurgence of natural colorants: a holistic view. *Natural Product* Research. 18: 59–84.
18. Jeeva S, Lyndem FB, Sawian JT, Laloo RC, Mishra BP. 2011. *Myrica esculenta* Buch-Ham. ex D. Don – A potential ethnomedicinal species in a subtropical forest of Meghalaya, northeast India. *Asian Pacific Journal of Tropical Biomedicine*. 1: S174–S177.
19. Pandey G, Sharma BD, Hore DK, Rao NK.1993.Indigenous minor fruits genetic resources and their marketing status in north-eastern hills of India. *Journal of Hill Research*. 6: 1–4.
20. Mallya SV, Nesari T, Sunil KN. 2016. Pharmacognostic standards of Katphala *(Myrica nagi* Hook.f.non-Thumb); A potent bark drug used in Indian systems of medicine. *Journal of Scientific and Innovative Research*. 5 (4): 135–137.
21. Sood P, Shri R. 2018. A review on ethnomedicinal, phytochemical and pharmacological aspects of *Myrica esculenta*. *Indian Journal of Pharmaceutical Sciences*. 80:2–13.
22. Bhatt ID, Dhar U. 2004. Factors controlling micropropagation of *Myrica esculenta* Buch-Ham. exD.Don: a high value wild edible of Kumaun Himalaya. *African Journal of Biotechnology*. 3: 534–540.
23. Bao J, Cai Y, Sun M, Wang G, Corke H. 2005. Anthocyanins, flavonols, and free radical scavenging activity of Chinese Bayberry (*Myrica rubra*) extracts and their color properties and stability. *Journal of Agricultural and Food Chemistry*. 53: 2327–2332.
24. Anonymous. 1999. *The Ayurvedic Pharmacopoeia of India, Part I*, 1st Edition. Government of India, Ministry of Health and Family Welfare, Department of Indian System of Medicine, and Homeopathy: New Delhi, India. Vol. III. pp. 92–93.
25. Chauhan, NS. 1999. *Medicinal and Aromatic Plants of Himachal Pradesh*. Indus Publishing Company, New Delhi. pp. 226.
26. Nainwal P, Kalra K. 2009. Study on the wound activity potential on the aqueous extract of the bark of *Myrica esculenta* Buch. & Ham. *International Journal of Pharmaceutical and Clinical Research*. 1: 85–87.
27. Rastogi RP, Mehrotra BN. 1995. *Compendium of Indian Medicinal Plants*, 4th Edition. Council of Scientific and Industrial Research Publication, New Delhi. pp. 490–492.
28. Chopra RN, Nayar SL, Chopra IC. 1986. *Glossary of Indian Medicinal Plants (Including the Supplement)*, 3rd Edition. Council of Scientific and Industrial Research Publication, New Delhi. pp. 203.
29. Pala NA, Negi AK, Todaria NP. 2019. Traditional uses of medicinal plants of Pauri Garhwal, Uttarakhand. *Natural Science*. 8: 57–61.
30. Mishra RN. 2011. Rasayan-the ayurvedic perspective. *Research Journal of Pharmaceutical, Biological and Che mical Sciences*. 2: 269–282.
31. Suresh P, Dhannapunei VK. 2007. *Rasendra Sara Sangrah of Sri Gopal Krishna Bhatt*, 1st Edition. Chaukhambha Sanskrit Sansthan, Varanasi.
32. Anonymous. 2007. *Ayurvedic Pharmacopoeia of India. Part* 1, V*ol* III. Ministry of Health and Family Welfare, Department of Indian System of Medicine and Homeopathy, New Delhi. pp. 90–96.
33. Pandey MM, Rastogi S, Khatoon S, Mehrotra S, Rawat AKS. 2013. Evaluation of Ayurvedic compound formulation 5-Katphaladi Churna. *Indian Journal of Traditional Knowledge*. 12: 295–299.
34. Kala CP. 2007. Prioritization of cultivated and wild edibles by local people in the Uttaranchal hills of Indian Himalaya. *Indian Journal of Traditional Knowledge*. 6: 239–243.
35. Srivastava B, Sharma VC, Pant P, Pandey NK, Jadhav AD. 2016. Evaluation for substitution of stem bark with small branches of *Myrica esculenta* for medicinal use-A comparative phytochemical study. *Journal of Ayurveda and Integrative Medicine*. 7: 218–223.
36. Gusain YS, Khanduri VP. 2016. *Myrica esculenta* wild edible fruit of Indian Himalaya: need a sustainable approach for indigenous utilization. *Ecology, Environment and Conservation*. 22: S267–270
37. Gangwar KK, Deepali GRS. 2010. Ethnomedicinal plant diversity in Kumaun Himalaya of Uttarakhand, India. *Nature and Science*. 8: 66–78.
38. Kumari P, Joshi GC, Tewari LM. 2011. Diversity and status of ethnomedicinal trees of Almora district in Uttarakhand, India. *International Journal of. Biodiversity and Conservation*. 3: 298–326.
39. Pandey NC, Joshi GC, Tiwari LM. 2016. Ethnobotanical plant diversity of Betalghat region, Kumaun Himalaya. Biolife. 4: 629–649.
40. Arya D, Khan AH, Adhikari M. 2014. Plant species used by locals as ethno-medicine in Kumaun region of Western Himalaya (India). *International Journal of Pharma Sciences and Research*. 5: 3128–3132.
41. Khan MY, Sagrawat H, Upmanyu N, Siddique S. 2008. Anxiolytic properties of *Myrica nagi* bark extract. *Pharmaceutical Biology*. 46: 757–761.
42. Maikhuri RK, Gangwar AK. 1993. Ethnobiological notes on the Khasi and Garo tribes of Meghalaya, Northeast India. *Economic Botany*. 47: 345–357.
43. Kayang H. 2007. Tribal Knowledge on wild edible plants of Meghalaya, Northeast India. *Indian Journal of Traditional Knowledge*. 6: 177–181.
44. Laloo D, Hemalatha S. 2011. Ethnomedicinal plants used for diarrhea by tribals of Meghalaya, Northeast India. *Pharmacognosy* Reviews. 5: 147–154.
45. Laloo RC, Kharlukhi L, Jeeva S, Mishra BP. 2006. Status of medicinal plants in the disturbed and the undisturbed sacred forests of Meghalaya, Northeast India: population structure and regeneration efficacy of some important species. *Current Science*. 90: 225–232.
46. Bhatt UVP, Negi GCS. 2006. Ethnomedicinal plant resources of Jaunsari tribe of Garhwal Himalaya. *Indian Journal of Traditional Knowledge*. 5: 331–335.
47. Chatterjee A, Pakrashi SC. 1994. *The Treatise on Indian Medicinal Plants*. : Publications and Information Directorate, New Delhi. Vol I. pp. 32–33.
48. Kirtikar KR, Basu BD. 1999. *Indian Medicinal Plants*, 2nd Edition. International Book Distributors, New Delhi. Vol. III. pp. 1699.
49. Nadkarni KM. 2002. *Indian Materia Medica*, 3rd Edition. Popular Book Depot, Mumbai. pp. 871.
50. 2007. Database on Medicinal Plants used in Ayurveda and Siddha. Volume VIII: CCRAS: New Delhi, India. p. 207.
51. Kabra A, Martins N, Sharma R, Kabra R, Baghel US. 2019. *Myrica esculenta* Buch-Ham. ex D. Don: a natural source for health promotion and disease prevention. *Plants*. 8: 149. https://doi.org 10.3390/plants8060149
52. Jones JR, Lebar MD, Jinwal UK, Abisambra JF, Koren J, Blair L, O'Leary JC, Davey Z, Trotter J, Johnson AG. 2011. The diarylheptanoid (+)-aR,11S-myricanol and two flavones from bayberry (*Myrica cerifera*) destabilize the microtubule-associated protein tau. *Journal of Natural Products*. 74: 38–44.

53. Semwal DK, Semwal R B. Combrinck S, Viljoen A. 2016. Myricetin; A dietary molecule with diverse biological activities. *Nutrients*. 8: 90.
54. Perkin AG, Hummel JJ. 1896. The coloring principle obtained in the bark of *Myrica nagi*. Part I. *Journal of the Chemical Society, Transactions*. 69: 1287–1294.
55. Zhang X, Zhang K, Wang Y, Ma R. 2020. Effect of myricitrin and relevant molecular mechanism. *Curr Stem Cell Res Ther*. 15(1): 11–17. doi: 10.2174/1574888X14666181126103338.
56. Yao Y, Lin G, Xie Y, Ma P, Li G, Meng Q, Wu T. 2014. Pre-formulation studies of myricetin: a natural antioxidant flavonoid. *Pharmazie*. 69: 19–26.
57. Perkin AG. 1902. Myricetin. Part II. *Journal of the Chemical Society, Transactions*. 81: 203–210.
58. Lin G B, Xie Y, Li GW. 2012. Research advances of myricetin. *Journal of International Pharmaceutical Research*. 39: 483–487.
59. Lin R D, Chin YP, Lee M H. 2005. Antimicrobial activity of antibiotics in combination with natural flavonoids against clinical extended-spectrum β-lactamase (ESBL)-producing Klebsiella pneumonia. *Phytotherapy Research*. 19: 612–617.
60. Song Y, Zhang YM, Xu J, Hua R. 2015. Periphery analgesic effect of myricetin on a rat model of inflammatory pain. *Chinese Pharmacological Bulletin*. 31: 1108–1111.
61. Smith C, Halliwell B, Aruoma OI. 1992. Protection by albumin against the pro-oxidant actions of phenolic dietary components. *Food and Chemical Toxicology*. 30: 483–489.
62. Hakkinen SH, Karenlampi SO, Mykkanen HM, Torronen AR. 2000. Influence of domestic processing and storage on flavonol contents in berries. *Journal of Agricultural and Food Chemistry*. 48: 2960–2965.
63. Yang Y, Choi JK, Jung CH, Koh HJ, Heo P, Shin JY, Kim S, Park WS, Shin HJ, Kweon DH. 2012. SNARE-wedging polyphenols as small molecular botox. *Planta Medica*. 78: 233–236.
64. Chen YH, Yang ZS, Wen CC, Chang YS, Wang BC, Hsiao CA, Shih TL. 2012. Evaluation of the structure-activity relationship of flavonoids as antioxidants and toxicants of zebrafish larvae. *Food Chemistry*. 134: 717–724.
65. Canada AT, Watkins WD, Nguyen TD. 1989. The toxicity of flavonoids to guinea pig enterocytes. *Toxicology and Applied Pharmacology*. 99: 357–361.
66. Seal T. 2011. Nutritional composition of wild edible fruits in Meghalaya state of India and their ethnobotanical Importance. *Research Journal of Botany*. 6: 58–67.
67. Chandra S, Saklani S, Mishra AP, Badoni PP. 2012. Nutritional evaluation, antimicrobial activity and phytochemical screening of wild edible fruit of *Myrica nagi* pulp. *International Journal of Pharmaceutical Sciences*. 4: 407–411.
68. Pant G, Prakash O, Chandra M, Sethi S, Punetha H, Dixit S, et al. 2014. Biochemical analysis, pharmacological activity, antifungal activity and mineral analysis in methanol extracts of *Myrica esculenta* and *Syzygium cumini*: the Indian traditional fruits growing in Uttarakhand Himalaya. *Indian Journal of Pharmaceutical and Biological Research*. 2: 26–34.
69. Pundir S, Tomar S, Upadhyay N, Sharma V. 2015. Antioxidant, anti-inflammatory and analgesic activity of bioactive fraction of leaves of *Myrica esculenta* Buch-Ham along with its pharmacognostic and chromatographic evaluation. *International Journal of Biology, Pharmacy and Al lied Sciences*. 4: 6509–6524.
70. Middha SK, Kumar GA, Talambedu U, Babu D, Misra AK, Prakash L. 2016. Evaluation of antioxidative, analgesic and anti-inflammatory activities of methanolic extract of *Myrica nagi* leaves – an animal model approach. Symbiosis. 13: 179–184.
71. Kabra A, Sharma R, Singla S, Kabra R, Baghel US. 2017. Pharmacognostic characterization of *Myrica esculenta* leaves. *Journal of Ayurveda and Integrative Medicine*. 10: 18–24.
72. Husain SR, Cillard J, Cillard P. 1987. Hydroxyl radical scavenging activity of flavonoids. *Phytochemistry*. 26: 2489–2491.
73. Afanaslev IB, Dorozhko A I, Bordskii AV. 1989. Chelating and free radicals scavenging mechanisms of inhibitory action of rutin and quercetin in lipid peroxidation. *Biochemical Pharmacology*. 38: 1763–1769.
74. Torel J, Cillard J, Cillard P. 1986. Antioxidant activity of flavonoids and reactivity with peroxy radical. *Phytochemistry*. 25: 383–385.
75. Patel T, Ladani K, Shah S. 2013. Anti-asthmatic activity of aqueous extract of *Myrica nagi* bark. *International Journal of Phytopharmacy Research*. 4: 40–45.
76. Patel KG, Bhalodia PN, Patel AD, Patel KV, Gandhi TR. 2008. Evaluation of bronchodilator and anti-anphylactic activity of *Myrica sapida*. *Iran Biomedical Journal*. 12: 191–196.
77. Rawal RS, Pandey B, Dhar U. 2003. Himalayan Forest Database-Thinking beyond dominants. *Current Science*. 84: 990–994.
78. Chapin FS, Zavaleta ES, Eviner VT, Naylor RL, Vitousek PM, Reynolds HL, Hooper DU, Lavorel S, Sala OE, Hobbie SE, Mack MC. 2000. Consequences of changing biodiversity. *Nature*. 405: 234–242.

18 *Nyctanthes arbor-tristis* (Patijat/Harsingar/Night Jasmine)

INTRODUCTION

Nyctanthes arbor-tristis Linn. (fam.: Oleaceae) is a fabulous plant rich in therapeutic ingredients, commonly known as night jasmine (English), har parijat (Sanskrit), and singhar (Hindi).[1] *N. arbor-tristis* is a native of India. It is flourishing wild in sub-Himalayan regions ranging from the Chenab to Nepal, Myanmar, Bengal, Assam, parts of central India (Madhya Pradesh, Rajasthan, and Chhattisgarh), and southwards to Godavari. It has highly fragrant flowers, so it is cultivated in many parts of India. The flowers of *N. arbor-tristis* open in the evening and drop at sunrise. In its natural habitat, it grows gregariously and covers dry, deep hillsides and rocky gardens.[2–4] The name *Nyctanthes* is derived from the Greek words 'Nykhta' and 'anthos' and means 'Night Flowering', and arbor-tristis means 'the sad tree', as it loses its brightness during the daytime. *N. arbor-tristis* is a shrub or small tree (10 m in height) with greenish or rough gray bark, and young branches are sharply quadrangular (Figure 18.1).[5] The fruit is heart-shaped to round, about 2 cm in diameter, with two sections, each containing a single seed. Its flowering season is from late September to December.[1] *N. arbor-tristis* plant is often planted near temples in India, Indonesia, Malaysia, and Sri Lanka.[1] Different Ayurvedic texts (Samhitas and Nighantus) have described the broad-spectrum medicinal uses of *N. arbor-tristis* and its different actions as medicine (Oushadhi) in detail. It is easily propagated through seeds and vegetative means.[1] Usually, it grows in black and red soils, with a pH of 5.6–7.5, and arid and semi-arid climatic conditions are most suitable.[6]

ETHNOBOTANY

N. arbor-tristis is an important medicinal plant that has had many medicinal uses since ancient times. Different parts of the plant have been used as folk and traditional medicines. It is utilized in Ayurveda, Siddha, and Unani systems of medicine as an antivenom, laxative, diuretic, digestive, tonic, expectorant, and mild bitter.[7] It has been used in folk medicine for antibilious, gynecological troubles and hepatoprotective activity since ancient times.[8] In central India, the tribal people use the various parts of the plant to relieve cough, hiccup, dysentery, snakebite, and sores.[9] In many parts of India, the leaves of *N. arbor-tristis* are used to cure diseases like malaria fever, diabetes, flu, HIV, and cancer.[10]

The mythological story reveals that the medicinal plant Parijat is a heavenly tree brought to earth by Lord Krishna, and a quarrel associated with its possession between Krishna's wives, Rukmini and Satyabhama. However, Krishna planted the tree in Satyabhama's courtyard in a way that the flowers fell into Rukmini's courtyard.[1] The etymology of Parijat is because of its origin in the ocean (samudra) as a result of extensive searching (paarinaha) (in Sanskrit, 'Paarinaha Samudrath jaatho va Parijatah').[11] Traditional pharmacological properties of Parijat are to cure ailments related to plasma (rasa), mental health (Guna: Sattva, Rajas, and Tamas), potency (virya), and the outcome of the biotransformation (vipaka), are per Ayurvedic literature.[12-14] Different Ayurvedic experts (Acharyas) have described different uses of Parijat, either alone or as an ingredient in multiple herbal formulations.

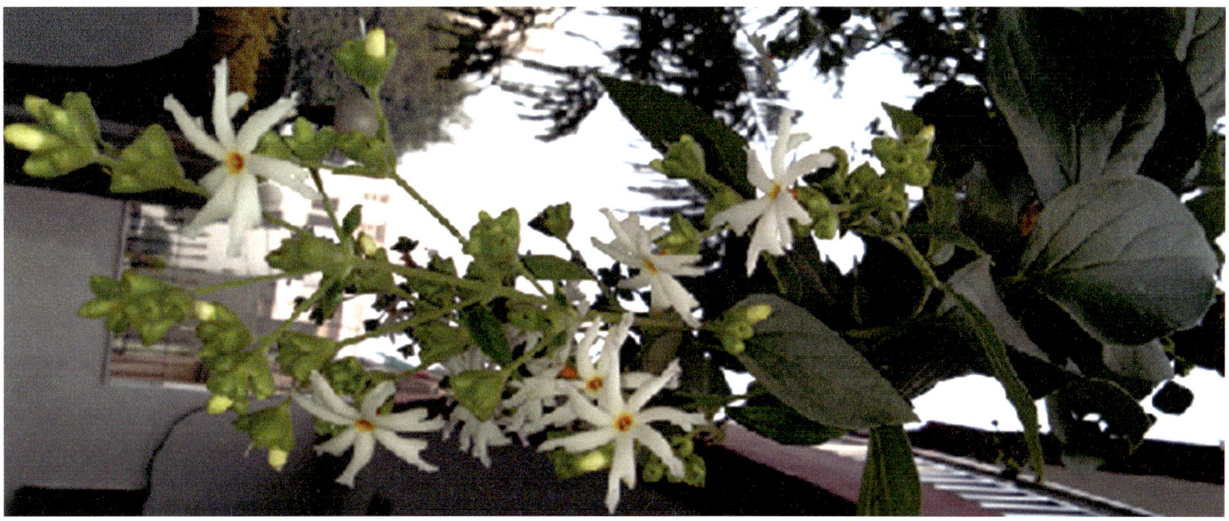

FIGURE 18.1 A branch of *Nyctanthes arbor-tristis* L. (picture at 9.45 pm).

DOI: 10.1201/9781003512868-20

The seed, root, leaf, and flower of Parijat are used in different forms like decoction, powder, juice, etc. to treat various diseases and conditions. It is specifically used to pacify the disease occurring due to vitiation of vata (i.e., dryness of skin, hair, ears, lips, joints, bloat, gas, constipation, dehydration, weight loss, dryness, and a lightness of the mind – restlessness, dizziness, feeling ungrounded, poor circulation, muscle spasm, asthma, pain, and aches) and kapha (increased fluid in the organism, such as in the nose, respiratory system, around the heart, localized in the mouth and tongue, spleen, stomach, nails, and hair).

The leaves of *N. arbor-tristis* are considered antibilious and expectorant. These are useful for treating fevers and rheumatism. The young leaves, when rubbed with ginger and water, are useful for the relief of intermittent fever. A decoction of the leaves, prepared over a gentle fire, is prescribed for sciatica and malaria among the Kondhs of southwestern Orissa and as a blood purifier (in skin disease) and febrifuge among the tribal inhabitants of southern Bihar. The expressed leaf juice is acrid and bitter. The juice is used as a laxative, diaphoretic, and diuretic. The leaf paste is used as an external application to treat ringworm, scabies, and eczema among the rural inhabitants of the Bhavnagar district of Gujarat and in southwestern Bengal. Mixed with honey, fresh leaf juice is taken to relieve chronic fever. The fresh juice of leaves is mixed with sugar and is given to children for the expulsion of intestinal threadworms and roundworms. The bark is used as an expectorant by residents of Konkan (coastal districts of Maharashtra) and in Ayurvedic practice. A decoction of roots, leaves, flowers, and bark is used in Ayurveda for treating enlargement of the spleen and excessive diuresis.[5]

The leaves are thermogenic, bitter, anti-inflammatory, acrid, antibacterial, anodyne, digestive, anthelmintic, depurative, sudorific, diuretic, and used as a tonic. These are used in vitiated conditions of kapha and vata, inflammation, dyspepsia, asthma, cough, pruritis, helminthiasis, constipation, hepatopathy, hemorrhoids, greyness of hair, and baldness. Leaves are also used as an antidote to reptile venom. About 5 grains of the bark are eaten with betel nut and leaf to promote the expectoration of thick phlegm.[5] Although the etymological meaning of the botanical name of Parijat seems to be 'tree of sorrow', for traditional healers, it seems to be a 'tree of joy'. It is a valuable medicinal as well as ornamental plant. In Southeast Asia, the natives have rich traditional medicinal knowledge of 'Parijat' and frequently use the herb to cure many diseases.[5]

Parijat is an integral component of home gardens in the Indian subcontinent. It is a common belief among the natives that the presence of the plant in the home gardens keeps the family tension-free. The natives also plant this herb to reduce the harmful effects of mango trees in home gardens. The natives use the fragrant flowers in many ways, including morning worship (Figure 18.2), either alone or with other flowers. The flowers are strung and worn as hair ornaments and necklaces. An orange-colored dye is obtained from the flowers and is used for coloring silk and cotton. Fresh flowers are added to water to be used for baths, resulting in smooth skin and being free from all skin-related troubles. It is also considered good for hair growth. The natives of Chhattisgarh, India, are very familiar with the folk medicinal uses of all parts of Parijat.[5] They use the seeds in the treatment of piles (Bavasir), typically administering one seed with water, and treatment is continued until

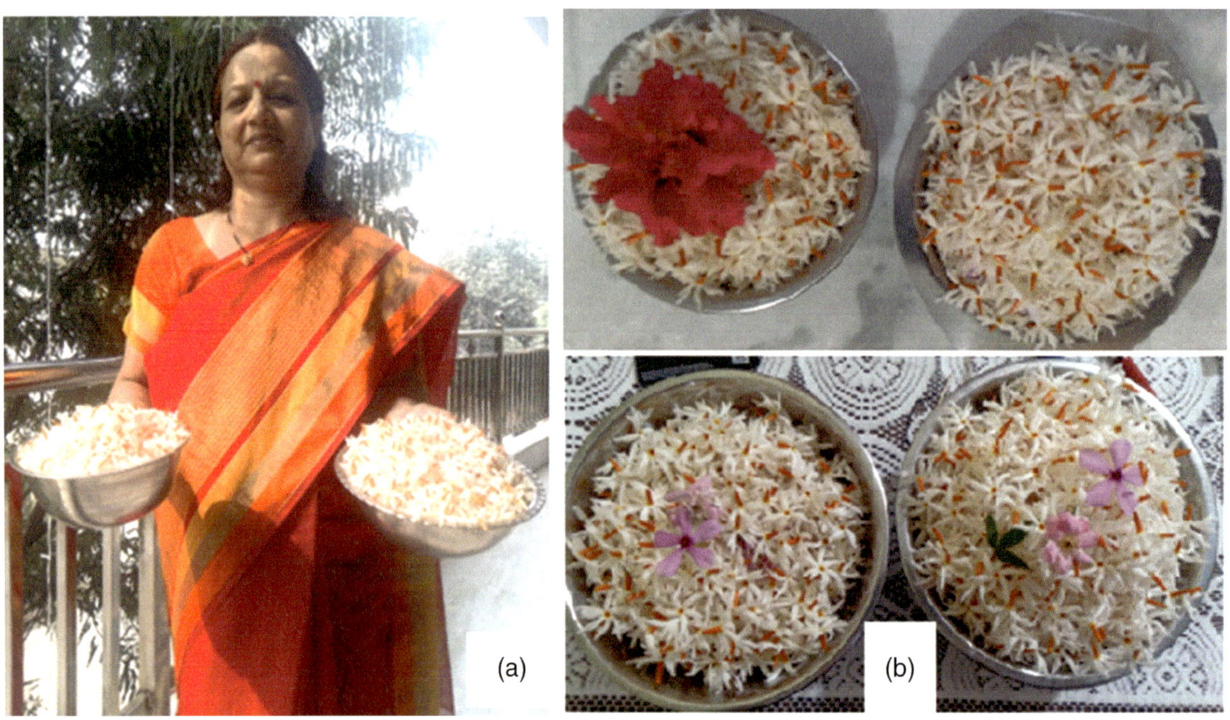

FIGURE 18.2 *N. arbor-tristis* flowers; (a) alone, (b) mixed with other flowers.

complete recovery. An aqueous paste is prepared from the crushed seeds for external applications. The decoction of Parijat flowers is used to treat gout and is prescribed for 1 week during the time of the attack. The juice of leaves with honey is orally used to treat dry cough.[5] The aqueous paste of leaves is applied externally to treat ringworm problems and other skin-related troubles. The natives of the Bastar region, India, prepare herbal oil by boiling fresh leaves in mustard oil (sarson ka tel) and use it externally to treat ringworm problems and skin ailments. The natives of Chhattisgarh use leaf juice with common salt for 7 regular days (once a day) to flush out all worms effectively.[5]

CHEMICAL COMPOSITION OF PARIJAT PLANT

Kiew and Baas have reported that leaves of *N. arbor-tristis* contain nyctanthin, mannitol, ascorbic acid, astringent principles, resinous substances, traces of the oily substance, sugar, and coloring matters.[4] Girach et al.[14] have reported that flowers of *N. arbor-tristis* have nyctanthin (the coloring matter), essential oils, mannitol, glucose, and tannin. The bark contains a glycoside and two alkaloids (one is hydrophilic, and the other one is hydrophobic in nature). *N. arbor-tristis* glycoside increases the amplitude of the frog's heart in small doses, but in higher quantities, the diastolic period is decreased till the heart stops with the A-V block. The *N. arbor-tristis* glycoside acts as a sedative to the CNS. The hydrophilic alkaloid stimulates the ciliary motility of the esophagus, but the hydrophobic alkaloid has no such action.[2]

Mathuram et al. have reported the presence of verbascoside in the leaves.[15] Srivastava et al. have described the presence of new benzoic esters of loganin and 6e-hydroxy-loganin in leaves.[16] Singh et al. have reported the presence of arborside in the leaves of *N. arbor-tristis* and named it O-benzoyl nyctanthoside.[17] 4-hydroxy hexahydrobenzofuran-7-one, a potential cytotoxic benzofuran derivative, has been isolated from flowers, which inhibits the cell growth by 43.27% but is found to have no significant cytotoxic effect on mice. Another benzofuran derivative [3-3a-,7, 7a-tetrahydro 3a-hydroxy-6 (2H) benzofuran] is reported from flowers, having potent antibacterial properties against both Gram-negative and Gram-positive bacteria.[18]

Flowers and leaves of *N. arbor-tristis* have mannitol.[4,19] Mannitol is applied clinically to reduce acutely raised intracranial pressure and is an osmotic diuretic agent. It is a weak renal vasodilator. Flowers and leaves are rich in polyphenolic compounds and are astringent and bitter. These polyphenolic compounds are used either to precipitate or bind and shrink proteins and various other organic compounds, including alkaloids and amino acids. Linoleic acid, an unsaturated omega-6 fatty acid, is beneficial in cystic fibrosis, has moisture-retentive properties, acts as an anti-inflammatory, and is acne-reductive when applied topically on the skin.[1]

In brief, flowers of *N. arbor-tristis* contain D-mannitol, nyctanthin, essential oil, carotenoid, glycosides, glucose, and tannin.[13] The essential oil of flowers consists of phenylacetaldehyde, α-pinene, L-hexanone, P-cymene, and 1-decanol.[13] Seeds contain arbortristoside A, arbortristoside B, glycerides of palmitic, stearic, oleic, linolenic, and myristic acids, nyctanthic acid, and a water-soluble polysaccharide fraction.[13] It also contains nyctanthic acid, ß-sitosterol, and 15% oil of a pale yellow-brown appearance.[13] Leaves of *N. arbor-tristis* have tannic acid, ß-sitosterol, methyl salicylate, ascorbic acid, carotene, nyctanthic acid, glycosides, mannitol, linoleic acid, 6-beta-hydroxyloganin, benzoic acid, triterpenoids, glucose, fructose, flavonol, and volatile oils in traces.[13] The stem of *N. arbor-tristis* has α-xylopyranoside, ß-sitosterols, and B-glucopyranosyl.[13] The *N. arbor-tristis* also has methyl-D-mannose, iridoid glycoside-nyctanthaside, alkaloids, methyl-D-glucose, arbortristoside (A, B, and C), and glycoside.[13]

The chemical classes of therapeutics vary in their properties, as the concentration varies in different parts of the plant; so, the therapeutic behavior also varies, as seen with alkaloids obtained from various plants. Alkaloids have important pharmacological roles such as anticancer, vasodilatory, antimalarial, antiarrhythmic, antiasthma, cholinomimetic, etc.[20] Flavonoids have antiviral, anti-inflammatory, antioxidant, anticancer, and antiallergic properties and are used to cure oxidative stress, wounds (scratches), cancer, inflammation, arteriosclerosis, ischemia, aging, and neurodegenerative disorders. The regular consumption of flavonoids reduces hyperpiesis, the risk of heart-related problems, and cures coronary diseases and mortality.[21]

Mannitol enhances the osmolarity of the glomerular filtrate, limits the tubular consumption of sodium, water, chloride, and other solutes, and promotes diuresis, blood plasma osmolarity, and flow of water from tissues into interstitial fluid and plasma.[22] ß-sitosterol, also known as 'plant sterol ester,' helps to reduce LDL-C (bad cholesterol) levels in the body. ß-sitosterol reduces cholesterol levels by limiting its absorption and has an anti-inflammatory function that binds to the prostate and reduces swelling.[23]

PHARMACOLOGICAL PROPERTIES

N. arbor-tristis plant has anticancer,[24] antiviral,[25] antimicrobial, antifungal,[26] anti-allergy,[27] antidiabetic,[28] anti-cholinesterase,[29] immunostimulant,[19] and hepatoprotective[25] properties effective against several diseases. The plant species has been reported to stimulate the immune system.[30] The leaf juice of the plant is used to cure many body disorders such as piles, loss of appetite and nausea, liver and bile-duct-related disorders, rheumatoid arthritis, obstinate sciatic nerve irritation, and as a diaphoretic. The bark of the *N. arbor-tristis* plant is useful to treat snakebites and asthma problems.[31]

The claimed folklore and traditional medicinal uses of *N. arbor-tristis* have been proved on a scientific basis using in vitro and in vivo investigations. Studies on the ethanolic, aqueous, and hydro-alcoholic extracts of the leaves have established the antibacterial activity against both antibiotic-resistant and non-resistant strains of *Staphylococcus aureus*.[32]

The water-soluble fraction of alcohol extract of leaves has been reported as effective in antihistaminic activity[33] and CNS tranquilizing properties. Ratnasooriya et al. have reported the sedative effect of a hot infusion of flowers of *N. arbor-tristis* in rats, attributing the sedation to antioxidant and membrane-stabilizing effects.[34] Alcoholic extract of the leaves has been reported to help in bypassing silica-induced fibrinogenesis of the lungs of mice.[35] The high phenolic and flavonoid contents and strong reducing power are responsible for the antioxidant activity of the plant species.[36] The powdered seeds of *N. arbor-tristis* are used as an application to relieve dandruff. Among the tribal inhabitants of eastern Bihar, the seed paste is applied for baldness; mixed with honey, the powdered seeds are given in the treatment of malaria.[36]

The young leaves of *N. arbor-tristis* are used as a tonic for patients having gynecological troubles, and they are advised to take three fresh leaves with five black peppers (Kali-Mirch). This combination is recommended up to 3 days a month. The natives of the Bagbahara region use the decoction of Parijat seeds as a hair tonic and wash their hair daily to get rid of dandruff and lice.[35] The natives of the Durg region, specifically from the Patan area, use the leaf juice as a safe purgative for infants, and they also use it in combination with other herbs to treat chronic fevers. The flowers are carminative, astringent, bitter, and stomachic and are used in ophthalmopathy, flatulence, inflammations, colic, greyness of hair, baldness, and dyspepsia.[37]

Due to the presence of numerous phytochemicals, the *N. arbor-tristis* plant exhibits various pharmacological actions, including analgesic, anti-inflammatory, antispasmodic, antiviral, antiallergic, antifungal, antibacterial, antipyretic, immune-modulator, insecticidal, respiratory stimulant, and antimalarial activities. In Malaysia, Indonesia, and India, flowers are used as medicine to provoke menstruation.[13] The bark of *N. arbor-tristis* is used to cure eye diseases and ulcers, and also serves as an expectorant. Bark decoction has been used as a remedy for bleeding gums.[13] The seeds, leaves, and flowers of *N. arbor-tristis* possess hepatoprotective, immune-stimulant, anti-leishmanial, antiviral, and antifungal activities.[13] The fresh leaves are in homeopathic medicines.[13]

COMMERCIAL APPLICATIONS

The *N. arbor-tristis* plant species is cultivated for its flowers, perfumes, and dyes. The dye is also used for coloring cotton cloth and coloring the sacred robes of Buddhist priests, a substitute for saffron. For dyeing, fabrics are immersed in a decoction of the corolla tubes, having alum or lime juice; the resulting color is moderately resistant to soap, light, alkalis, and acid. The stem bark is used as a tanning material, and the leaves are used to polish the ivory and substitute sandpaper to polish wood.[1]

FUTURE SCOPE

N. arbor-tristis is a wonder tree and hub of medicinal properties. There is a wide scope for research professionals to validate its ethnomedicinal applications using modern molecular knowledge and advanced technologies to decipher the mechanisms of action of the different therapeutic ingredients found in the *N. arbor-tristis* plant.

Presently, the COVID-19 crisis reflects the future need for an herbal composition offering higher protection against various infections and a cell-mediated immune system to protect from different viral, bacterial, and fungal infections with no/lower toxic effects. Herbal formulations have very high therapeutic potential with high efficacy, low toxicity, and cost-effectiveness. *N. arbor-tristis, Withania somnifera*, *Tinospora cordifolia*, *Punica granatum*, and others possess excellent anti-inflammatory, antitumor, oxidant-inhibiting, immunomodulatory, and carcinoma-preventive properties. These herbs, due to different therapeutic compounds, secure the body from cumulative damage by oxidation and diseases. Food supplements of herbal origin and/or medicine that help boost the immune system during such a pandemic are equally as needful as a vaccine.

Herbs have been used as medicines and to increase immunity since the prehistoric era to cure several diseases, such as cough, cancer, the common cold, diabetes, malaria, viral fevers, etc. Many types of multi-herbal compositions of plant products (*Withania somnifera*, *Nyctanthes arbor-tristis*, *Ocimum sanctum*, *Curcuma longa*, *Piper nigrum*, etc.) are used by medicine men in Indian villages to cure the aforesaid diseases. Recently, the key role of withanone present in *W. somnifera* in blocking viral replication has been reported, providing strong validation for its traditional application.[38]

In many parts of India, people are using *N. arbor-tristis* leaves to cure many diseases like diabetes, malarial fever, HIV, flu, and cancer. There is scientific support for utilizing the leaves of *N. arbor-tristis* to boost the immunity power.[10] All plant parts of *N. arbor-tristis* have been used for different medicines for more than thousands of years to better health. Due to the broad-spectrum uses of *N. arbor-tristis* in health management, its specifications (identification, morphology, sources, availability, dose, and therapeutic use) are described in all ancient literature. On chemical and phytochemical screening, the plant is reported to have active principles and biomarkers such as ß-sitosterol, nyctanthic acid, tannic acid, linoleic acid, D-mannitol, and oleic acids, which are richly found in the leaves and are responsible for their high therapeutic efficacy. Similarly, multiple active ingredients present in other parts of the plant may contribute to its broad-spectrum therapeutic applications. It is proven that linoleic acid has an anti-inflammatory effect. Overall, *N. arbor-tristis* is a very important herbal medicine now and then, even during the pandemic.

Ayurveda, the world's most ancient healing science, has used herbs and herbals since its inception for both diet and medicine as per need. Ancient medicine men (Acharyas) have felt the enormous therapeutic potential of every plant when used judiciously. *N. arbor-tristis* is a preferred choice to cure certain disease conditions like chronic fever and worm infestations. The plant *N. arbor-tristis* is a rich source of medicinally important phytochemicals and has been widely studied by scientists. So far, most of the research has been conducted on the seeds and leaves of the *N. arbor-tristis* plant, although there are reports about using bark powder and root extract in folk medicine.

The main aim of the present text is to encourage entrepreneurship among youth. As literature reveals, the leaf extract of *N. arbor-tristis* has been extensively studied, but there is also a need to pay attention to the flowers, stem, and unripened green seeds.

REFERENCES

1. Hiremath V, Hiremath BS, Mohapatra S, Das AK. 2016. Literary review of Parijata (*Nyctanthus arbor-tristis* Linn.); An herbal medicament with special reference to Ayurveda and botanical literatures. *Biomedical & Pharmacology Journal*. 9 (3): 1019–1025.
2. Anonymous. 1997. *Wealth of India. A Dictionary of Indian Raw Materials and Industrial Products*. National Institute of Science Communication, CSIR, New Delhi. Vol. VII. pp. 69–70.
3. Kirtikar KR, Basu BD. 2000. *Indian Medicinal Plants*. Sri Satguru Publications, New Delhi. Vol. VII. pp. 2110–2113.
4. Kiew R, Baas P. 1984. *Nyctanthes* is a member of Oleaceae. *Proceedings of the Indian National Science Academy (Plant Science)*. 93 (3): 349–358.
5. Bhosale AV, Abhyankar MM, Pawar SJ, Khan S, Patil N. 2009. *Nyctanthes arbortristis*: A pharmacognostic review. *Research Journal of Pharmacognosy and Phytochemistry*. 1 (2): 91–97.
6. Latha PG, Suja SR, Shyamal S, Rajasekharan S. 2005. Some hepatoprotective garden plants. *Natural Product Radiance*. 4 (4): 278–279.
7. Rangika BS, Dayananda PD, Peiris DC. 2015. Hypoglycemic and hypolipidemic activities of aqueous extract of flowers from *Nyctanthes arbor-tristis* L. in male mice. *BMC Complementary and Alternative Medicine*. 15 (1): 1–9.
8. Kumari TDS, Madhuri TDS, Charya MAS, Rao KS. 2012. Antioxidant and anticancer activities of *Nyctanthes arbor-tristis*. *International Journal of Pharmacy and Pharmaceutical Science*. 4 (4): 452–454.
9. Jain P K, Pandey A. 2016. The wonder of Ayurvedic medicine-*Nyctanthes arbor-tristis*. *International Journal of Herbal Medicine*. 4 (4): 9–17.
10. Mousum SA, Ahmed S, Gawali B, Kwatra M, Ahmed A, Lahkar M. 2018. *Nyctanthes arbor-tristis* leaf extract ameliorates hyperlipidemia- and hyperglycemia-associated nephrotoxicity by improving antioxidant and anti-inflammatory status in high-fat diet–streptozotocin-induced diabetic rats. *Inflammopharmacology*. 26: 1415–1428.
11. Acharya Sharma PV. 2004. *Priya Nighantu*, 1st Edition. Chowkhamba Surabharati Prakashana, Varanasi. Haritakyadi Varga, Verse 190–192. pp. 42/192.
12. Mishra AB. 2006. *Bhava Prakasha Nighantu*, Commentary by Dr. K. C. Chunekar and Ganga Sahay Panday, Guduchyadi Verga, Chowkhamba Bharati Academy, Varanasi. Reprint. pp. 335.
13. Anonymous. 2002. Central Council for Research in Ayurveda and Siddha, *Data Base on Medicinal Plants used in Ayurveda*. Publication Department of CCRAS, Govt. of India. Vol. 4: pp. 470–483
14. Girach R D, Aminuddin S A, Siddiqui PA, Khan SA. 1994. Ethnomedicinal studies on Harsinghar (*Nyctanthes arbor-tristis* L.); A less known medicinal plant in Unani medicine. *Hamdard Medicines*. 37 (2): 60–66.
15. Mathuram V, Rao RB, Haldar S, Banerji A, Kundu AB. 1994. Occurrence of desrhamnosylverbascoside in *Nyctanthes arbortristis* and NMR studies of its acetate. *Indian Journal of Chemical Society*. 71: 215–217.
16. Shrivastav V, Rathor A, Ali S, Tandon JS. 1990. New benzoic esters of loganin and 6ß-hydroxy loganin from *Nyctanthes arbortristis*. *Journal of Natural Products*. 53 (2): 303–308.
17. Singh KL, Roy R, Srivastava V, Tandon JS, Mishra A. 1995. Arborside D; A minor iridoid glucoside from *Nyctanthes arbortristis*. *Journal of Natural Products*. 58 (10): 1562–1564.
18. Khatune NA, Islam Md E, Rahman Md A, Mosaddik Md A, Haque Md E. 2003. In vivo cytotoxic evaluation of a new benzofurane derivative isolated from *Nyctanthes arbortristis* L. on Ehrlich Aschite Carcinoma Cells (EAC) on mice. *Journal of Medical Sciences*. 3(2): 169–173.
19. Rathee JS, Hassarajani SA, Chattopadhyay S. 2007. Antioxidant activity of *Nyctanthes arbor-tristis* leaf extract. *Food Chemistry*. 103: 1350–1357.
20. Lu JJ, Bao JL, Chen XP, Huang M, Wang YT. 2012. Alkaloids isolated from natural herbs as the anticancer agents. *Evidence-Based Complementary and Alternative Medicine*. 2012. https://doi.org/10.1155/2012/485042
21. Shukla R, Pandey V, Vadnere GP, Lodhi S. 2019. Role of Flavonoids in Management of Inflammatory Disorders. In: *Bioactive Food as Dietary Interventions for Arthritis and Related Inflammatory Diseases*, 2nd Edition. Watson R. R., Preedy V. R. (Eds.) Academic Press. pp. 293–322. https://doi.org/10.1016/C2017-0-00605-5
22. Nissenson AR, Weston RE, Kleeman CR. 1979. Mannitol. *Western Journal of Medicine*. 131: 277–284.
23. Valerio M, Awad AB. 2011. β-sitosterol down-regulates some pro-inflammatory signal transduction pathways by increasing the activity of tyrosine phosphatase SHP-1 in J774A.1 murine macrophages. *International Immunopharmacology*. 11: 1012–1017.
24. Shrivastava R, Bharadwaj AK. 2018. *Nyctanthes arbortristis* an important medicinal plant of Madhya Pradesh State-A review. *UK Journal of Pharmaceutical Biosciences*. 6 (6): 10–15.
25. Srivastava P, Trivedi D, Shukla G, Srivastava P. 2018. *Nyctanthes arbor-tristis*: A wonder Indian herbal drug needs healthcare attention. *Biomedical Journal of Scientific & Technical Research*. 5: 4527–4530.
26. Patil M, Khan A. 2015. Antibacterial activity of leaves of *Nyctanthus arbor-tristis* L, *Hibiscus rosa-sinensis* L. and *Sapindus emerginatus* Vahl. *Science Park Research Journal*. 2: 1–5.
27. Kalyana SI, Sarangi DD, Sundararajan V, George S, Sheik MS. 2018. Poly herbal formulation with anti-elastase and antioxidant properties for skin anti-aging. *BMC Complementary and Alternative Medicine*. 18(1): 33. doi: 10.1186/s12906-018-2097-9
28. Mathur C, Gupta R. 2018. A review on medicinal plants of Rajasthan having antidiabetic activity. *Asian Journal of Pharmaceutical and Clinical Research*. 11 (12): 33–39.
29. Pattanayak C, Datt, PP, Chauhan AK, Firdoush KA, Prasad A, Panda P. 2012. Hypoglycemic effect of *Nyctanthes arbor-tristis* leaf extract on alloxan induced diabetic rabbits. *American Journal of PharmTech Research*. 2: 380–387.

30. Godse CS, Tathed PS, Talwalkar SS, Vaidya RA, Amonkar AJ, Vaidy AB, Vaidya ADB. 2016. Antiparasitic and disease-modifying activity of *Nyctanthes arbor-tristis* Linn. in malaria: An exploratory clinical study. *Journal of Ayurveda and Integrative Medicine*. 7: 238–248.
31. Agrawal J, Pal A. 2013. *Nyctanthes arbor-tristis* Linn-A critical ethnopharmacological review. *Journal of Ethnopharmacology*. 146: 645–658.
32. Khandelwal KR, Kadam SS, Singhama SS. 1999. Antibacterial activity of the leaves of *Nyctanthes arbortristis* Linn. *Indian Journal of Natural Products*. 15: 18–20.
33. Saxena RS, Gupta B, Lata S. 2002. Tranquillizing, antihistaminic, and purgative activity of *Nyctanthes arbortristis* leaf extract. *Journal of Ethnopharmacology*. 81 (3): 321–325.
34. Ratnasooriya WD, Jayakody JRAC, Hettiarachchi ADI, Dharmasiri MG. 2005. Sedative effects of hot flower infusions of *Nyctanthes arbortristis* on rats. *Pharmaceutical Biology*. 43 (2): 140–146.
35. Venkatanarasimhan M, Kundu AB, Banerjee S, Patra A. 1991. Occurrence of two new esters of 6-hydroxyloganin in *Nyctanthes arbortristis*. *Journal of Indian Chemical Society*. 68: 581–584.
36. Singh BR. 1991. Structural study of water soluble glucomannan from *Nyctanthes arbortristis* seeds. *Polish Journal of Chemistry*. 65 (2–30): 353–359.
37. Singh BR. 1992. Structure of non-ionic seeds polysaccharide from *Nyctanthes arbortristis*. *Acta Ciencia Indica*. 18 (1): 57–60.
38. Balkrishna A, Pokhrel S, Singh J, Varshney A. 2020. Withanone from *Withania somnifera* may inhibit novel coronavirus (COVID-19) entry by disrupting interactions between viral S-protein receptor binding domain and host ACE2 receptor. *Research Square*. 2020. https://doi.org/10.21203/rs.3.rs-17806/v1

19 *Prunus cerasoides* (Padmaka/Panyyan)

INTRODUCTION

Prunus cerasoides D. Don (Hindi: Padmaka), also called the Himalayan cherry tree, is an Ayurvedic medicinal plant (Figure 19.1). It is distributed mainly in the temperate regions of the northern hemisphere.[1] In India, the species is found in the montane and sub-montane Himalayas (1,500–2,400 MSL) and is abundantly available in hilly zones of Uttarakhand State (Pauri, Chamoli, Uttarkashi, Tehri Garhwal, Champawat, Pithoragarh, and Almora).[2,3]

P. cerasoides is a sacred plant of Hindu culture and is used to cure many body ailments such as asthma, burning sensations, leprosy, leukoderma, erysipelas, etc. Locally, it is known as 'Panyyan' in Uttarakhand.[4] It blooms at the beginning of the winter in certain patches of the hilly regions and imparts a spring-like appearance from October to mid-December with its pinkish-white flowers. The flowers are a rich source of pollen and nectar for bees during a season with minimum flowers, which hardly fulfills the needs of honeybees. Beekeepers have a hard period and are compelled to use artificial feeding for bees;[4] hence, *P. cerasoides* helps beekeepers and checks the starvation of the nearby surrounding *P. cerasoides* plants.

P. cerasoides is a middle-sized plant; horizontal stripes appear on its stem at the bark (Figure 19.2), and peeling off it appears with pale redwood.[4] Its fruits are edible and important food items in traditional diets, rich in nutrients, and a source of therapeutic compounds,[1] more so than conventionally eaten crops.[4] *Prunus*, a genus of trees and shrubs, consists of about 430 species. The family Rosaceae plays a leading role among all temperate fruits of the Northern Hemisphere.[5,6] It produces fleshy fruits, relatively large, with a single hard-coated seed, commonly known as stone fruit.[7] *P. cerasoides* is one of the plants identified as an excellent framework species for

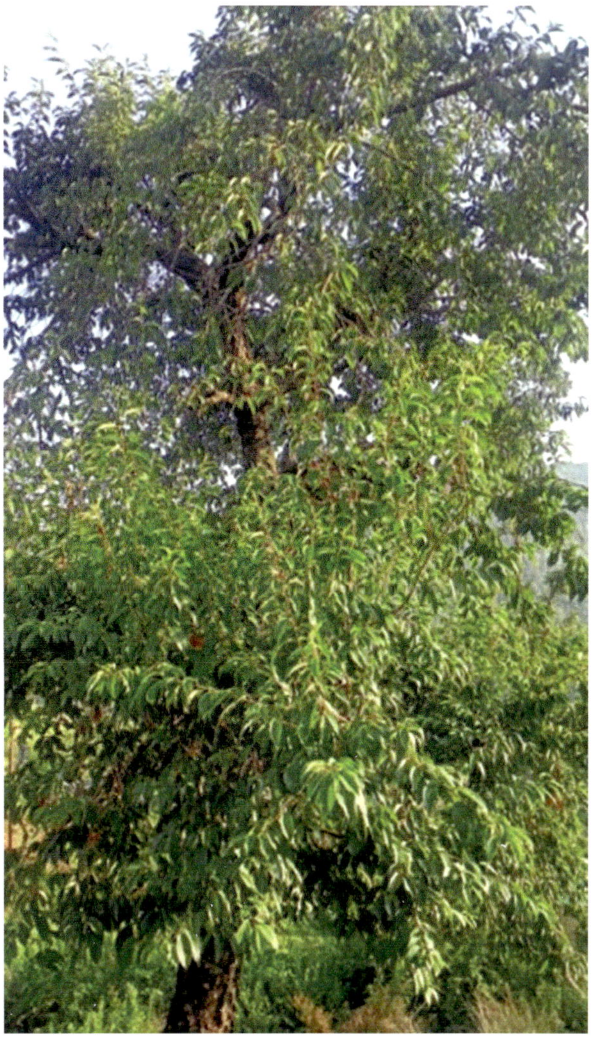

FIGURE 19.1 *P. cerasoides* tree.

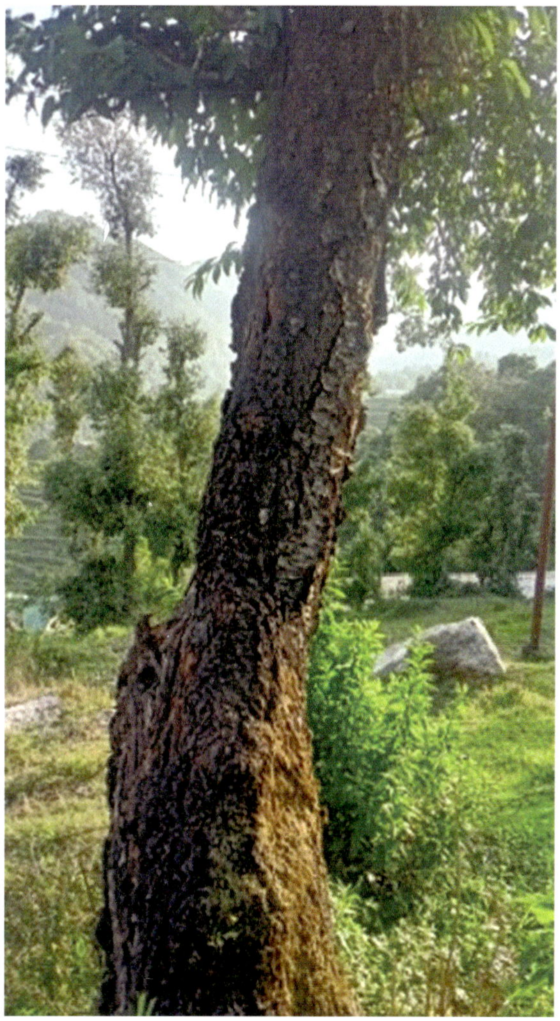

FIGURE 19.2 *P. cerasoides* stem.

DOI: 10.1201/9781003512868-21

restoring evergreen forests in seasonally dry tropical forestlands.[8,9] *P. cerasoides* is a useful plant for the upliftment of low-economic-status local people, as it is one of 31 identified multipurpose species used as a medicinal plant in the Himalayan region.[10] Relevant information and literature on *P. cerasoides* are available in electronic databases such as Google Scholar, Academic Journals, Google, ScienceDirect, Web of Science, etc., covering its ethnomedicinal value, traditional uses, phytopharmacological, and toxicological aspects.

It is worshipped on all auspicious occasions by the Himalayan inhabitants, and they never cut the whole tree. Only the twigs are used in rituals, as the wood is forbidden to be used as fuel or burned; so, adequately, quite old trees of *P. cerasoides* are often found in the Uttarakhand Himalaya.[11] *Prunus* species have been introduced in various parts of the world because of their considerable value as ornamental plants, food, and folk medicine.[2]

ETHNOPHARMACOLOGY

The fruit, seed, and gum of *P. cerasoides* have a range of traditional medicinal applications.[12] Ripped fruits are edible, though occasionally eaten raw due to their astringent taste; they are cooked and used to make cherry brandy and sauces.[13] Both cooked and raw seeds are also eaten. Gum exuding from branches and trunk is chewed and used as a substitute for gum tragacanth, and it is used by honeybees as honeydew.[2] *P. cerasoides* wood is strong, durable, moderately hard, and aromatic, so it is used by locals in several rituals, including ornamental furniture. The root suckers, branches, and wood make excellent walking sticks and umbrella crooks. The young twigs are used as toothbrushes, and leaves are used as fodder.[14] A dark greenish dye is extracted from the fruits, and the leaves are also used as a source of green dye. The bark of *P. cerasoides* is a source of tannins.[15] The seeds are used in rosaries and as beads in necklaces.[3] The tree is mainly used as a rootstock for cherry cultivation and has immense apicultural importance. The flowers are a useful source of bee forage and are rich in pollen and nectar.[16–18] The bark, twigs, leaves, and seed kernels are used medicinally,[19,20] and *P. cerasoides* is recognized as a pioneer species in reforestation.[21]

The bark paste is applied on the forehead to cure hemicrania[2] and is used as plaster for fractured bones,[22,23] painful outgrowths below the tongue, indigestion, fever, burns, dislocations, and foot-and-mouth disease.[24] The bark's paste has wound-healing properties and is also applied as a bandage on the back.[26] In folk tradition, an amulet made from the bark is tied to the arm or waist of a child for their well-being.[25] Bark juice is applied externally to treat backaches. The bark is extracted with oil and is used on the head for good-quality hair.[26] The bark paste is beneficial in neuralgia and is prescribed to check over sweating in the body.[27] The branches and stems are used to treat gravel on kidneys, asthma, stone problems, thirst, leukoderma, vomiting, and leprosy. The stem is reported to be useful in vomiting, thirst, asthma, leprosy, and leukoderma. The stem bark decoction concentrated at a low temperature is used to cure joint pains. Heartwood is aromatic, antipyretic, strong, acrid, astringent, refrigerant, tonic, and moderately hard. It is useful in vitiated conditions of pitta and is used to cure burning sprains, sensations, ulcers, wounds, stomach troubles, seminal weakness, skin discolorations, and leprosy. It is beneficial in leukoderma, hallucinations, erysipelas, hiccough, thirst, asthma, diarrhea, cardiac debility, and vomiting.[28–30] The fruit is digestive and astringent. Seed kernel is used in the treatment of stones and gravel in the kidney;[31] seeds are chewed to cure kidney stones[32] and are used for burning sensations, bleeding disorders, and skin diseases.[20] The decoction of crushed smaller branches is used orally to stop abortion[29] and is beneficial in scorpion stings.[33] Charcoal of powdered shell is used as tooth powder. The species is used with other fragrant herbs as a medicated smoking wick.[8] The honey from flowers of *P. cerasoides* is slightly bitter, but it has medicinal properties and is used to treat eye ailments.[34] The natives of Punjab (India) believe the fruits to be useful as an acaricide. In Indo-Chinese folk medicine, the bark is used for edema. The flowers are considered diuretics and laxatives. The seeds are used as an anthelmintic. In Malaya and China, its kernels are given for blood disease, cough, and rheumatism. In Ayurveda, the plant is called the 'Padmaka' and is used to treat skin diseases and is said to enhance complexion. The leaf extract of the species is used in prostate and urinary disorders.[29,35]

P. cerasoides, as a whole plant and its various parts, is traditionally used as important ingredients in several formulations of Ayurveda. These formulations include Arista and Asava (Chandanasava, Dashmoolarista, Mritasanjivani sura, Sarivadyasava, Usirasava), Arka (Karpuradyarka), Kvatha Churna (Draksadi Kvatha churna, Guduchyadi ghana Kvatha churna), Ghrita (Brihat chagaladya ghrita, Kasisadi ghrita, Maha Kalyanaka ghrita, Satavaryadi ghrita), Churna (Sudarshana churna), Taila (Arimedadi taila, Ashvagandha taila, Bala taila, Bhringaraja taila, Chandanadi taila, Jatyadi taila, Guduchyadi taila, Kumkumadi taila, Madhuyashtyadi taila, and Triphaladi taila), Vati and Gutika [Khadiradi Gutika (Mukharoga)].

Chandanadi taila (taila means oil) is used to treat dizziness, burning sensation, and nasal bleeding; Mahabhringaraj oil treats headache, hair fall, stiffness of the neck, and pain. Jatyadi oil is beneficial in the treatment of ulcers and wounds. Triphaladi oil is used for external application to treat sinusitis, neck pain, and hair fall. Bala oil is used to treat Vata diseases (cold, cough, vomiting, wounds, emaciation, asthma, etc.), and Grahani mihira oil for cough, diarrhea, fever, etc.[36,37] Stanyajanana rasayana, an ayurvedic formulation having *P. cerasoides*, is used to benefit lactating mothers by increasing breast milk, body strength, and immunity. Kernel extract of *P. cerasoides* is used in beautification creams such as sun creams, etc., to make the skin fairer.[38]

PHYTOPHARMACOLOGY

The *P. cerasoides* plant is reputed for its high therapeutic value. The heartwood of the plant is acrid, bitter, refrigerant, demulcent, anodyne, antipyretic, constipating, vulnerary, and causes flatulence.[29,30] It is a diuretic, depurative, anti-abortifacient, emmenagogue, carminative, analgesic, conceptive, febrifuge, tonic, and expectorant. Different ingredients are aromadendrin, chrysin, dihydrotectochrysin, dihydrowogonin, kaempferol, pinocembrin, naringenin, quercetin, taxifolin, carasinone, carasidin, and carasin.[39] The sapwood has a flavone glycoside, puddumin A, prunetin, genistein, triacontane, n-pentacosane, β-sitosterol, octacosanol, ursolic acid, oleic acid, palmitic acid, stearic acid, afzelin, naringenin, kaempferitrin, and β-sitosterol-β-D-glucoside.[40]

The stem, stem bark, and branches of *P. cerasoides* have medicinal value and are used as antipyretics and refrigerants. Its tender branches have spasmolytic and anthelminthic properties. Branches and stems have prunasin and amygdalin and, on hydrolysis, produce hydrocyanic acid, a poison found mainly in the seed, bark, and leaves, and readily identified by its bitter taste.[41] The young shoots and seeds have cyanogenic glycosides, especially prunasin and amygdalin, which, on ingestion, break down and release cyanide in the digestive tract, so they are used in very small quantities in both traditional and conventional therapies, resulting in improved digestion, stimulated respiration, and feelings of well-being, but they are exceedingly poisonous compounds. In higher concentrations, cyanide causes spasms, weakness, gasping, pupil dilation, coma, excitement, convulsions, and respiratory failure leading to death.[42] The stem bark is an anti-inflammatory and contains prunetin, genistein, genkwanin, and sakuranetin.[43] Its fruits are astringent and digestive,[44] and seed oil is emollient.[31,33] Fruits have nar ingenin-5-O-α-L-rhamnopyranoside, 4′-Omethyl-liquirit igenin-7-O-α-L-rhamnopyranoside, naringenin 4′-methylether 7-xyloside, and β-sitosterol-3-O-D-galactopyranos ide. [45] The root bark has glucogenkwanin, ursolic acid, prunetinoside, stigmasterol, etc.[46]

SCOPE FOR BIOTECHNOLOGICAL INTERVENTIONS

The occurrence of different chemical classes of secondary metabolites in *P. cerasoides* is indicative of its therapeutic and biological significance against several diseases. A high concentration of flavonoids and diterpenes in *P. cerasoides*, which are most effective against yeast strains, Gram-negative, and Gram-positive bacteria, can be further used to develop potent therapeutic products to control resistant pathogens by excreting an antimicrobial effect by binding with the extracellular proteins of the bacterial cell wall. The diverse ethnomedicinal uses of this species suggest it could be a promising candidate for developing new drug formulations with synergistic combinations. However, there is a significant gap in pharmacological studies needed to validate its traditional claims. Addressing this knowledge gap is essential to ensure the species can be used more beneficially for society.

Different products from *P. cerasoides* are applied externally (paste as refrigerant, anti-pruritic, and complexion enhancer) and internally (to stimulate appetite, as an analgesic, cardiotonic, aphrodisiac, and anti-dermatosis agent). Its uses in bleeding, breathlessness, abortion, leukoderma, whooping cough, irregular menstruation, as a laxative, for stomachache, as a diuretic highlight the need to develop validated products with proper specifications to achieve its medicinal benefits for society.

Barks are generally treated as a waste product, and there are limited studies on their utilization, so it is necessary to explore modern green medicines from their bark. Exploration of appropriate preservation and processing techniques for the bark is a prerequisite to combat the seasonal and limited availability. Simultaneous research on the cost-effective processes for the extraction and utilization of pigments, pure phytochemicals, and nutraceuticals from *P. cerasoides* is necessary to meet the global demand. Deforestation, a most serious environmental problem of the current time, causes drought, floods, worsens rural poverty, and leads to biodiversity loss. The plantation of *P. cerasoides* and its other species may serve as an excellent alignment for regional reconstitution into an evergreen forest in dry tropical forestland.

REFERENCES

1. Anonymous. 1997. *The Wealth of India. Publications, and Information*. Directorate CSIR, Hillside Road, New Delhi. Reprint. Vol 7. pp. 250.
2. Gaur RD. 1999. *Flora of the District Garhwal Northwest Himalaya (with Ethnobotanical Notes)*. Trans Media, Srinagar Garhwal, India. pp: 226.
3. Polunin O, Stainton A. 1984. *Flowers of the Himalaya*. Oxford University Press, Delhi, India.
4. Tiwari C, Chubey S, Kurule R, Nautiyal R. 2016. A review on Padmaka *(Prunus cerasoides* D. Don): Different species and their medicinal uses. *Ayushdhara*. 4 (1):1051–1055.
5. ITIS (Integrated Taxonomic Information System), Online Database *Prunus cerasoides* https://www.itis.gov/, as on 22nd June 2022.
6. Kirtikar KR, Basu BD. 1989. *Indian Medicinal Plants*, 2nd Edition. Published by Lalit Mohan Basu, Allahabad, India. Vol. 2. pp. 959–960.
7. Vagbhatt A. 2013. *Astang Hridyam*. Vol II. Chikitsa sthan: 164–167, English translation by Prof. K.R. Srikantha Murty, Reprint edition, Chawkhamba Krishnadas Academy, Varanasi. pp: 105.
8. Vaidya BG. 2002. *Nighantu Adarsa*, 3rd Edition. Chaukhamba Bharati Academy. Vol. I. pp: 527. Varanasi.
9. Chunekar KC. 2013. *Bhavaprakash Nighantu Commentary*. Late Dr Pandey G. S. (Ed.) Chaukhamba Bharti Academy, Varanashi. pp. 193.
10. Sharma AP. 2006. *Kaiydeva Nighantu (Pathyapatyvibodhakha) Commentary*, 2nd Edition. Chaukhamba Oriyantalia. pp. 259. Varanasi.
11. Pratap U. 1997. *Bee Flora of the Hindukush Himalaya. Inventory and Management*. International Centre for Integrated Mountain Development (ICIMOD), Kathmandu, Nepal.

12. Anonymous. 2000. *The useful plants of India*, Reprinted edition. National Institute of Science Communication, Council of Scientific and Industrial Research, New Delhi. pp. 289.
13. Tanaka T, Nakao S. 1976. *Tanaka's Cyclopedia of Edible Plants of the World*. Keigaku Publishing, Tokyo.
14. Singh M, Nautiyal S. 1991. *Prunus cerasoides* (Himalayan wild cherry) – A promising winter tree for fodder. Indian Forester Ind For. 117 (7): 580–581.
15. Grae I. 1974. *Nature's Colors - Dyes from Plants*. MacMillan Publishing Co., New York.
16. Gaur RD, Nawani P. 1989. A melissopolynological analysis of apiary honey from Pauri Garhwal, U.P. India. *Indian Bee Journal*. 51 (1): 12–14.
17. Tiwari P, Tiwari JK, Ballabha R. 2009. *Prunus cerasoides* D. Don (Himalayan Wild Cherry): a Boon to Hill – Beekeepers in Garhwal Himalaya. *Nature and Science*. 7 (7): 21–23.
18. Awasthi P, Ram R, Reddy SG, Nadda G, Zaidi AA, Hallan V. 2015. Himalayan wild cherry (*Prunus cerasoides*) as a new natural host of Cherry necrotic rusty mottle virus (CNRMV) and a possible role of insect vectors in their transmission. *Annals of Applied Biology*. 166: 402–409.
19. Dolui AK, Sarma HK. 2001. Traditional medicinal plants in Mizoram. *Fitoterapia*. 72: 141–161.
20. Khare CP. 2007. *Indian Medicinal Plants: An Illustrated Dictionary*. Germany: Springer Science & Business Media, LLC.
21. Pakkad G, Elliott S, Blakesley D. 2004. Selection of *Prunus cerasoides* D. Don seed trees for forest restoration. *New Forests*. 28: 1–9.
22. Singla C, Drabu S, Verma R, Dhiman A, Sharma A. 2011. Recent update on proficient bone fracture revivifying herbs. *International Research Journal of Pharmacy*. 2 (11): 3–5.
23. Thakur S, Sidhu MC. 2014. Phytochemical screening of some traditional medicinal plants. *Research Journal of P harmaceutical, Biological and Chemical Sciences*. 5 (4): 1088–1097.
24. Pande PC, Tiwari L, Pande HC. 2007. Ethnoveterinary plants of Uttaranchal – a review. *Indian Journal of Traditional Knowledge*. 6 (3): 444–458.
25. Singh P, Attri BL. 2014. Survey on traditional uses of medicinal plants of Bageshwar valley (Kumaun Himalaya) of Uttarakhand, India. *International Journal of Conservation Science*. 5 (2): 223–234.
26. Uniyal MK. 1989. *Medicinal Flora of Gharwal Himalayas*, 1st Edition. Published by Baidyanath Ayurved Bhavan Pvt Ltd, Nagpur.
27. Rastogi RP, Mehrotra BN. 2001. *Compendium of Indian Medicinal Plants (*1980–1984*)*. Central Drug Research Institute Lucknow and Publications and Information Directorate, New Delhi. Vol IV. pp. 600.
28. Pullaiah T. 2006. *Encyclopaedia of World Medicinal Plants*. Regency Publication West Patel Nagar, New Delhi., Vol 1. pp. 1615.
29. Kirtikar KR, Basu BD. 2005. *Indian Medicinal Plants*. International Book Distributors, Dehradun. Vol. 1. pp. 951–964.
30. Chopra RN, Chopra IC, Varma BS. 1986. *Glossary of Indian Medicinal Plants*. Publications and Information Directorate, New Delhi. pp. 204.
31. Chatterjee A, Pakrashi SC. 1992. *The Treatise on Indian Medicinal Plants*. Publications and Information Directorate, CSIR, New Delhi. Vol 2. pp. 13–14.
32. Mehra A, Bajpai O, Joshi H. 2014. Diversity, utilization, and sacred values of ethno-medicinal plants of Kumaun Himalaya. *Tropical Plant* Research. 1 (3): 80–86.
33. Nadakarni KM. 2002. *Indian Materia Medica*. Reprint. Bombay Popular Prakashan, Mumbai. Vol. I. pp. 10–16.
34. Dhiman KS, Dhiman K, Puri S, Ahuja D. 2010. A comprehensive review of cataract (*Kaphaja linganasa*) and its surgical treatment in Ayurvedic literature. *AYU (An International Quarterly Research Journal in Ayurveda*. 31 (1): 93.
35. Anonymous. 2003. *The Wealth of India-Raw Materials*, 1st supplement series. National Institute of Science Communication, CSIR, New Delhi. Vol IV. J-Q. pp. 405.
36. 1978. *The Ayurvedic Formulary of India*, 1st edition. Ministry of Health and Family Welfare, Department of ISM & H, Government of India, New Delhi.
37. 2000. *The Ayurvedic Formulary of India*, Part-II. Ministry of Health and Family Welfare, Department of ISM & H, Government of India, New Delhi.
38. Esfahlan AJ, Jamei R, Esfahlan RJ. 2010. The importance of almond (*Prunus amygdalus* L.) and its by-products. *Food Chemistry*. 120 (2): 349–360.
39. Singh VK, Ali ZA. 1998. *Herbal Drugs of Himalaya (Medicinal Plants of Garhwal and Kumaon Regions of India)*. Today and Tomorrow's Printers and Publishers, New Delhi. pp. 163.
40. Rhodes L, Pollard RP, Maxted N. 2017. *Cerasus cerasoides*. The IUCN Red List of Threatened Species 2016: e.T50026860A50670270. 2016, as on 14th June 2022.
41. Joseph N, Anjum N, Tripathi YC. 2018. *Prunus cerasoides* D. Don: A review on its ethnomedicinal uses, phytochemistry and pharmacology. *International Journal of Pharmaceutical Sciences Review and Research*. 48 (1): 62–69.
42. Bown D. 1995. *Encyclopaedia of Herbs and their Uses*. Dorling Kindersley, London.
43. Manandhar NP. 2002. *Plants and People of Nepal*. Timber Press. Oregon.
44. 2001. *The Ayurvedic Pharmacopoeia of India*, 1st Edition, Part 1. Ministry of Health and Family Welfare, Department of ISM & H, Government of India, New Delhi. Vol III. pp. 145–146.
45. Chakravarti D, Ghosh RP. 1942. Isolation of a new flavone from the bark of *Prunus puddum* (N.O. Rosaceac). *Science and Culture*. VIII (II): 463.
46. Chakravarti D, Bhar CN. 1942–43. Isolation of a new isoflavone from the bark *of Prunus puddum* (N.O. Roseceae). *Science and Culture*. VIII (XII): 498.

20 *Prunus persica* (Aaru/Peach)

INTRODUCTION

Prunus persica (Linn.) Batsch., a plant of the subfamily Amygdaloideae (family: Rosaceae),[1–3] has stony nut-bearing fruits and is distributed worldwide.[2] The stone fruits are soft at maturity and hardy in comparison to pome. Fruits are much preferred as fresh because of their outstanding taste and flavor. These fruits have a very short storage life compared to others and can be consumed dried, like plums and apricots.[2,4] Genus *Pyrus* has its origin in the Asian continent.[5] The Rosaceae, or in other words, the rose family, includes some large genera like *Prunus* (peach), *Pyrus* (apple), etc., which has about 90–125 genera and 3,370–3,500 species[1,6,7] of trees, shrubs, and herbs. It has a worldwide distribution,[8] ranging from cosmopolitan[1] to sub-cosmopolitan, though it varies in distribution.[2]

P. persica, known as 'Aaru' in Hindi[9] (English name: Peach, and Ayurvedic name: Aaruka),[10] has been extensively consumed worldwide. Its fruits have many nutritional ingredients and can be used in fresh, dried, or processed forms. *P. persica* fruits are nutritionally beneficial and economically cheap, so they have an identity as one of the most popular fruits consumed worldwide.[9] There is a wide variety of fruits of *P. persica*, where flesh color ranges from yellow to red, and different shapes (Figure 20.1) contribute to its uniqueness.[2,11] *P. persica* fruits are rich in phenolic compounds.[12,13]

Aadu is a deciduous tree (see Figure 20.3) up to 10 m in height,[14] naturally distributed throughout temperate regions, from Southern Europe to Asia.[15,16] Generally, its bark is grayish or ashy, acuminate, and glabrous,[15,17] and is used as an expectorant (in chronic bronchitis and whooping cough), demulcent, antiscorbutic, sedative, diuretic, and stomachic.[15] Its flowers are pinkish-white, sessile, short, and pedicellate. Leaves are green in color and are used as diuretics, febrifuges, astringents, demulcents, expectorants, laxatives, parasiticides, and sedatives.[17,18] Fresh leaves are anthelmintic, and powdered leaves are externally styptic.[10] The fruit of these species is botanically known as a drupe (i.e., a fleshy fruit having thin skin and a stony seed at the center)[19] and has antiscorbutic and stomachic action biologically.[10] The fruits usually have a clear ventral suture (Figure 20.2), do not retain floral residues next to the pedicel, and are characterized by a membranous exocarp[20] with an outer fleshy mesocarp,[21] consisting mainly of parenchyma cells.[22] The mesocarp surrounds a shell (the pit or stone) formed by a hardened endocarp (Figure 20.3) with a seed inside (see Figures 20.4–20.6). For this reason, the *P. persica* species is also known as a 'stone fruit'.

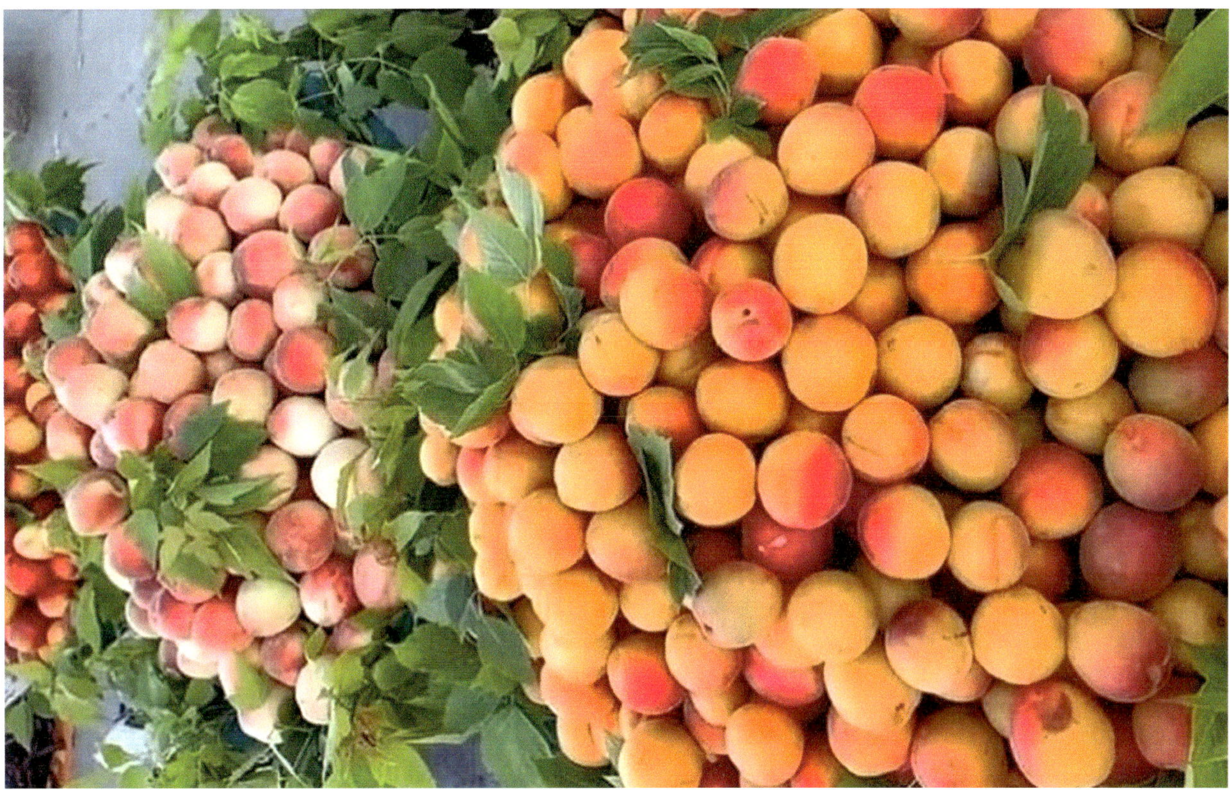

FIGURE 20.1 *P. persica* fruits at market, Nainital, Uttarakhand, India.

DOI: 10.1201/9781003512868-22

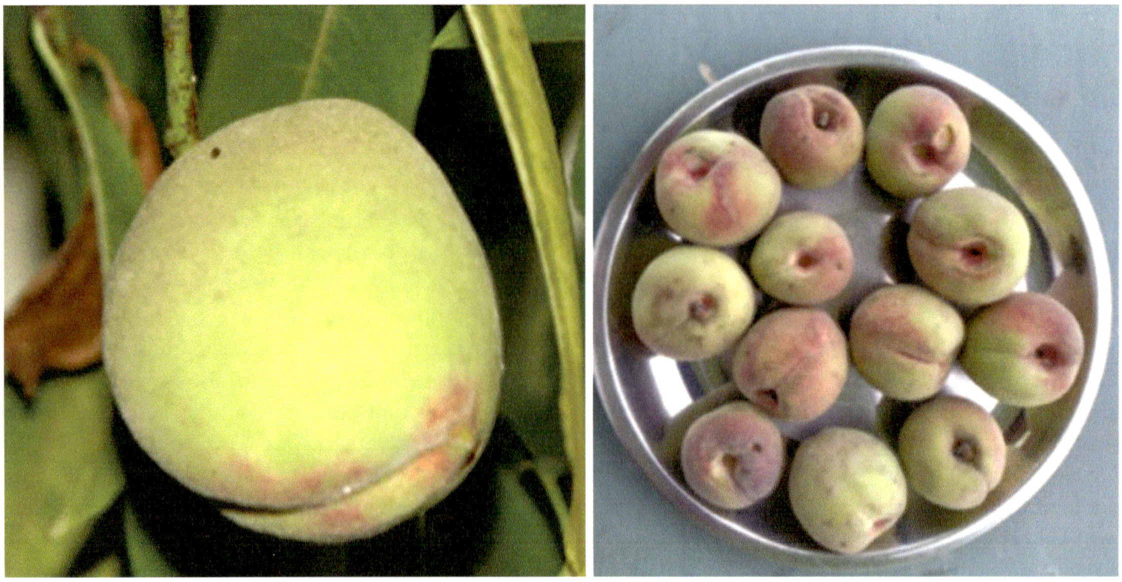

FIGURE 20.2 *P persica* semi-ripen fruits.

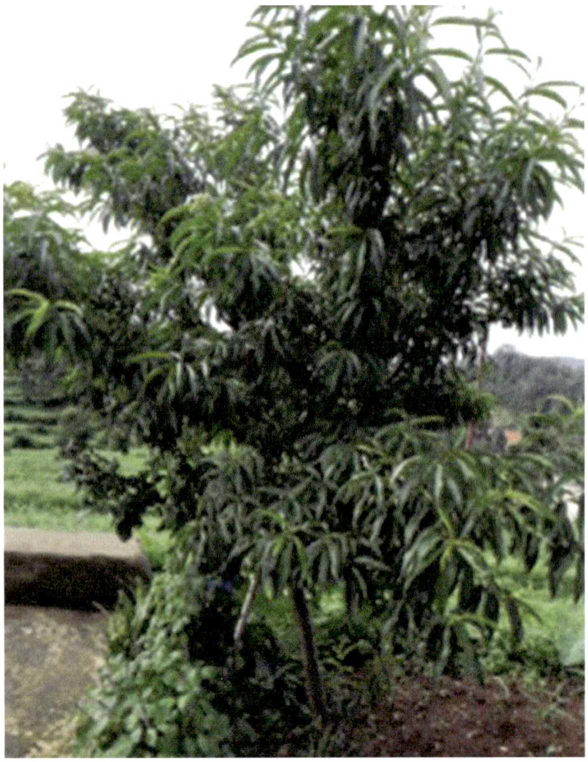

FIGURE.20 3 *P. persica* plant.

Most *Prunus* fruits and seeds are commonly used for roasting or canning[4] and jam production and are regularly consumed year-round. Among stone fruits, *P. persica* has the highest phenolics.[23] *P. persica* fruit varies in low, medium, or high acid concentrations.[19,24] Despite these general features, both the quantitative and qualitative profiles of phenolics vary markedly depending on the variety.[16,25,26] Fruits of *P. persica* are rich in vitamin C (ascorbic acid), provitamin A (carotenoids), and phenolic compounds, a good source of antioxidants.[24,27]

P. persica is commonly cultivated in the Himalayas and India up to an altitude of 1,000 ft,[1] as well as in West Asia and Europe.[1] Nearly 200 species are cultivated for their edible fruits and seeds.[28,29] *P. persica* varieties are grouped based on flesh color (yellow and white), stone adhesion to the flesh (freestone, semi-clingstone, and clingstone), melting nature of flesh (melting and non-melting), and chilling requirement.[30] In India, the Gene Bank of NBPGR (National Bureau of Plant Genetic Resources), Regional Station, Shimla (India), has about 22 indigenous and 27 exotic accessions;[31] such a huge range of cultivars provides important genetic resources for the evaluation of the phenolic profile. Phytochemical screening of *P. persica* reveals the presence of more than 100 compounds in the species.[32] A wide range of pre- and post-harvest conditions can alter the synthesis and emanation of volatile compounds from harvested plant products,[33] which may be associated with ripening, flavor, and other factors impacting quality or storage duration. The volatile composition of fruits has been thoroughly studied and has identified more than one hundred volatile compounds. The most abundant compounds are C 6 compounds (benzaldehyde, linalool, and ester terpenoids) and C 13 compounds (ketones, nor-isoprenoids, and lactones).[34] The flowering properties derive from lactones and particularly γ & δ-decalactones, with smaller contributions from C6 aldehydes, alcohols, and terpenoids.[35] The chemical composition of the volatile compound varies in the different parts of the fruit. In the pulp, volatile compounds such as C 6 compounds, C13 nor-isoprenoids, and benzaldehydes are more concentrated than in the inner mesocarp.[36] During the ripening process, the composition alters differently: C6 compound levels decrease drastically, while the contents of benzaldehyde, lactones, linalool, phenylalanine derivatives, and nor-isoprenoids increase.[37] The volatiles and their composition in fruits are also affected by the storage conditions and storage duration.[38]

ETHNOBOTANY

The leaves of *P. persica* are traditionally used as an anthelmintic, diuretic, insecticide, vermicide, demulcent, sedative, and expectorant and are used to treat leukoderma and piles.[28] A paste made from leaves is used to kill worms in wounds and treat fungal infections. The treatment of chronic bronchitis, whooping cough, and gastritis is carried out internally using leaves.[39]

The flowers are used as a diuretic and laxative, and to cure constipation and edema.[18] The fruit is used as a stomachic, demulcent, and antiscorbutic. Fruit, being antipyretic and an aphrodisiac, acts as a brain tonic, enhances the blood, removes bad smells from the mouth, and has antitumor properties.[40] The seeds are used as an emmenagogue and anthelmintic.[41] The oil extracted from seeds is used as an abortifacient and is good for deafness, earache, stomach troubles of children, and piles.[18] The kernel oil is applied to impetigo. The bark is used to treat jaundice and leprosy.[18]

In China and Malaysia, kernels are used to cure menstrual disorders, coughs, blood diseases, and rheumatism. The kernel oil (Figures 20.4–20.6) is applied to impetigo. The bark is used for leprosy and jaundice.[42] *P. persica* is used in traditional Chinese medicine to treat blood stasis.[43]

Roots of *P. persica* are also described as an important ingredient in traditional Chinese medicine to treat diseases like hemorrhoids, hematemesis, jaundice, amenorrhea, and tinea.[43] The phytopharmacological investigations reveal that the roots of *P. persica* have anti-inflammatory activity.[44] In the Garhwal-Himalayan region, the infusion of leaves and bark is used to relieve coughs and colds.[45]

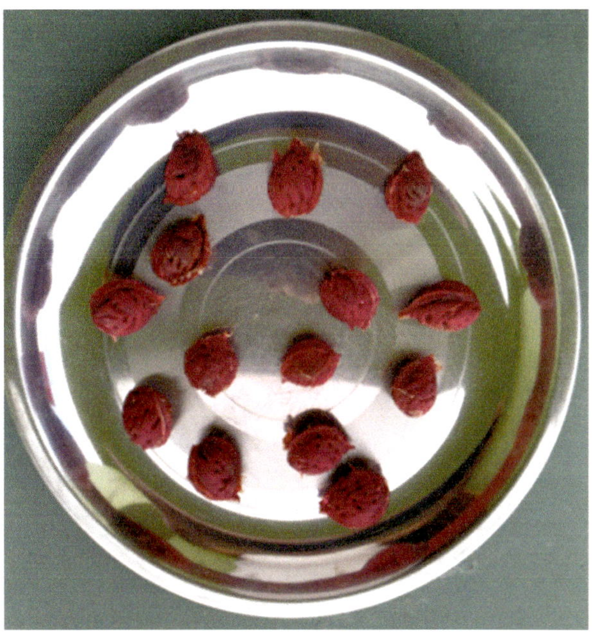

FIGURE 20.4 *P. persica* Kernel.

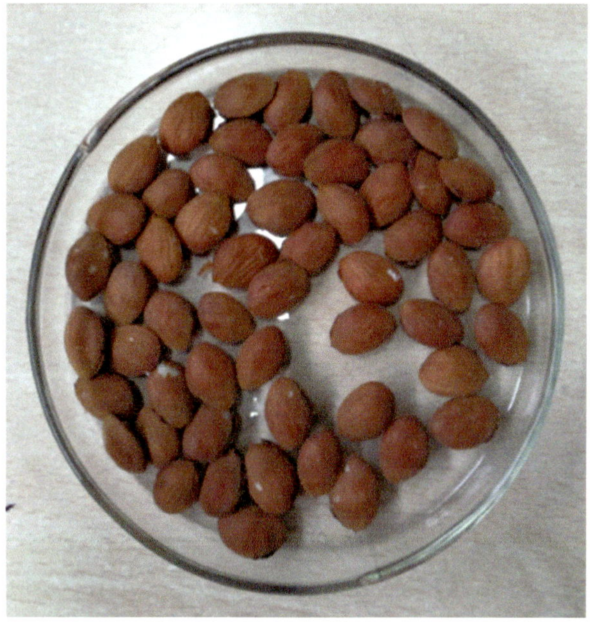

FIGURE 20.5 *P. persica* kernels.

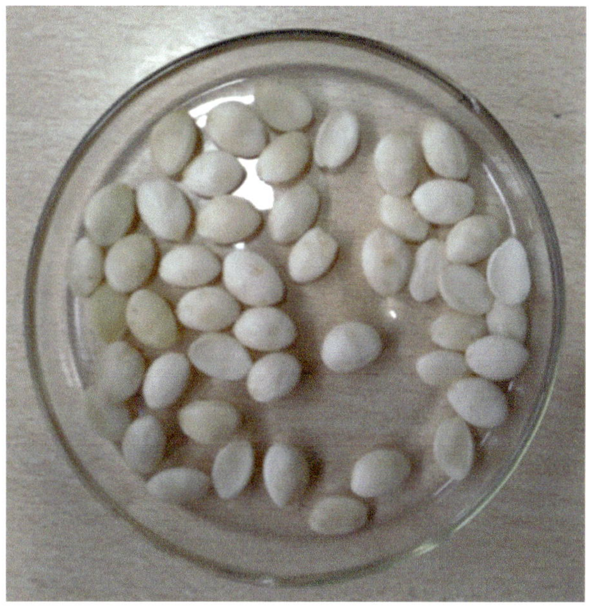

FIGURE 20.6 Blanched kernels.

PHYTOCHEMICAL SCREENING

Traditionally, each part of the plant *P. persica* is known to treat certain body ailments, more specifically to prevent diseases. Fruits of *P. persica* have been reported to be rich in carotenoids, tocopherols, and phenolic compounds, although research on their potential benefits for human health is still nascent. *P. persica* fruits are one of the most prevalent fruits enjoyed throughout the world by different cultures for their nutritional and economic value.[4] Green leaves are used as a diuretic, astringent, laxative, demulcent, parasiticide, febrifuge, expectorant (chronic bronchitis, whooping cough, and cough), antiscorbutic, demulcent, sedative, diuretic, and stomachic.

P. persica species have amygdalin, cyanogenetic glycosides, and prunasin along with glycerides and sterols as the main therapeutic compounds of the seeds. Rho et al. have identified an alkaloidal compound that is isolated from the methanolic extract of seeds.[46] The stem bark of the plant contains 8-O-β-D-galactopyranoside, crysophenol, 6-hydroxy4-methoxy 2-O-β-D-glucopyranoside, quercetin, and β-sitosterol.

The leaves of the plant contain ursolic acid, kaempferol, chlorogenic acid, caffeic acid, p-coumaric acid, quercetin-3-glycoside, quercetin, quercetin-3-rhamnoside, zeaxanthin, and tannin. *P. persica* essential oil is a mixture of 130 compounds, of which limonene, 3-carene, 1-methylhydrazine, benzaldehyde, and 4-ethenyl-1,4-dimethyl cyclohexene are the most significant.[47,48]

PHARMACOLOGY

The leaves are sedative, diuretic, anthelmintic, insecticidal, demulcent, vermicide, and expectorant, and are used to treat piles and leukoderma.[28] Paste of leaves is used to kill worms in wounds and fungal infections. The treatment of whooping cough, gastritis, and chronic bronchitis is carried out internally using leaves[39] and has been reported to have anti-inflammatory and antioxidant properties.[49,50]

The flowers of *P. persica* have laxative and diuretic properties and are used to treat edema and constipation. Its fruits are used as an antiscorbutic, demulcent, and stomachic. Fruits are used to remove bad smells from the mouth and have been reported to have antitumor properties.[40] *P. persica* seeds have anthelmintic and emmenagogue properties.[41] The oil extracted from seeds is good for deafness and is used as an abortifacient to treat piles, stomach troubles of children, and earaches. Its kernels are used to treat menstrual disorders, blood diseases, coughs, and rheumatism in Malaysia and China.[42] The consumption of *P. persica* juice and its by-products during juice preparation are used to cure hyperglycemia in obese rats,[51] revealing the potential of its fruits for preventing diabetes.

P. persica flowers are used to treat skin cancer effectively and skin damage caused by UV radiation, either alone or in a mixture with other pharmacologically active drugs.[52]

SCOPE AND OPPORTUNITIES

P. persica fruits are one of the most popular fruits consumed worldwide. Economically, these fruits are cheap and nutritionally valuable. There are more than 3,000 cultivars of *P. persica* that have been reported in the world today.[11] The health benefits of *P. persica* fruits are due to the high content of bioactive components, mainly phenolics.[53] Phenolic compounds affect the digestive enzymes involved in the hydrolysis of dietary carbohydrates.[54,55] α-Glucosidase is one of the key enzymes responsible for the hydrolysis of dietary carbohydrates.[56] Phenolic-rich fruits can inhibit the α-glucosidase activity and may offer a natural dietary approach for preventing type 2 diabetes mellitus.

The α-glucosidase inhibitory activity of *P. persica* fruits has been reported in cultivars grown in Poland and Portugal.[57,58] However, no extensive investigation of the α-glucosidase inhibitory activity of Chinese cultivars or those from other regions/countries has been carried out. Furthermore, the chemical composition of *P. persica* fruits, which leads to the difference in activity, is still not clear.

Recently, the polyphenolic fraction from *P. persica* fruits has been reported to inhibit the proliferation of in vitro breast cancer cells, as well as in vivo breast tumor growth and lung metastasis.[59,60] The *P. persica* fruit and its polyphenolic extract have a chemoprotective role against cancer through modulating in vivo xenobiotic-metabolizing enzymes.[61] Fukuda et al. have reported that glycosides from *P. persica* seeds have antitumor activity both in vitro and in vivo.[40]

Biological screening of extracts of *P. persica* bark was carried out by Sumaira Aziz and Habib-ur-Rahman (2013) using methanolic extract and its various fractions, namely chloroform, dichloromethane, ethyl acetate, and petroleum ether.[28] The methanolic extract has antibacterial activity against *Klebsiella pneumoniae* and *Enterococcus faecalis*. The petroleum ether fraction has antibacterial activity against *Escherichia coli* and *Staphylococcus aureus*. The dichloromethane fraction inhibits the growth of *E. coli* and *K. pneumoniae*. The chloroform fraction has no significant activity against *E. coli*, *K. pneumonia*, and *Bacillus subtilis*. The ethyl acetate fraction has activity against *E. faecalis*. Among the tested fungal species, *Aspergillus flavus*, *Fusarium solani*, and *Microsporum canis* were more susceptible to dichloromethane, chloroform, and methanol fractions. The methanol extract has moderate phytotoxic activity at high doses, while other fractions have low activity.[28]

Overall, variations in metabolites in *P. persica* juice and pulp extracts, respectively, reflect the need for detailed investigation for each cultivar of the species and standardized markers for future research and investigations on therapeutic properties. Furthermore, *P. persica* cultivars rich in phenolics have a high potential as a natural dietary source for preventing the postprandial hyperglycemic condition in type 2 diabetes mellitus patients.

REFERENCES

1. Judd W, Cambell C, Kellogg E, Stevens P, Donoghue M. 1999. *Plant Systematics: A Phylogenetic Approach*. Sinauer Associates, Sunderland, USA.
2. Hummer KE, Janick J. 2009. *Genetics and Genomics of Rosaceae, Plants Genetics and Genomics: Crop and Models-Book*. Germany: Springer Science Business Media, LLC.
3. Rasheed HM, Khan T, Wahid F, Khan R, Shah AJ. 2015. Chemical composition and vasorelaxant and antispasmodic effects of essential oil from *Rosa indica* L. petals. *Evidence-Based Complementary and Alternative Medicine*. 2015. Article ID 279247, 9 pages. https://doi.org/10.1155/2015/279247

4. Poonam V, Raunak, Kumar G, Reddy CSL, Jain R, Sharma SK, Prasad AK, Parmar VS. 2011. Chemical constituents of the genus *Prunus* and their medicinal properties. *Current Medicinal Chemistry*. 18: 3758–3824.
5. Bastos C, Barros L, Dueñas M, Calhelha RC, Queiroz MJ, Santos-Buelga C, Ferreira IC. 2015. Chemical characterization and bioactive properties of Prunus avium L.: the widely studied fruits and the unexplored stems. *Food Chemistry*. 173: 1045–1053.
6. Potter D, Eriksson T, Evans RC, Oh S, Smedmark JE, Morgan DR, Kerr M, Robertson KR, Arsenault M, Dickinson TA, Campbell CS. 2007. Phylogeny and classification of Rosaceae. *Plant Systematics and Evolution*. 266: 5–43.
7. Potter D, Gao F, Bortiri PE, Oh SH, Baggett. 2002. Phylogenetic relationships in rosaceae inferred from chloroplast matK and trnL-trnF nucleotide sequence data. *Plant Systematics and Evolution*. 231: 77–89.
8. Pigg M L, De V, Robertson K B. 2007. A brief review of the fossil history of the family Rosaceae. *Plant Systematics and Evolution*. 266: 45–57.
9. Zhao X, Zhang W, Yin X, Su M, Sun C, Li X, Chen K. 2015. Phenolic composition and antioxidant properties of different peach [Prunus persica (L.) Batsch] cultivars in China. *International Journal of Molecular Science*. 16: 5762–5778.
10. Khare CP. 2007. *Indian Medicinal Plants*. Germany: Springer, Science Business Media, LLC.
11. Faust M, Timon B. 1995. Origin and dissemination of peach. *Horticultural* Reviews. 17: 331–379.
12. Tomás-Barberán, Gil FA, Cremin MI, Waterhouse P, Hess-Pierce ALB, Kader AA. 2001. HPLC-DAD-ESI-MS analysis of phenolic compounds in nectarines, peaches, and plums. *Journal of Agricultural and Food Chemistry*. 49: 4748–4760.
13. Scordino M, Sabatino L, Muratore A, Belligno A, Gagliano G. 2012. Phenolic characterization of Sicilian yellow flesh peach (*Prunus persica* L.) cultivars at different ripening stages. *Journal of Food* Quality. 35: 255–262.
14. Lurie S, Carlos HC. 2005. Chilling injury in peach and nectarine. *Postharvest Biology and Technology*. 37: 195–208.
15. Gaur RD. 1999. *Flora of the District Garhwal Northwest Himalayas*. Transmedia, Srinagar Garhwal. pp. 227.
16. Ariel RV, George AM, Luis CZ, Carlos HC. 2011. *Health-Promoting Properties of Fruit and Vegetables*. Terry LA. (Eds.) (pp. 238–259). CABI Digital Library, CABI Global CAB International.
17. Raturi R, Sati SC, Singh H, Sati MD, Bahuguna P, Badoni PP. 2011, Chemical examination, and anti-inflammatory activity of Prunus persica steam bark. *International Journal of Pharmacy and Pharmaceutical Sciences*. 3: 315–317.
18. Kritikar KR, Basu BD. 1984. *Indian Medicinal Plants*. Bishen Singh Mahendra Pal Singh, Dehradun.
19. Brady CJ. 1993. Stone fruit. In: *Biochemistry of Fruit Ripening*. Seymour GB, Taylor JE, Tucker GA. (Eds.) Chapman & Hall. pp. 379–404. ISBN: 0412408309.
20. Lingdi L, Cuizhi G, Chaoluan L. Alexander C, Bartholomew B, Brach AR, Spongberg SA. 2003. Rosaceae. *Flora of China*. 9: 46–434.
21. Kim HR, Kim ID, Dhungana SK, Kim MO, Shin DH. 2014. Comparative assessment of physicochemical properties of unripe peach (Prunus persica) and Japanese apricot (Prunus mume). *Asian Pacific Journal of Tropical Biomedicine*. 4 (2): 97–103.
22. Romani RJ, Jennings WG. 1971. Stone fruits. In: *The Biochemistry of Fruits and Their Products*. Hulme AC (Ed.) Academic Press, New York. Vol. 2. pp. 411–436.
23. Vicente AR, Manganaris GA, Sozzi GO, Crisosto CH. 2009. Nutritional quality of fruits and vegetables. In: *Postharvest Handling: A Systems Approach*, 2nd Edition. Florkowski WJ, Shewfelt RL, Brueckner B, Prussia SE (Eds.). Academic Press. pp. 58–106. ISBN: 978-0-12-374112-7.
24. Lurie S, Crisosto CH. 2005. Chilling injury in peach and nectarine. *Postharvest Biology and Technology*. 37: 195–208.
25. Ruiz D, Reich M, Bureau S, Renard CMG, Audergon JM. 2008. Application of reflectance colorimeter measurements and infrared spectroscopy methods to rapid and nondestructive evaluation of carotenoids content in apricot (*Prunus armeniaca* L.). *Journal of Agricultural and Food Chemistry*. 56: 4916–4922.
26. Díaz-Mula HM, Zapata PJ, Guillén F, Castillo S, Martinez-Romero D, Valero D, Serrano M. 2008. Changes in physicochemical and nutritive parameters and bioactive compounds during development and on-tree ripening of eight plum cultivars: a comparative study. *Journal of the Science of Food and Agriculture*. 88: 2499–2507.
27. Byrne DH. 2002. Peach breeding trends. *Acta Horticulturae*. 592: 49–59.
28. Aziz S, Rahman H. 2013. Biological activities of *Prunus persica* L. *Batch*. 7 (15): 947–951.
29. Rheder A. 1940. *Manual of Cultivated Trees and Shrubs Hardy in North America*. Macmillan Company, New York. pp. 425–481.
30. Wang ZH, Zhuang EJ. 2001. *China Fruit Monograph-Peach Flora*. China Forestry Press, Beijing. pp. 42–51.
31. Sharma BD, Rana JC, Yadav SK. 2001. *A Glance at Temperate Fruits Gene Bank*. NBPGR, Regional Station, Shimla. Vol. 4. pp. 1–20.
32. Aubert C, Gu-nata Z, Ambid C,Baumes R. 2003.Changes in physicochemical characteristics and volatile constituents of yellow and white-fleshed nectarines during maturation and artificial ripening. *Journal of Agricultural and Food Chemistry*. 51: 3083–3091.
33. Kays SJ, Paull RE. 2004. *Postharvest Biology*. Exon Press, Athens, GA.
34. Horvat RJ, Chapman GW. 1990. Comparison of volatile compounds from peach fruit and leaves (cv. Monroe) during maturation. *Journal of Agricultural and Food Chemistry*. 38 (7): 1442–1444.
35. Spencer MD, Pangborn RM, Jennings WG. 1978. Gas-chromatographic and sensory analysis of volatiles from cling peaches. *Journal of Agricultural and Food Chemistry*. 26 (3): 725–732.
36. Aubert C, Milhet C. 2007. Distribution of the volatile compounds in the different parts of a white-fleshed peach (*Prunus persica* L. Batsch). *Food Chemistry*. 102 (1): 375–384.
37. Eduardo I, Chietera G, Bassi D, Rossini L, Vecchietti A. 2010. Identification of key odor volatile compounds in the essential oil of nine peach accessions. *Journal of the Science of Food and Agriculture*. 90 (7): 1146–1154.
38. Zhang B, Xi WP, Wei WW, Shen JY, Ferguson I, Chen KS. 2011. Changes in aroma-related volatiles and gene expression during low temperature storage and subsequent shelf-life of peach fruit. *Postharvest Biology and Technology*. 60 (1): 7–16.

39. Kirtikar KR, Basu BD. 2001. *Indian Medicinal Plant*, IInd Edition. International Book Distributors, Dehradun.
40. Fukuda T, Mukainaka T, Tokuda H, Nishino H, Yoshida T. 2003. Anti-tumor promoting effect of glycosides from Prunus persica seeds. *Biological and Pharmaceutical Bulletin*. 26 (2): 271–273.
41. Suh SJ, Koo BS, Jin UH, Hwang MJ, Lee IS, Kim CH. 2006. Pharmacological characterization of orally active cholinesterase inhibitory activity of Prunus persica L. Batsch in rats. *Journal of Molecular Neuroscience*. 29 (2): 101–107.
42. Bankole AE, Adekunle AA, Sowemimo AA, Umebese CE, Abiodun O, Gbotosho GO. 2016. Phytochemical screening and in vivo antimalarial activity of extracts from three medicinal plants used in malaria treatment in Nigeria. *Parasitology Research*. 115: 299–305.
43. Kim DH, Lee SM, Leeetal YJ. 2017. Effect of Paeotang on tumor necrosis factor α-induced vascular inflammation in human umbilical vein endothelial cells. *Chinese Journal of Integrative Medicine*. 1–10. https://doi.org/10.1007/s11655-017-2759-3
44. Xia J, Huagang L. 2006. Experimental study of anti-inflammation activity of root of Prunus persica. *Journal of Chinese Me*dicinal Materials. 29 (8): 821–823.
45. Bhandari BS, Riaz T, Panwar R, Gusain P. 2016. Indigenous traditional knowledge of healthcare system adopted by the Bhotia tribe and other inhabitants in the part of Garhwal Himalaya. *World Journal of Pharmacy and Pharmaceutical Sciences* 5 (12): 802–816.
46. Rho JR, Jun CS, Ha Y, Yoo MJ, Cui MX, Baek HS, Lim JA, Lee YH, Chai KY. 2007. Isolation and characterization of a new alkaloid from the seed of *Prunus persica* L. and its anti-inflammatory activity. *Bulletin of the Korean Chemical Society*. 28(8): 1289–1293.
47. Gilani AH, Aziz N, Ali SM, Saeed M. 2000. Pharmacological basis for the use of peach leaves in constipation. *Journal of Ethnopharmacology*. 73 (1–2): 87–93.
48. Vicente AR, Manganaris GA, Cisneros-Zevallos L, Crisosto CH. 2011. Chapter 13: Prunus. In: Health Promoting Properties of Fruits and Vegetables. Leon Terry (Ed.). pp. 238–259. https://www.researchgate.net/publication/235724103
49. Deb L, Gupta R, Dutta AS, Yadav A, Bhowmik D, Kumar KPS. 2010. Health promoting properties of Prunus species In: *Health promoting properties of fruits and vegetables*, Leon Terry (Ed.) (pp. 238–259) CABI.
50. Shin TY, Park SB, Yoo JS, Kim IK, Lee HS, Kwon TK, Kim MK, Kim JC, Kim SH. 2010. Anti-allergic inflammatory activity of the fruit of *Prunus persica*: role of calcium and NFkappa. *Journal of Food and Chemical Toxicology*. 48 (10): 2797–2807.
51. Rodriguez-Gonzalez S, Perez-Ramirez IF, Amaya-Cruz DM, Gallegos-Corona MA, Ramos-Gomez M, Mora O, Reynoso-Camacho R. 2020. Polyphenol-rich peach (*Prunus persica* L.) by-product exerts a greater beneficial effect than dietary fiber-rich by-product on insulin resistance and hepatic steatosis in obese rats. *Journal of Functional Foods*. 45: 58–66.
52. Heo MY, Kim SH, Yang HE, Lee SH, Jo BK, Kim HP. 2001. Protection against ultraviolet B-and C-induced DNA damage and skin carcinogenesis by the flowers of *Prunus persica* extract. *Mutation Research/Genetic Toxicology and Environmental Mutagenesis*. 496 (1–2): 47–59.
53. Crozier A, Jaganath IB, Clifford MN. 2009. Dietary phenolics; Chemistry, bioavailability and effects on health. *Natural Product Reports*. 26: 1001–1043.
54. Hanhineva K, Torronen R, Bondia-Pons I, Pekkinen J, Kolehmainen M, Mykkanan H, Poutanen K. 2010. Impact of dietary polyphenols on carbohydrate metabolism. *International Journal of Molecular Science*. 11: 1365–1402.
55. Xiao J, Kai G, Yamamoto K, Chen X. 2013. Advance in dietary polyphenols as -glucosidases inhibitors: a review on structure-activity relationship aspect. *Critical Reviews in Food Science*. 53: 818–836.
56. Podsedek A, Majewska I, Redzynia M, Sosnowska D, Koziolkiewicz M. 2014. In- vitro inhibitory effect on digestive enzymes and antioxidant potential of commonly consumed fruits. *Journal of Agricultural and Food Chemistry*. 62: 4610–4617.
57. Nowicka P, Wojdylo A, Laskowski P. 2020. Inhibitory potential against digestive enzymes linked to obesity and type 2 diabetes and content of bioactive compounds in 20 cultivars of the peach fruit grown in Poland. *Plant Foods for Human Nutrition*. 73: 314–320.
58. Bento C, Goncalves AC, Silva B, Silva LR. 2020. Assessing the phenolic profile, antioxidant, antidiabetic and protective effects against oxidative damage in human erythrocytes of peaches from Fundao. *Journal of Functional Foods*. 43: 224–233.
59. Noratto G, Porter W, Byrne D, Cisneros-Zevallos L. 2014. Polyphenolics from peach (Prunus persica var. Rich Lady) inhibit tumor growth and metastasis of MDA-MB-435 breast cancer cells in-vivo. *The Journal of Nutritional Biochemistry*. 25 (7): 796–800.
60. Vizzotto M, Porter W, Byrne D, Cisneros -Zevallos L. 2014. Polyphenols of selected peach and plum genotypes reduce cell viability and inhibit proliferation of breast cancer cells while not affecting normal cells. *Food Chemistry*. 164:363–370.
61. Canistro D, Vivarelli F, Cirillo S, Costa G, Andreotti C, Paolini M. 2016. Comparison between two peach (Prunus persica L. Batsch) supplementation and its polyphenolic extract on rat liver xenobiotic metabolizing enzymes. *Food and Chemical* Toxicology. 97: 385–394.

21 *Punica granatum* (Dadim)

INTRODUCTION

Punica granatum Linn. (Sanskrit name: Dadim, Eng.: Pomegranate) is wild as well as cultivated globally, especially in Afghanistan, Baluchistan, Central Asia, the Mediterranean, and Iran, in tropical and subtropical areas.[1,2] It is crowned as a fruit crop plant and as an ornamental one, with the specific character of drought-resistant species. The *P. granatum* plant can adapt to adverse environmental conditions and can be grown in dry, arid, and semiarid regions.[3] It is a deciduous shrub or small tree (Figure 21.1) that grows up to 12–16 ft tall. *P. granatum* plants are either naturally scattered along the borders or planted in fruit orchards, as reported in many Mediterranean countries, regions where their fruits are very popular in local markets. It is cultivated both for fruit production and as an ornamental tree in Central Asia, the USA, China, Russia, and Japan. *P. granatum* can tolerate summer heat and winter as low as 10°F. It requires full sun and can tolerate alkaline soils.[4] *P. granatum* fruits are large and globose, having many seeds separated by a membranous pericarp. Seed are angular, brown, and wedge-shaped, with a sweetish-sour taste. As the tree ages, its bark turns gray.[5]

Fruits (Figure 21.2) at the ripe stage change color and make a metallic sound when tapped. Fruits are harvested before over-maturity, as they tend to crack open, particularly when rained on.[5] Descriptions of *P. granatum* have been found since the Vedic period, including the Rigvedic regime. Aacharya Sushruta described Dadim (Dadim, the Sanskrit name of *P. granatum*) as 'Shrestha Phalavarga', i.e., the best fruit.[6–8] In Europe, its fruits have been praised since ancient times for their medicinal properties and are considered sacred by the major religions. Dadim seeds are considered the best-known contraceptive in Greek mythology and are described in the Bible and Babylonian Talmud.[4] Greek mythology describes *P. granatum* fruits as sacred as life and used for rejuvenation and marriages.[9–11] A fruit of *P. granatum* has a total of 613 seeds in number, which represents each of the Bible's 613 directives along with abundance, sanctity, and fertility.[12]

In Buddhism, *P. granatum* fruit symbolizes the occurrence of favorable influences,[13] while the Chinese consider it a symbol of a prosperous future.[14] It is considered a sign of revival in Christianity,[15] and in Islamic mythologies, fruit has a distinct role in the ritual of marriages among

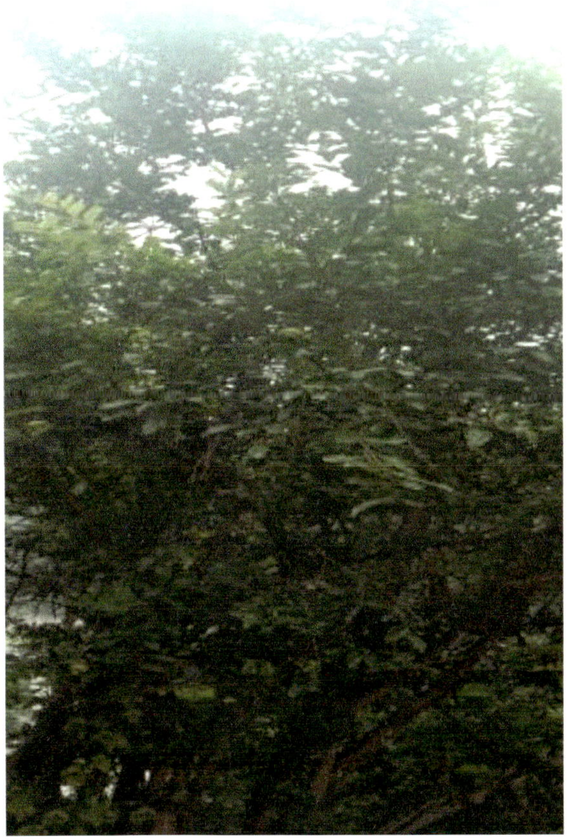

FIGURE 21.1 *P. granatum* plant.

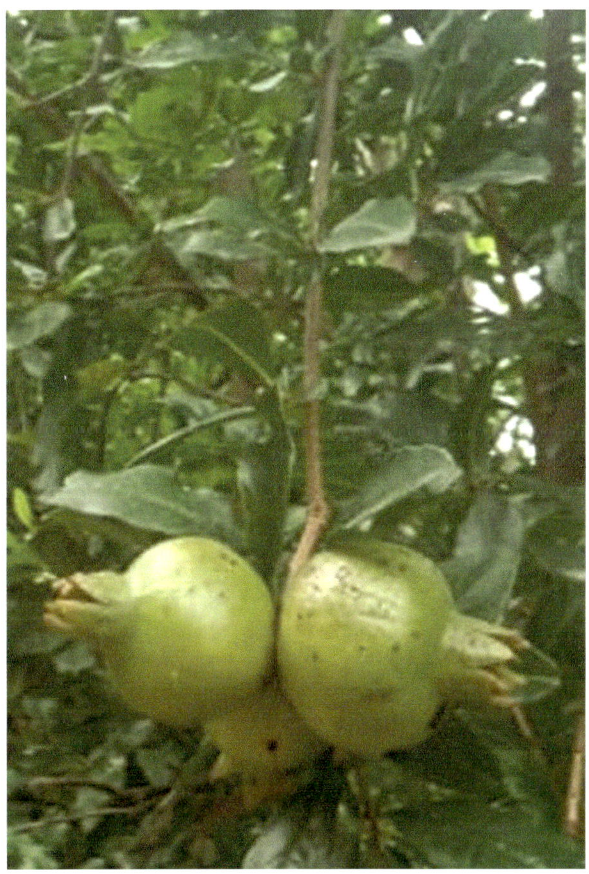

FIGURE 21.2 *P. granatum* unripen fruits.

DOI: 10.1201/9781003512868-23

the Bedouins of the Middle East.[16] In India, it is called 'Beejpur' in Sanskrit and is related to the earth goddess and Lord Ganesha.[17,18]

P. granatum, as a whole, is described as a medicinal plant that uses its fruit rind, fruit, bark, root, seeds, floral seed oil, and bud for therapeutic applications.[19]

The edible fruit is a berry with a thick reddish skin, measuring 5–12 cm in diameter, and has a rounded hexagonal shape. Each seed, the edible part of the fruit, is surrounded by a water-laden pulp (aril) ranging in color from purple to deep red or white. The seeds are embedded in a spongy, white, astringent pulp.[20] According to the holy Quran, *P. granatum* grows in the gardens of paradise and is praised as God's good creation twice a day. The fruit has been extensively used in different traditional healing practices against microbial infections, diarrhea, hemorrhage, acidosis, helminth infection, dysentery, and respiratory pathologies.[21] Seeds of *P. granatum* are known to contain estrogenic compounds.[21] The dried pericarp and fruit juice are beneficial to treat menorrhagia, colic, colitis, acne, headaches, piles, oral diseases, and allergic dermatitis.[22] Current molecular studies also support the various traditional applications of the species.[22]

ETHNOBOTANY

P. granatum fruits have been described in the Old Testament of the Bible, the Babylonian, and the Talmud, the Jewish Torah, as a sacred fruit conferring powers of good luck, fertility, and abundance.[23]

P. granatum has been traditionally used for healing practices since ancient times in different countries. The ashes of the fruit peels are used as protection against skin infection in Turkey. In Iran, its flowers are used as an antiviral, antifungal, astringent, hemostatic, and antibacterial remedy for dermally infected wounds, cut wounds, diarrhea, bronchitis, re-constituted men's sex power, digestive problems, and diabetes. In China, flowers are used to treat injuries from falls and gray hairs.[24] In Ayurvedic medicine, *P. granatum* is advised as a pharmacy unto itself and is used as an anti-parasitic agent,[25] blood tonic,[26] and to heal ulcers.[27]

PHYTOCHEMISTRY AND FUNCTIONAL COMPONENTS

The highly therapeutic *P. granatum* ingredients (Tables 21.1 and 21.2) are ellagitannins, ellagic acid, flavonoids, punicic acid, anthocyanins, anthocyanidins, estrogenic compounds, and flavones. Ellagic acid has potent anti-carcinogenic and antioxidant properties, the cause of the forefront research on the species. Commercially available extracts of *P. granatum* are standardized against the ellagic acid (not less than 40% or more). Lansky and Newman have warned about the lack of understanding of other ingredients in the species regarding their biological properties.[28]

TABLE 21.1
Therapeutic Ingredients in *P. granatum*[5,19]

Plant Components	Constituents
P. granatum fruit juice	Ascorbic acid, anthocyanins, ellagic acid, caffeic acid, quercetin, gallic acid, rutin, catechin, glucose, etc. with minerals
P. granatum seed oil	Fatty acids ellagic acid, sterols, and punicic acid
P. granatum pericarp (peel and rind)	Gallic acid, catechin, quercetin, rutin, flavones, and punicalagins
P. granatum leaves	Tannins (punicafolin and punicalin) and flavone glycosides mainly luteolin and apigenin
P. granatum flower	Triterpenoids, gallic acid, maslinic acid, asiatic acid, and ursolic acid
P. granatum roots and bark	Piperidine-type alkaloids, punicalagin, punicalin, and ellagitannins

TABLE 21.2
Nutritional Ingredients (100 g) of the Edible Portion in *P. granatum*[2]

Compositions	Units	Quantity
Water	g	80–82.3
Energy	kcal	63–78
Protein	g	0.5-0.95
Fat	g	0.3–09
Carbohydrates	g	16.4
Fiber	g	0.2-0.6
Ash	g	0.5
Phosphorus	mg	8.0
Iron	mg	0.3
Potassium	mg	259
Calcium	mg	3.0
Sodium	mg	3.0
Manganese	mg	3.0
Zinc	mg	0.12
Magnesium	mg	0.15
Copper	mg	0.07
Selenium	mg	0.6
Pantothenic acid	mg	0.59
Vitamin B1	mg	0.03
Vitamin B2	mg	0.03
Vitamin B3	mg	0.03
Vitamin C	mg	4–6

P. granatum juice has antihypertensive, antiaging, anti-atherosclerotic, and potent antioxidative properties. Its seed oil is mainly composed of sterols and punicic acid and is known for its nephron-protective properties. The other ingredients are ascorbic acid, anthocyanins, caffeic acid, gallic acid, ellagic acid, glucose, catechin, quercetin, epigallocatechin, rutin, amino acids, and iron. The pericarp (peel, rind) has punicalagin, flavones, flavanones, and other flavanols, and is known to possess antimutagenic, antifungal, and anti-inflammatory activities. Leaves are potent antioxidants and known for the presence of flavone glycosides (apigenin and luteolin) and tannins (punicafolin and punicalin) as major ingredients.[17,29] The flowers contain ursolic acid and triterpenoids (maslinic acid and asiatic acid), which possess antioxidant and hepatoprotective properties, and are used as a remedy for diabetes mellitus.[17,30] Piperidine, ellagitannins, and alkaloids are present in its roots and bark. The bark has molluscicide properties.[17] The bark and roots are known for their anthelmintic and vermifuge properties.[27] The most therapeutic ingredients of *P. granatum* are anthocyanidins, anthocyanins, estrogenic flavones, flavonoids, ellagitannins, and punicic acid.[17]

PHARMACOLOGICAL PROPERTIES

P. granatum is a commonly available fruit in markets all over the world and is known for various promising therapeutic properties, such as anti-inflammatory, antitumor, immunomodulatory, antibacterial, wound-healing effects, that have been attributed to the various constituents of its bark, seeds, pericarp, and juice.[31]

1. **Anti-carcinogenic activity**: Investigations on mice have revealed the anti-carcinogenic properties of *P. granatum* in treating prostate cancer, due to its inhibitory action on the growth of prostate cancer cells via cell cycle disruption and induced apoptosis.[32,33,34, 35 36,37] Ephraim et al. have studied the seed, flower, leaf, bark, roots, peels, and juice of *P. granatum* and concluded that the juice, peel, and oil have anticancer activity.[38]

   Dahlawi et al. conducted an in vitro investigation on the fruit juice extract of *P. granatum* with leukemia cells. They observed that juice has a potent effect on the leukemia cells due to inhibition. The *P. granatum* juice induces apoptosis in all cell lines, including non-tumor control cells, but lymphoid and myeloid cells show a better response. The 4′,6-diamidino-2-phenylindole analysis and the count for leukemia cells indicated that *P. granatum* juice has the potential to inhibit the cell cycle and concluded that *P. granatum* juice has potent ingredients to treat and control leukemia.[39]

   The aqueous extract of the flower and peel of *P. granatum* has been reported to improve insulin sensitivity and reduce blood glucose levels in alloxan-induced diabetic rats due to inhibition of α-glucosidase activity and regeneration of pancreatic ß-cells.[40,41] An in vitro study has revealed the potent anti-nociceptive and anti-inflammatory activity of *P. granatum* species.[42]
2. **Hepatoprotective action**: Kaur et al. and Xu et al. have reported that *P. granatum* flowers significantly reduce liver fatty acids.[43,44]
3. **Cardioprotective properties**: Bhandari has studied the effect of daily intake of *P. granatum* for 3 months and concluded that *P. granatum* juice is effective in reducing stress-induced myocardial ischemia on daily consumption. The effect was postulated due to the presence of antioxidants (tannins, polyphenols, and anthocyanins, either alone or in their synergistic action) present in the juice.[17] In another study, *P. granatum* juice has been reported to inhibit serum angiotensin-converting enzyme (ACE) activity, resulting in a reduction of cardiovascular diseases and blood pressure.[45] The concentrate of *P. granatum* juice is reported to increase fecal cholesterol excretion, decrease cholesterol absorption, and improve the activity of cholesterol-metabolizing enzymes, PPAR-gamma, etc., resulting in improved total HDL and LDL:HDL cholesterol ratio.[46]
4. **Skin health management**: Polyphenol-rich herbals have been proven to be a protective and efficient factor to treat skin damage due to UV radiation. *P. granatum* fruit is a rich source of polyphenols with anti-carcinogenic, anti-inflammatory, and antioxidant properties. An in vitro study on the effect of *P. granatum* fruit juice on UV-A- and UV-B ray-induced skin damage has reported it as a healing agent.[47] It has been observed that pomegranate juice extract (PJE) protects the human skin fibroblasts and reduces cell death. From these results, researchers have concluded that the *P. granatum* fruit extract has a potent protective effect against UVA- and UVB-induced cell damage and is recommended for topical applications.[47]

   Bae et al. have reported on the role of ellagic acid in the skin healing process.[48]

   Further, studies based on ellagic acid and anti-wrinkle activity in animal models have reported *P. granatum* fruit juice as a promising source to treat skin wrinkles due to damage caused by UV exposure, aging, or photoaging.[48]
5. **Gastro-protective properties**: Alam et al. reported that the aqueous methanolic extract of *P. granatum* fruits is effective in the treatment of gastric ulcers.[49]
6. **Obesity prevention**: *P. granatum*-based medicines have been proven effective in treating obesity. A study by Al-Muammar and Khan on *P. granatum* fruit extract in obesity concluded that fruit extract exhibits significant results in the reduction of fat in obese patients and concluded that the beneficial effect was due to the presence of tannins, anthocyanins, flavonoids, and polyphenols.[50]
7. **Activity against** ***Trichomonas vaginalis***: The antifungal drug metronidazole is used worldwide

to treat gynecological ailments caused by *T. vaginalis*, and many cases of metronidazole resistance have been reported with unpleasant adverse effects and repeated infection. In vitro and in vivo studies have revealed that *P. granatum* juice is effective in completely curing infections and is a promising medicine against *T. vaginalis* infections.[51]

8. **Treatment of erectile dysfunction**: El-Sherbini et al.[51] studied 53 male patients with mild to moderate erectile dysfunction who received *P. granatum* juice orally for 4 weeks using a placebo. The results of the study have revealed improved scores during the treatment compared to the placebo.[52]
9. **Antiviral properties**: Haidari et al. have isolated the four major polyphenols of the *P. granatum*, namely ellagic acid, luteolin, punicalagin, and caffeic acid, to conduct an in-vitro study against the influenza virus and observed that out of these polyphenols, punicalagin efficiently blocked the replication of RNA of the influenza virus. Punicalagin has also been reported to inhibit the agglutination of RBCs of chicken caused by the influenza viruses and replication of human influenza A/Hong Kong (H3N2) in the above experiment.[53] De Siqueira et al. reported *P. granatum* as a potent virucidal drug in an in vitro study.[54] *P. granatum* juice has also been reported to have antiviral properties.[55]
10. **Anti-osteoporotic properties**: Studies on postmenopausal osteoporosis and tissue-selective estrogen agonists and antagonists for the anti-osteoporotic action of various drugs,[56–58] including *P. granatum* methanol-soluble extract (PME), have revealed the control of accelerated bone turnover.[59-60] Further, it concluded that PME played an efficient and protective role in hormone deficiency-related osteoporosis and had bone-preserving effect.[61]
11. **Chemotherapy-induced toxicity**: Synthetic anticancer drugs frequently have hepatotoxicity and nephrotoxicity. Research on *P. granatum* has shown that its seed extract can help counteract the harmful effects of synthetic drugs, particularly by reducing oxidative stress caused by Cisplatin-induced injury to the kidneys and liver. The extract has demonstrated a significant protective effect on liver and kidney cells by lowering the levels of lipid peroxidation.[17] Cayir et al. concluded that *P. granatum* seed extract is an essential dietary supplement for patients taking chemotherapy medications.[62]
12. **Immunomodulatory activity**: *P. granatum* used in an in vivo study in rabbits at the oral dose of 100 mg/kg of fruit rind powder has shown that fruit rind powder caused an increase in antibody titer to typhoid-H antigen and an increase in inhibition of leukocyte migration.[63]

Monica Amelia et al. have reported the anthelmintic activity of *P. granatum* peel extract.[64] Methanolic extract of fruits of *P. granatum* has a potent antidiarrheal effect.[65]

SCOPE AND OPPORTUNITIES

The fruit of *P. granatum* has impactful therapeutic properties in several diseases and serves as a nutritive dietary supplement even to subside the side effects of chemotherapy. It is a highly praiseworthy fruit used since ancient times in different traditional healing practices. Results of different in vitro and in vivo studies have supported the protective effects of *P. granatum* on the cardiovascular system, including a reduction in blood glucose levels, lowering lipid peroxidation, reduction in oxidative stress, vasodilatory effects, and decreasing blood pressure via inhibition of ACE activity. It also exhibits antidiarrheal activity, wound-healing properties, antiulcer activity, antimicrobial properties, anthelmintic activity, hepatoprotective and immunomodulatory activity, and much more. Besides these, in numerous preclinical and clinical studies, *P. granatum* has been proven effective in chronic vaginal infections, in male infertility cases such as erectile dysfunction, as an antinociceptive drug, and as an antiviral drug. *P. granatum* has been proven to be an effective medication therapy for diabetes, osteoporosis, obesity, and even leukemia. *P. granatum* has been proven effective in various skin diseases like UV skin damage, wrinkles, and photoaging; hence, it is used in the form of topical ointments and can serve as a promising drug in rising skin illnesses. Consequently, *P. granatum* is a natural medicine that has potential uses in various chronic diseases.

P. granatum and its ingredients have been utilized for centuries without any side effects.[66] Data collected from folk and traditional applications of *P. granatum* as a medicine did not indicate any toxic effects.[67] *P. granatum* powdered extracts, oil, or juice can be consumed by healthy individuals without any risk. No adverse effects on liver or renal function have been recorded in humans upon administration of up to 1,420 mg/day of its fruit extract tablets.[68] As P450 enzymes have a pivotal role in the metabolism of various drugs, *P. granatum* inhibits this enzyme, resulting in altered drug pharmacokinetics of carbamazepine, pentobarbital, and tolbutamide.[69–71] There are no data on the bioavailability (IC_{50}) of the different products obtained from *P. granatum*.

Nevertheless, the kinetics involved in the therapeutic and toxic effects of many *P. granatum* ingredients are not fully understood even today. Detailed investigations and trials are to be extensively used as a possible therapy to prevent and treat several types of diseases, including colon cancer, prostate cancer, lung cancer, breast cancer, leukemia, skin cancer, hyperlipidemia, anti-atherosclerosis, myocardial ischemia, infection, hypertension, diabetes, myocardial perfusion, oral inflammation, male infertility, neonatal hypoxic-ischemic brain injury, anti-erectile dysfunction, and obesity.

REFERENCES

1. Facciola S. 1990. *Cornucopia: A Source Book of Edible Plants*. Kampong Publications, Vista, CA. pp 166.
2. Akhlaghi M, Band B. 2009. Mechanisms of flavonoid protection against myocardial ischemia reperfusion injury. *Journal of Molecular and Cellular Cardiology*. 46: 309–317.
3. Sheidai M, Khandan M, Nasre ES. 2007. B-chromosomes in Iranian pomegranate (*Punica granatum*) cultivars. *Pakistan Journal of Botany*. 39: 85–91.
4. Garachh D, Patel A, Chakraborty M, Kamath JV. 2012. Phytochemical and pharmacological profile of *Punica granatum*; An overview. *International Research Journal of Pharmacy*. 3 (2): 65–68.
5. Jurenka J. 2008. Therapeutic applications of Pomegranate (*Punica granatum* L.): a review. *Alternative Medicine* Review. 13: 128–144.
6. Sushrut, Sushrut samhita vol I sutrasthan, Adhyay 46, Annapanavidhi, Verse 336, Reprint 2010. Shastri Kaviraj Ambikadutta (Ed.) Chaukhamba Sanskar Sanstan, Varanasi. pp. 270.
7. Vagbhat, Astanga samgraha, Sutrasthan, Adhyay 15, Mahakashaya, Verses 7. Reprint 2016. Dr. Sharma Shivprasad (Ed.) Chaukhamba Sanskrit Series Office, Varanasi. pp. 130–131.
8. Yogratnakar, Dhanyadiphalakandashaka guna, Reprint 2014. Versus 68 by Vaidya Laxmipati shastri. Sastri Bhisagratna Bramhasanskar (Ed.) pp. 30. UP, India
9. Langley P. 2000. Why a pomegranate? Trees at the Chelsea Physic Garden, London. BMJ. 321: 1153–1154. https://doi.org/10.1136/bmj.321.7269.1153
10. Modi JJ. 1922. *The Religious Ceremonies and Customs of the Parsees*. British India Press, Bombay.
11. Curtis VS. 1996. *Persian Myths*. British Museum Press, London. pp. 54.
12. Good A, Nurock M. 1968. *The Fruits of the Holy Land*. Israel Universities Press, Jerusalem.
13. Hall J. 1995. *Hall's Illustrated Dictionary of Symbols in Eastern and Western Art*. John Murray, London.
14. Cooper JC. 1995. *An Illustrated Encyclopaedia of Traditional Symbols*. Thames and Hudson, London. pp. 134.
15. Cherry J. 1995. *Mythical Beasts*. British Museum Press, London. pp. 47–52.
16. Herodotus. 1996. *The Histories*. Penguin, London. pp. 389.
17. Bhandari PR. 2012. Pomegranate (*Punica granatum* L). Ancient seeds for modern cure? Review of potential therapeutic applications. *International Journal of Nutrition, Pharmacology, Neurological Diseases*. 2 (3): 171–184.
18. Ward C. 2003. Pomegranates in eastern Mediterranean contexts during the Late Bronze Age. *World Archaeology*. 34: 529–541.
19. Shribhavamishra. 2015. Bhavprakash Nighantu, Haritkyadi varga, Verses 101, Reprint Edition. Padmashree Pro. Krushnachandra Chunekar (Ed.) Chaukhamba Bharati Academy, pp. 570. UP, India.
20. Stover E, Mercure EW. 2007. The pomegranate: a new look at the fruit of paradise. *Horticultural Science*. 42: 1088–1092.
21. Kim YH, Choi EM. 2009. Stimulation of osteoblastic differentiation and inhibition of interleukin-6 and nitric oxide in MC3T3-E1 cells by pomegranate ethanol extract. *Phytotherapy Research*. 23: 737–739.
22. Ricci D, Giamperi L, Bucchini A, Fraternale D. 2006. Antioxidant activity of *Punica granatum* fruits. *Fitoterapia*. 77: 310–312.
23. Mars M. 2000. Pomegranate Plant Material: Genetic Resources and Breeding, A Review. https://www.researchgate.net/publication/286496230_Pomegranate_plant_material_Genetic_resources_and_breeding_a_review, as on 28th June 2021.
24. Lansky EP, Newman RA. 2007. *Punica granatum* and its potential for prevention and treatment of inflammation and cancer. *Journal of Ethnopharmacology*. 109: 177–206.
25. Pirbalouti AG, Koohpayeh A, Karimi I. 2010. The wound healing activity of flower extracts of *Punica granatum* and *Achillea kellalensis* in wistar rats. *Acta Polonia Pharmaceutics Drug Research*. 67 (1): 107–110.
26. Lad V, Frawley D, Santa FE. 1986. *The Yoga of Herbs*. Lotus Press, New Maxico. pp. 135–136.
27. Naqvi SA, Khan MS, Vohora SB. 1991. Antibacterial, antifungal, and antihelminthic investigations on Indian medicinal plants. *Fitoterapia*. 62: 221–228.
28. Lansky EP, Newman RA. 2007. *Punica granatum* and its potential for prevention and treatment of inflammation and cancer. *Journal of* Ethnopharmacology. 109: 177–206.
29. Viuda-Martos M, Fernández-López J, Pérez-Álvarez JA. 2010. Pomegranate and its many functional components as related to human health: a review. *Comprehensive Reviews in Food Science and Food Safety*. 9: 635–654.
30. Saxena A, Vikram NK. 2004. Role of selected Indian plants in management of type 2 diabetes: a review. *Journal of Alternative and Complementary Medicine*. 10: 369–378.
31. Saeed M, Naveed M, Bibi J, Kamboh AA, Arain MA, Shah QA, Alagawany M, El-Hack ME, Abdel-Latif MA, Yatoo MI, Tiwari R. 2018. The promising pharmacological effects and therapeutic/medicinal applications of *Punica Granatum L*. (Pomegranate) as a functional food in humans and animals. *Recent Patents on Inflammation & Allergy Drug Discovery*. 12 (1): 24–38.
32. Malik A, Afaq F, Sarfaraz S, Adhami VM, Syed DN, Mukhtar H. 2005. Pomegranate fruit juice for chemoprevention and chemotherapy of prostate cancer. *Proceedings of the National Academy of Sciences of the United States of America*. 102: 14813–14818.
33. Malik A, Mukhtar H. 2006. Prostate cancer prevention through pomegranate fruit. *Cell Cycle*. 5: 371–373.
34. Lansky EP, Jiang W, Mo H, Bravo L, Froom P, Yu W, Harris NM, Neeman I, Campbell MJ. 2005. Possible synergistic prostate cancer suppression by anatomically discrete pomegranate fractions. *Investigational New Drugs*. 23: 11–20.
35. Albrecht M, Jiang W, Kumi-Diaka J, Lansky EP, Gommersall LM, Patel A, Mansel RE, Neeman I, Geldof AA, Campbell MJ. 2004. Pomegranate extracts potently suppress proliferation, xenograft growth and invasion of human prostate cancer cells. *Journal of Medicinal Food*. 7: 274–283.
36. Schubert SY, Lansky EP, Neeman I. 1999. Antioxidant and eicosanoid enzyme inhibition properties of pomegranate seed oil and fermented juice flavonoids. *Journal of Ethnopharmacology*. 66: 11–17.
37. Bando H, Ramachandran C, Melnick SJ, Imai A, Fife RS, Carr RE, Oikawa T, Lansky EP. 2003. Preliminary studies on the anti-angiogenic potential of pomegranate fractions in vitro and in vivo. *Angiogenesis*. 6: 121–128.
38. Lansky EP, Robert A. 2006. Newman, *Punica granatum* (Pomegranatum) and its potential for prevention & treatment of inflammation & cancer. *Journal of Ethanopharmacology*. 6: 1–30.

39. Dahlawi H, Jordan-Mahy N, Clench MR, Le Maitre CL. 2012. Bioactive actions of pomegranate fruit extracts on leukemia cell lines in vitro hold promise for new therapeutic agents for leukemia. *Nutrition and Cancer.* 64: 100–110.
40. Huang TH, Peng G, Kota BP, Li GQ, Yamahara J, Roufogalis BD, Li Y. 2005. Anti-diabetic action of *Punica granatum* flower extract: activation of PPAR-gamma and identification of an active component. *Toxicology and Applied Pharmacology.* 207: 160–169.
41. Khalil EA. 2004. Antidiabetic effect of an aqueous extract of pomegranate (*Punica granatum* L) peels in normal and alloxan diabetic rats. *Egyptian Journal of Hospital Medicine.* 16: 92–99.
42. Ouachrif A, Khalki H, Chaib S, Mountassir M, Aboufatima R, Farouk L, Benharraf A, Chait A. 2012. Comparative study of the anti-inflammatory and antinociceptive anti-inflammatory and antinociceptive effects of two varieties of *Punica granatum. Pharmaceutical Biology.* 50: 429–438.
43. Kaur G, Jabbar Z, Athar M, Alam MS. 2006. *Punica granatum* (pomegranate) flower extract possesses potent antioxidant activity and abrogates Fe-NTA induced hepatotoxicity in mice. *Food and Chemical Toxicology.* 44: 984–993.
44. Xu KZ, Zhu C, Kim MS, Yamahara J, Li Y. 2009. Pomegranate flower ameliorates fatty liver in an animal model of type 2 diabetes and obesity. *Journal of Ethnopharmacology.* 123: 280–287.
45. Aviram M, Dornfeld L. 2001. Pomegranate juice consumption inhibits serum angiotensin converting enzyme activity and reduces systolic blood pressure. *Atherosclerosis.* 158: 195–198.
46. Esmaillzadeh A, Tahbaz F, Gaieni I, Alavi-Majd H, Azadbakht L. 2006. Cholesterol-lowering effect of concentrated pomegranate juice consumption in type II diabetic patients with hyperlipidemia. *International Journal for Vi tamin and Nutrition Research.* 76: 147–151.
47. Pacheco-Palencia LA, Noratto G, Hingorani L, Talcott ST, Mertens- Talcott SU. 2008. Protective effects of standardized pomegranate (*Punica granatum* L.) polyphenolic extract in ultraviolet- irradiated human skin fibroblasts. *Journal of Agricultural and Food Chemistry.* 56: 8434–8841.
48. Bae JY, Choi JS, Kang SW, Lee YJ, Park J, Kang YH. 2010. Dietary compound ellagic acid alleviates skin wrinkle and inflammation induced by UV-B irradiation. *Experimental Dermatology.* 19: 182–190.
49. Alam MS, Alam MA, Ahmad S, Najmi AK, Asif M, Jahangir T. 2010. Protective effects of *Punica granatum* in experimentally induced gastric ulcers. *Toxicology Mechanisms and Methods.* 20: 572–578.
50. Al-Muammar MN, Khan F. 2012. Obesity; The preventive role of the Pomegranate (*Punica granatum*). *Nutrition.* 28:595–604.
51. El-Sherbini GM, Ibrahim KM, El Sherbiny ET, Abdel-Hady NM, Morsy TA. 2010. Efficacy of *Punica granatum* extract on *in-vitro* and *in-vivo* control of *Trichomonas vaginalis. Journal of the Egyptian Society of Parasitology.* 40: 229–244.
52. Forest CP, Padma-Nathan H, Liker HR. 2007. Efficacy and safety of pomegranate juice on improvement of erectile dysfunction in male patients with mild to moderate erectile dysfunction: a randomized, placebo-controlled, double-blind crossover study. *International Journal of Impotence Research.* 9: 564–567
53. Haidari M, Ali M, Casscells SW, Madjid M. 2009. Pomegranate (*Punica granatum*) purified polyphenol extract inhibits influenza virus and has a synergistic effect with oseltamivir. *Phytomedicine.* 16: 1127–1136.
54. De Siqueira RS, Dodd CE, Rees CE. 2006. Evaluation of the natural viricidal activity of teas for use in the phage amplification assay. *International Journal of Food Microbiology.* 111: 259–262.
55. Neurath AR, Strick N, Li YY, Debnath AK. 2005. *Punica granatum* (pomegranate) juice provides an HIV-1 entry inhibitor and candidate topical microbicide. *Annals of the New York Academy of Sciences.* 1056: 311–327.
56. Jordan VC, Phelps E, Lindgren JU. 1987. Effects of antiestrogens on bone in castrated and intact female rats. *Breast Cancer Research and Treatment.* 10 (1): 31–35.
57. Ke HZ, Paralkak VM, Grasser WA, Crawford DT, Qi H, Simmons HA, Pirie CM, Chidsey-Frink KL, Owen TA, Smock SL, Chen HK. 1998. Effects of CP- 336, 156, a new, non-steroidal estrogen agonist/antagonist, on bone, serum cholesterol, uterus, and body composition in rat models. *Endocrinology.* 139 (4): 2068–2076.
58. Lerner LJ, Jordan VC. 1990. Development of antiestrogens and their use in breast cancer: eighth Cain memorial award lecture. *Cancer Research.* 50 (14): 4177–4189.
59. Kim YY, Kim SH, Oh S, Sul OJ, Lee HY, Kim HJ, Kim SY, Choi HS. 2010. Increased fat due to estrogen deficiency induces bone loss by elevating monocyte chemoattractant protein-1 (MCP-1) production. *Molecules and Cells.* 29 (3): 277–282.
60. Neerup TSR, Stahlhut M, Petersen JS, Daugaard JR, Jensen JE, Peng Z, Morko J, Thorkildsen C. 2011. ZP2307, a novel, cyclic PTH (1–17) analog that augments bone mass in ovariectomized rats. *Bone.* 48 (6): 1319–1327.
61. Sreeja S, Santhosh Kumar TR, Lakshmi BS, Sreeja S. 2012. Pomegranate extract demonstrate a selective estrogen receptor modulator profile in human tumor cell lines and in-vivo models of estrogen deprivation. *The Journal of Nutritional Biochemistry,* 23 (7): 725–732.
62. Cayir K, Karadeniz A, Simşek N, Yıldırım S, Karakuş E, Kara A, Akkoyun HT, Şengül E. 2011. Pomegranate seed extract attenuates chemotherapy-induced acute nephrotoxicity and hepatotoxicity in rats. *Journal of Medicinal Food.* 14: 1254–1262.
63. Gracious Ross R, Selvasubramanian S, Jayasundar S. 2001. Immunomodulatory activity of *Punica granatum* in rabbits; A preliminary study. *Journal of Ethnopharmacology.* 78: 85–87.
64. Amelia M, Jasaputra DK, Tjokropranoto R. 2017.Effects of Pomegranate Peel (*Punica granatum* L.) extract as an anthelmintic. *Journal of Medicine and Health.* 1: 409–416.
65. Akter S, Sarkar A, Hossain Md S. 2013. Anti-diarrhoeal activity of rind of *Punica granatum. International Current Pharmaceutical Journal.* 2(5): 101–104.
66. Jurenka JS. 2008. Therapeutic applications of Pomegranate (*Punica granatum* L.): a review. *Alternative Medicine Review.* 13: 128–144.
67. Prakash CVS, Prakash I. 2011. Bioactive chemical constituents from Pomegranate (Punica granatum) juice, seed, and peel-a review. *International Journal of Research in Chemistry and Environment.* 1: 1–18.

68. Viladomiu M, Hontecillas R, Lu P, Bassaganya-Riera J. 2013. Preventive and prophylactic mechanisms of action of pomegranate bioactive constituents. *Evidence-Based Complementary and Alternative Medicine*. 2013, Article ID 789764. https://doi.org/10.1155/2013/789764
69. Nagata M, Hidaka M, Sekiya H, Kawano Y, Yamasaki K, Okumura M, Arimori K. 2007. Effects of pomegranate juice on human cytochrome P450 2C9 and tolbutamide pharmacokinetics in rats. *Drug Metabolism and Disposition* 35: 302–305.
70. Hidaka M, Okumura M, Fujita K, Ogikubo T, Yamasaki K, Iwakiri T, Setoguchi N, Arimori K. 2005. Effects of pomegranate juice on human cytochrome P450 3A (CYP3A) and carbamazepine pharmacokinetics in rats. *Drug Metabolism and Disposition*. 33: 644–648.
71. Faria A, Monteiro R, Azevedo I, Calhau C. 2007. Pomegranate juice effects on cytochrome P450S expression: in vivo studies. *Journal of Medicinal Food*. 10: 643–649.

22 *Pyracantha crenulata* (Ghingharu)

INTRODUCTION

Pyracantha crenulata (D. Don) M. Roem., Syn *Crataegus crenulata* Roxb, is commonly known as Himalayan firethorn. It is an evergreen thorny shrub species (family: Rosaceae) that grows between 900 and 2,400 MSL, extending from Myanmar to southwest China and Himalayan regions.[1] The species grows up to a height of 2 m and occurs near cultivated areas such as shrubberies on open slopes. In Uttarakhand, India, the ripened fruits are eaten directly by the local communities, where they are known as 'Ghingharu'.[2] *P. crenulata* is reported for many ethnomedicinal and traditional applications. It is used to treat cardiac, skin, stomach, and hepatic diseases.[3,4] Molecular biological investigations on its fruits have revealed their diuretic,[5] anti-inflammatory,[3] antihypertensive,[6] and antibacterial properties.[7] *P. crenulata* fruits are a potent source of natural antioxidants,[8] and a herbal beverage named 'Hridyamrit' (nectar for the heart) is a value-added product from the fruits of *P. crenulata*.[6] Its wood (stems and branches) is used for making walking sticks.[9] Its tender twigs and leaves are browsed by sheep and goats, and the plant is traditionally used for fencing around the agricultural fields and orchards by the local people in the hilly areas of the state of Uttarakhand, India (Figures 22.1 and 22.2). The species has the potential to restore the landslide-affected sites in the Himalayan region due to its wide adaptability and rapid growth.[10] The fruits of *P. crenulata* are eaten by apes[9] and different species of birds[11] and have an important role in the food chain in Himalayan forest ecosystems.

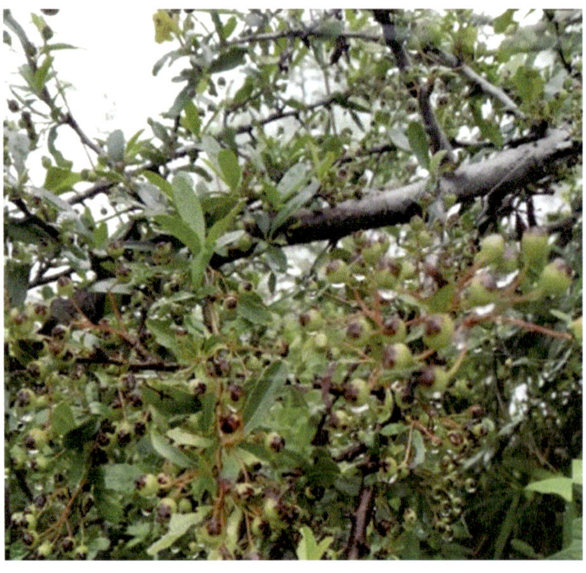

FIGURE 22.1 *P. crenulata* plant.

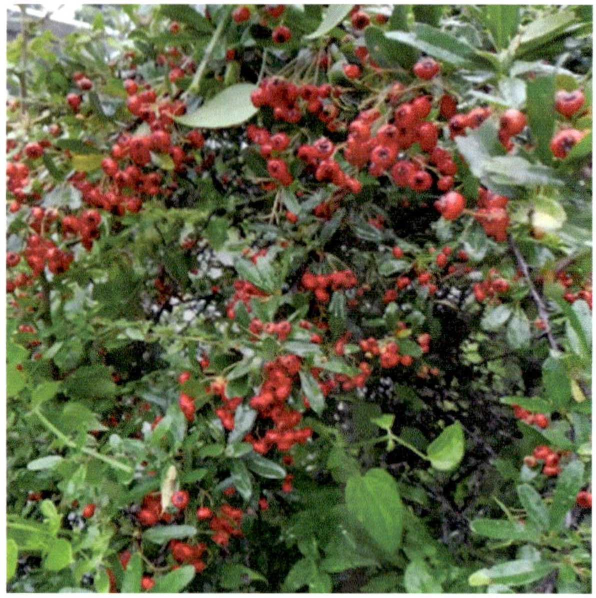

FIGURE 22.2 *P. crenulata* ripen fruits.

Medicinal plants are a source of drugs to treat animal and human diseases. The fruits of *P. crenulata* are used to treat diabetes, heart disorders, blood pressure, angina, and hypertension in the Garhwal Himalayan region.[12] The leaves have immunomodulatory, antioxidant, and anti-inflammatory properties and are used to make herbal tea. Its fruits are orange-red in color and rich in nutrients[13] compared to the cultivated berry fruits. 500 g of *P. crenulata* fruits have been reported to have enough nutrients required per day by a healthy person.[14]

It is well adapted to a wide range of soil types and can tolerate extreme drought and frost. The fences of the species are ideal for the protection of the farmlands from intruders and wild animals. Branches of the plants are used for preparing tool handles and walking sticks.[6]

The leaves of *P. crenulata* are used to make herbal tea, locally, and have a dark green, smooth surface ranging from 2.5 to 4.0 cm in length with 1.0 to 2.2 cm width, having tapering ends.[6]

The fruits of *P. crenulata* are small berries, and approximately 4,000 ± 32 fruits weighing 1 kg. The average weight of a berry is 250 mg, which has 25% juice (wt./wt.). Phytochemical screening of fruit juice reveals 0.11% ± 0.015% protein, 0.022% ± 0.001% magnesium, 0.08% ± 0.001% calcium, 73% ± 2% moisture, 0.43% ± 0.03% potassium, 1.006% ± 0.04% flavonoids, 1.2 ± 0.03 mg/100g vitamin C, 101 ± 9 μg/100g vitamin B12, 0.38 ± 0.02 mg/100g vitamin A, and 17.5 ± 1.02 mg/100g vitamin E.[6] A few heavy metals have been detected but were below the permissible limit.[6] The fruits are full of medicinal properties.[15]

DOI: 10.1201/9781003512868-24

Its bark is useful in the prevention of heavy bleeding during the menstrual cycle.[13] In Ayurveda, *P. crenulata* is depicted as useful to cure stomach, hepatic, and skin diseases. It is described as having anti-rheumatic, anti-inflammatory, cardiotonic, depurative, diuretic, tonic, hypotensive, hypoglycemic, and lithotriptic properties.[3,4,16–18]

ETHNOBOTANY

P. crenulata is traditionally used for its cardioprotective properties. It is also listed in the pharmacopeias of some Asian and European countries. Oligomeric pro-anthocyanidins and flavonoids have been reported as therapeutic ingredients of *P. crenulata* and are used to treat heart ailments. Conventionally, it is used in the Himalayan region for fencing, making sticks and tool handles, and as a firewood. Its berries are sometimes casually chewed by locals just for fun and to change the taste. Decomposed leaves under the shrubs are used by local farmers for mulching their fields, and their sticks are sold in the local market.[19] Ghingharu wood is hardy, so no major insect pests and diseases are reported to cause damage to the plant, except by larvae of *Agalope javana* rarely.[20]

The fruits are a good source of food for birds, langurs (*Presbytis* spp.), and wild animals in the rainy season. Ghingharu is the best folk remedy to reduce the risks of arteriosclerosis, hypertension, heart failure, Buerger's disease, and paroxysmal tachycardia.[16] The dried fruit powder with yogurt is used to cure bloody dysentery, while freshly ripened fruits are eaten as such. The plant is commercially harvested from forest areas for the preparation of different Ayurvedic medicines, such as tinctures, liquid extracts, and infusions of dried fruits.[1]

The *P. crenulata* plant is used as an excellent hedge and a good soil binder to stabilize slopes and degraded areas that are prone to landslides. The species generally prefers sun-facing hill slopes and grows in moist and fertile land.[21] Its propagation is carried out by spreading its seeds and sending out suckers.[22] The bioflavonoids in most *Pyracantha* species are used to overcome the malfunctioning of the blood circulatory system and heart.[23] *P. crenulata* fruits also have diuretic, sedative, vasodilatory, and antispasmodic properties. The hypotensive properties of flowers and fruits of the species are used to treat high blood pressure cases.[24]

PHARMACOLOGY

P. crenulata is a multipurpose medicinal plant, and every part is used to cure certain body ailments. Since the 18th century, its fruits are in practice to treat respiratory illnesses and circulatory disorders. Bioflavonoids present in fruits are used to treat cardiac ailments. *P. crenulata* fruits have sedative, vasodilatory, antispasmodic, and diuretic properties. The fruits and flowers of the species have hypotensive properties, so they are used to cure high blood pressure.[25] A few important medicinal applications of *P. crenulata* are described below.

P. crenulata berries reduce free radical impact,[26] and berries are used as a potential heart tonic to normalize heart rhythm in hypertensive patients.[27] Its regular use has been reported to strengthen the heart and its muscles. The flowers and berries of the plant are used to treat heart failure, irregular heartbeat, chest pain, high blood pressure, and hardening of the arteries.[28] It is commonly used for manifestations of old age, arteriosclerosis, nervous heart problems, and inflammation. *P. crenulata* berries are used to enhance memory. A mixture of *P. crenulata* and *Ginkgo biloba* (Ginkgo) leaves enhances brain cell activity and memory.[29] The leaves of *P. crenulata* are used as tisane[30] and a natural source of substantial health. A decoction of the bark and shoots of *P. crenulata* stops excess menstrual flow, while stem extract is used to cure fevers. Bark extract is applied externally to protect sunburned skin and all body organs from frostbite. *P. crenulata* fruit juice has a hypoglycemic effect, so it is used to treat type 2 diabetes mellitus[31] and is effective in curing hypertension.[29,32] *P. crenulata* leaves have anti-inflammatory, antioxidant, and immunomodulatory properties. The *P. crenulata* plant is effective in curing various diseases, more particularly cardiovascular disease, and a major cause of death per year globally.[32]

The nutraceutical and pharmaceutical attributes of *P. crenulata* are in the form of modern herbal medicine, the Hridyamrit, an herbal beverage made from *P. crenulata* fruits, which are highly energizing, refreshing, and nutritious.[6] It is rich in minerals, antioxidants, proteins, and vitamins. There are no synthetic flavors or artificial colors, as the fruit pulp has its natural color and flavor.[33] Results of clinical trials using the 'Hridyamrit' have revealed a lowering of blood cholesterol levels with significant improvement in heart patients.[34]

To prepare 'Hridyamrit', the mature and healthy fruits of *P. crenulata* were collected from their natural habitat in the Himalayan hills of Uttarakhand and processed into an herbal beverage as per good manufacturing practices. Before processing to juice, an equal amount of fruit juice and water (v/v) was taken in a separate container with 70% sugar (70 g sugar + 30 mL water) and heated to just the boiling point. The mixture was mixed with sodium benzoate solution (700 ppm) after attaining room temperature. The beverage so prepared is stored in airtight clear PET bottles in a cool place.[6]

The chemical analysis of the beverage was evaluated by estimation of flavonoids, moisture, protein content, vitamins, and minerals, including heavy metals (lead, cadmium, mercury, and arsenic), which were reported below the permitted levels.[6]

SCOPE AND OPPORTUNITIES

There is a standardized propagation technique for *P. crenulata*,[1] a multipurpose plant species, with the potential for various pharmaceutical and nutraceutical products. Its fruits are a rich repository of bioactive compounds, and various food products, such as herbal energy bars, jams, fruit juice, beverages, powder, and many more items, may be formulated.

The *P. crenulata* plant has environmental importance owing to its extensive root system, which is useful to prevent soil erosion on fragile hill slopes, and as a medicinal herb for pharmaceutical industries. The leaves can be utilized for tisane as a cardiotonic and have immense potential for the formulation of nutraceutical products as a food supplement to fight malnutrition. Because of its thorny nature, a bio-fence for agricultural fields and a sustainable source of its leaves as a beverage for cardiac health may improve the socio-economic conditions of the hilly marginal farmers, and *P. crenulata*-based products have a wide scope of commercial trade.

REFERENCES

1. Singh R, Negi PS, Arya MC, Ahmed Z. 2012. Propagation techniques of *Crataegus crenulata*. *Indian Forester*. 138 (2): 169–172.
2. Kala CP. 2007. Prioritization of cultivated and wild edibles by local people in the Uttaranchal hills of Indian Himalaya. *Indian Journal of Traditional Knowledge*. 6 (1): 239–243.
3. Otsuka H, Fujioka S, Komiya T, Goto M, Hiramatsu Y, Fujimura H. 1981. Studies on anti-inflammatory agent s. V. A new anti-inflammatory constituent of *Pyracantha crenulata* Roem. *Chemical and Pharmaceutical Bulletin*. 29 (11): 3099–3104.
4. Khare CP. 2004. *Indian Herbal Remedies: Rational Western Therapy, Ayurvedic and Other Traditional Usages, Botany*. Springer Verlag, Berlin Heidelberg.
5. Bahuguna YM, Rawat MSM, Juyal V, Gusain K. 2009. Evaluation of *Pyracantha crenulata* Roem for anti-urolithogenic activity in albino rats. *African Journal of Urology*. 15 (2): 159–166.
6. Negi PS, Singh R, Dwivedi SK. 2018. Evaluation of anti-hypertensive effect of fruit beverage of *Crataegus crenulata* Roxb.: a wild shrub of Himalayan hills. *Defence Life Science Journal*. 3 (2): 146–150.
7. Saklani S, Chandra S. 2014. In vitro antimicrobial activity, nutritional value, antinutritional value and phytochemical screening of *Pyracantha crenulate* fruit. *International Journal of Pharmaceutical Sciences Review and Research*. 26 (1): 1–5.
8. Bhatt ID, Rawat S, Badhani A, Rawal RS. 2017. Nutraceutical potential of selected wild edible fruits of the Indian Himalayan Region. *Food Chemistry*. 215: 84–91.
9. Shah S, Tewari B, Bisht S, Tewari A. 2006. Seed maturation indictors in *Pyracantha crenulata* Roxb. in Kumaun Central Himalaya. *New Forests*. 32: 1–7.
10. Chaudhry S, Singh SP, Singh JS. 1996. Performance of seedlings of various life forms on landslide-damaged forest sites in Central Himalaya. *Journal of Applied Ecology*. 33 (1): 109–117.
11. Palita SK, Ponkshe AV, Dhar U. 2011. Habitat enrichment and its impact on avian diversity: a study at GBPIHED, Kosi-Katarmal, Uttarakhand, India. *Current Science*. 100 (11): 1681–1689.
12. Singh R, Negi PS, Ahmad Z. 2010. Himalaya Red Berry- Wonder Heart Tonic. Spectrum, Science Reporter. September: 16–18.
13. Pal RS, Kumar RA, Agrawal PK, Baatt JC. 2013. Antioxidant capacity and related phytochemicals analysis of methanolic extract of two wild edible fruits from north Wester Indian Himalaya. *International Journal of Pharma and Bio Sciences* 4 (2): 113–123.
14. Saklani S, Chandra S. 2011. Evaluation of nutritional profile, medicinal value and qualitative estimation in different parts of *Pyrus pashia*, *Ficus palmata* and *Pyracantha crenulata*. *Journal of Global Trends in Pharmaceutical Science*. July–Sept.: 350–354.
15. Mehra A. 2014. Diversity; Utilization and sacred values of ethno-medicinal plants of Kumaun Himalaya. *International Journal by Society for Tropical Plant Research*. 1 (3): 80–86.
16. Chauhan NS. 1999. *Medicinal and Aromatic Plants of Himachal Pradesh*. Indus Publishing Co. FS-5, Tagore Garden.
17. Gaur RD. 1999. *Flora of the District Garhwal Northwest Himalaya*, 1st Edition. Trans-Media, Srinagar Garhwal, India.
18. Fern K. 2008. *Plants of a Future*. Plants of a Future Species, Database, England.
19. Singh B, Peter KV. 2018. New Age Herbals. Springer Nature Singapore Pvt Ltd. https://doi.org/10.1007/978-981-10-8291-7_7, as on 16th July 2022.
20. Patade VY, Singh N, Bala M. 2022. Agalope javana: threat for Ghingaru (*Pyracantha crenulata*), An economically important Himalayan medicinal plant. *National Academy Science Letters*. https://doi.org/10.1007/s40009-020-00960-w, as on 18th July 2022.
21. Gamble JS. 1972. *A Manual of Indian Timbers: An Account of the Growth, Distribution, and Uses of the Trees and Shrubs of India and Ceylon, with Descriptions of Their Wood-Structure*. Bishen Singh Mahendra Pal Singh Publication, Dehradun.
22. Barnes BV, Zak DR, Denton SR, Spurr SH. 1998. *Forest Ecology*. Wiley, New York.
23. Peschel W, Bohr C, Plescher A. 2008.Variability of total flavonoides in *Crataegus* –Factor evaluation for the monitored production of Industrial starting material. *Fitoterapia*. 79: 6–20.
24. Anonymous. 2011. *Annual Report*. Defence Institute of Bio-Energy Research (DRDO), Haldwani.
25. Walker AF, Marakis G, Simpson E, Hope JL, Robinson PA, Hassanein M, Simpson HCR. 2006. Hypotensive effects of hawthorn for patients with diabetes taking prescription drugs. *British Journal of General Practice*. 56: 437–443.
26. Anna S, Oszmian J, Aneta W. 2007.Antioxidant activity of phenolic compounds of Hawthorn, pine, skullcap. *Food Chemistry*. 103: 853–859.
27. Chang Q, Zuo Z, Harrison F, Chow MSS. 2002. Comparison of the pharmacokinetics of Hawthorn phenolics in extract versus individual pure compound. *Journal of Clinical Pharmacology* 42: 605–612.
28. Tassell MC, Kingston R, Gilroy D, Lehane M, Furey A. 2010. Hawthorn (*Crataegus* spp.) in the treatment of cardiovascular disease. *Pharmacognosy Reviews*. 4: 32–41.
29. Guven K, Yucel E, Cetintas F. 2006. Antimicrobial activities of fruits of *Crataegus* and *Pyrus* species. *Pharmaceutical Biology*. 44: 79–83.

30. Kunkel G. 1984. *Plants for Human Consumption: An Annotated Checklist of the Edible Phanerogams and Ferns*. Koeltz Scientific Books, Koenigstein. pp. 393.
31. Andrade-Cetto A, Heinrich M. 2005. Mexican plants with hypoglycaemic effect used in the treatment of diabetes. *Journal of Ethnopharmacology*. 99: 325–348.
32. Wagner H, Grevel J. 1982. Cardio-active drugs IV. *Planta Medica*. 6: 98–110.
33. Sheat WG. 1948. *Propagation of Trees, Shrubs and Conifers*. MacMillan and Co., London. pp. xii+479 pp. ISBN 19501602763.
34. Tenorio fA, Valledel L, Gonzalez A, Pastelin G. 2005. Vasodilator activity of the aqueous extract of *Viscum album*. *Fitoterapia*. 76 (2): 204–209.

23 *Pyrus pashia* (Mehal)

INTRODUCTION

Pyrus pashia Buch.-Ham. ex. D. Don. (fam.: Rosaceae) is a medium-size fruiting tree (Figure 23.1), known locally as 'Indian Wild Pear',[1] Himalayan Pear, Batangi, Tangai, and Mehel.[2,3] It generally grows on sandy loamy soil at a temperature range from 10°C to 35°C. The leaves of the plant are known for various physiological properties and have many useful polyphenol ingredients such as chlorogenic acids, arbutin, flavan-3-ols, etc.[2] The extract from leaves is used as a tonic for hair loss, and woods are a major fuel source in the central Himalayan region. The hot tisane of leaves is consumed by Monpa communities of Twang, Arunachal Pradesh, India.[3] The indigenous people of the Jammu and Kashmir and Ladakh divisions of India use twinges of the species to treat toothache.[4] *P. pashia* fruits are used to treat gastrointestinal disorders, headaches, dehydration, hysteria, epilepsy, and fever.[5] Flowers are used to cure certain cancers and cardiovascular diseases. These healing properties of flowers are attributed to the presence of phenolic compounds.[6] Chemical investigation on *P. pashia* reveals the presence of triterpenoids, alkaloids, sterols, flavonoids, and phenolic compounds.[7]

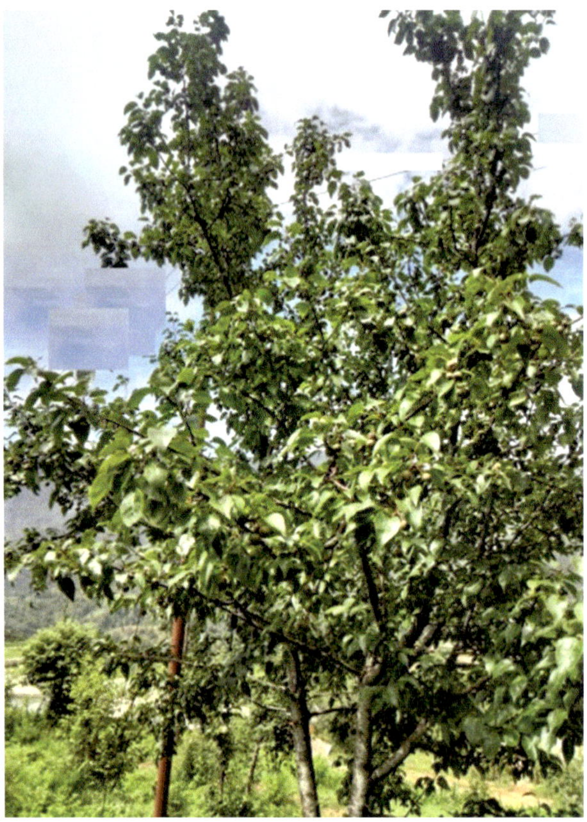

FIGURE 23.1 *Pyrus pashia* plant.

ETHNOBOTANY

The local population of the mid-Himalayas utilizes *P. pashia* leaf extract for treating infection of the toe finger, particularly during the rainy season. The juice of ripe unripe fruits (Figure 23.2) of the species is used to treat mouth sores and eye injury, respectively.[8] Barks, fruits, and leaves are traditionally used as food supplements and as medicine.[9] Strong antioxidant activity with free radical scavenging properties has been attributed to the flower extract of *P. pashia*.[10]

Traditionally, crushed fruits and leaves are used to treat fungal infections, cuts, and wounds.[11] Fruits, leaves, wood, and twigs are used to cure mouth infections and eye problems.[12,13] In the Garhwal region of Uttarakhand, India, fruits of *P. pashia* are used to treat digestive disorders.[14]

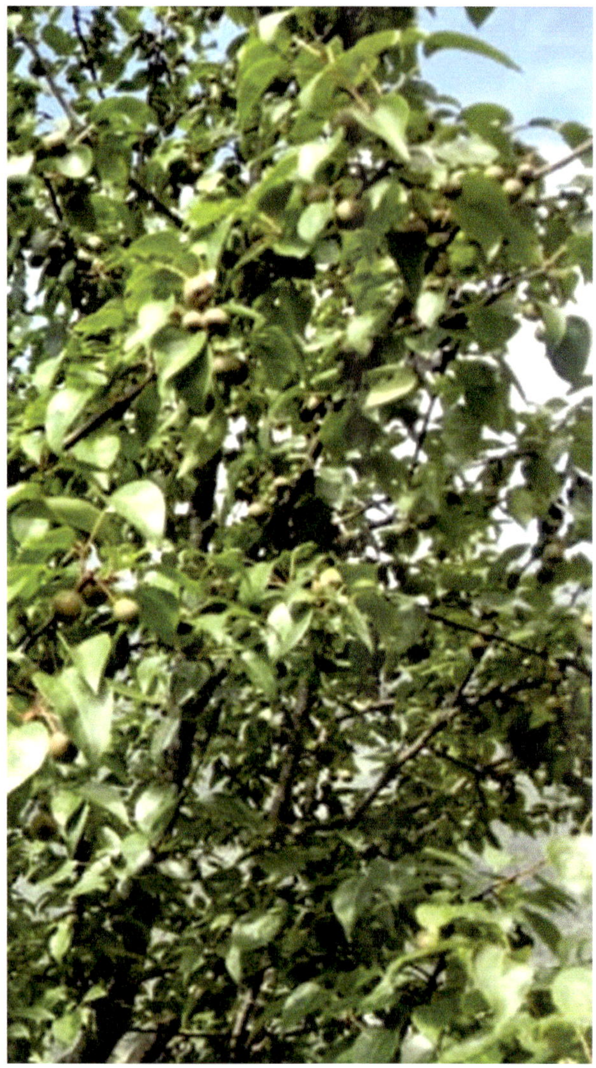

FIGURE 23.2 *P. pashia* branches with fruits.

DOI: 10.1201/9781003512868-25

The ripened fruits are edible, while twigs and tender leaves are used as fodder. In the central Himalayan region, the leaf extract is applied as a tonic for hair loss, and wood is used as a source of fuel.[15–17] The leaves are used as tisane in Arunachal Pradesh (India) by the Monpa Community, Tawang. In the Ladakh, Kashmir, and Jammu regions of India, twigs of the plant are used to cure toothache.[18] Crushed fresh leaves are used for staining nails, feet, and palms.[19] Constipation is treated by eating the ripened fruits of *P. pashia*.[20] In Khanabad village of Pakistan, fruits are a popular home medicine and are used as an astringent, sedative, and febrifuge[21] and are prescribed to treat asthma.[22] Fruits have been reported as having potent antimicrobial activity against *Escherichia coli*, *Shigella flexneri*, and *Klebsiella pneumoniae*.[23] Ripened fruits are eaten by tribes.[24–27] *P. pashia* has been used conventionally by many communities in the Himalayan region for the management of vascular complications and gastrointestinal and respiratory problems. The plant species is well known for its therapeutic and nutritional values. The leaves are used as a tisane and serve as fodder for sheep and goats.[4,28] On boiling with water, leaves of *P. pashia* produce a red color like the tea of *Camellia sinensis*, which is served as traditional tea among the Monpa community.[28] The fresh leaves have been reported to possess laxative, febrifuge, sedative, astringent, and cosmetic properties.[6] The fruits are tasty and eaten to cure constipation,[20] minimize thirst,[29] manage dysentery,[30] leishmaniasis[31] eye problems,[32] anemia, irritability, sore throat, digestive disorders, and abdominal pain.[33] Molecular biology-related studies have revealed the stomachic, antioxidant, hypoglycemic, and antimicrobial activities of fruit.[7,34] The decoction of dry fruits with other plant parts is used to improve the spleen and stomach functions.[35] Fruits are given to cattle to enhance milk production.[36] The bark of the tree possesses laxative, febrifuge, anthelmintic, and astringent properties[37] and is traditionally used to cure digestive disorders.[38] The barks have tonic and astringent properties and are used to cure peptic ulcers, sore throats, gastric ulcers, fever,[39,40] and typhoid fever.[41]

P. pashia cell sap is used to treat conjunctivitis.[42] Fruits are used for headaches, sweating of the body, gastrointestinal disorders, fever, epilepsy, and hysteria. It is mostly used as a laxative, febrifuge, and sedative.[2,43]

The plant species contain pectin, which lowers the low-density lipids (bad cholesterol), triglycerides, and very-low-density lipids (i.e., bad form of cholesterol), thereby reducing the risk of high cholesterol. Arbutin, a skin-whitening agent, is present in *P. pashia* leaves, which decreases the melanin in the facial skin.[44] Fruit juice is diuretic and astringent, managing eye problems, anemia, and dysentery. The bark is used as an astringent, laxative, and anthelmintic, and to treat peptic ulcers, typhoid fever, and gastric ulcers. Fresh leaves are used as a laxative, astringent, sedative, and febrifuge. Leaf extract is used as a tonic for hair loss. Fruits are used for dehydration and digestive ailments. The plant is used to reduce fever, headache, sweating of the body, hysteria, and epilepsy.[45] The paste of young twigs and fresh leaves is used to treat fungal infection of the toe.[46]

PHYTOPHARMACOLOGY

Phytopharmacological investigations of *P. pashia* fruits have revealed the presence of tannins, steroids, flavonoids, alkaloids,[47] lupeol, β-sitosterol, and β-sitosterol-β-D-glucoside.[31] Fruits are known for their antimicrobial activity.[47] Leaves have been reported for pectin, phlorizin, tannins, amygdalin, arbutin,[48] chlorogenic acids, flavan-3-ols, and arbutin.[26] Leaves are used as a source of antioxidant, antimutagenic, and anticarcinogenic compounds.[26] The plant species is used as a remedy for multiple ailments, and it is a rich source of phytochemicals like alkaloids, flavonoids, sterols, triterpenoids, and phenolic compounds in different plant parts (Tables 23.1 and 23.2).

TABLE 23.1
Therapeutic Compounds of *P. pashia*[7,34]

Chemical Class	Chemical Name	Plant Part
Alkaloids	Caffeic acid and genistein	Leaves and fruit
Flavonoids	Quercetin-3-o-β-D-glucopyranoside phloridzin and kaempferol-3-β-D-(6-o-cis-p-coumaroyl) gluco-pyranoside	Leaves
Phenolic glycoside	4-O-Z-coumaroyl arbutin and arbutin (hydroquinone-β-D-glucopyranoside)	Flower
Sterols	β-sitosterol, β-sitosterol-3-D glucoside	Fruit
Triterpenes	Lupeol	Fruit

TABLE 23.2
Pharmacological Activity of *P. pashia* Plant

S. No	Therapeutic Activity	Used Part	Solvent Used
1	Hepatoprotective[49]	Areal parts	Aqueous
2	Antidepressant activity[50]	Leaves	Methanol
3	In vivo anti-inflammatory activity[51]	Leaves	Methanol
4	In vivo anti-inflammatory activity[52]	Fruits	Methanol
5	Disinfectant[53]	Leaves	Water
6	Antioxidant and antiproliferative[54]	Fruit	Methanol and acetone
7	Antioxidant activity[5]	Leaves	Chloroform
8	Spasmolytic, bronchodilator, and vasoconstrictive activities[55]	Fruit	Aqueous ethanol
9	Antimicrobial activity[47]	Bark and fruit	Ethanol

Case Studies for Deciphering Therapeutic Ingredients

CASE STUDY 1

Arya et al. have studied the plant *P. pashia* to evaluate its medicinal uses, especially in the treatment of digestive ailments.[15] To understand the therapeutic properties of the different plant parts, various parameters like extractive values, foreign organic matter content, ash values, moisture content, foaming index, swelling index, analysis of powdered drug reaction with different chemical reagents, fluorescence analysis, etc., were studied. The powdered crude herb was extracted using a Soxhlet apparatus with different solvents of increasing polarity from n-hexane, chloroform, acetone, n-butanol, and water. Chemical screening of these extracts revealed the presence of different chemical classes, such as saponins, flavonoids, carbohydrates, phenolics, tannins, and steroids in some extracts, which later were also confirmed by thin layer chromatography (TLC) analysis.[15]

The physicochemical, morphological, chromatographic, and microscopic results were documented against the reference standard for authentication, identification, and distinguishing the plants from adulterants.[15]

Qualitative analysis for each extract was carried out by employing standard methods, particularly by TLC.[15] After the solvent distillation and drying of each extract in a vacuum desiccator, the phytoconstituents were identified by the TLC using different spot-detecting reagents. The test extract was dissolved in an appropriate solvent at a concentration of 1 mg/mL and spotted on a silica gel TLC plate. A total of four solvent systems were used as mobile phase, namely, n-hexane-EtOAc (8:2), $CHCl_3$-MeOH-H_2O (8:2:0.2), EtOAc-$CHCl_3$-MeOH-H_2O (12:8:8:2), and $CHCl_3$-MeOH-H_2O (65:35:10). Spots were detected by using both non-destructive (UV light, iodine chamber) and destructive visualization techniques [spraying reagents (anisaldehyde sulfuric acid and vanillin-sulfuric acid)]. Various extracts were applied with the help of a microcapillary, just 2 cm above the bottom of the TLC plate. The spots were equally sized, dried, and developed, and finally, the retention factor (R_f) values were calculated.[15]

These data are helpful for the preparation of a *P. pashia* monograph and its inclusion in various pharmacopeias. The bark of *P. pashia* has been reported to be rich in saponins, fats, flavonoids, steroids, carbohydrates, and tannins. The TLC results of the n-butanol, acetone, n-hexane, chloroform, and aqueous extract revealed the presence of at least four different constituents in each extract of *P. pashia* stem bark.[15]

Arbutin, chlorogenic acids, flavan-3-ols, etc., have been reported as the main compounds of the plant *P. pashia*. These compounds are well known for antioxidant, antimutagenic, and anticarcinogenic effects. *P. pashia* has been employed as herbal medicine and used to treat digestive ailments.[15]

CASE STUDY 2

Hemalatha et al. have studied the *P. pashia* fruits to ensure their safety and quality, as traditionally acclaimed.[56] The fresh fruits of *P. pashia* were phytochemically screened as per WHO guidelines, and the ethanolic extract was standardized to total phenolic and flavonoid content, followed by quantification using lupeol as a marker by the HPLC analysis. Fruit's microscopy reveals the characteristics of a berry, with a thick fleshy pericarp differentiated into a thin epicarp and a thick mesocarp along wide radiating carpel chambers with one or two seeds attached to the axile placenta. Further, an analysis of physicochemical parameters like water-soluble ash, total-ash value, loss on drying, acid-insoluble ash, fluorescence analysis, % of heavy metal, and pesticide residue contents was performed to define safety. Further, the ethanolic extract of *P. pashia* obtained by cold maceration and its phytochemical screening using liquid-liquid partitioning revealed the presence of various secondary metabolites such as steroids, flavonoids, triterpenoids, glycosides, phenols, etc. The whole investigation concluded that fruits are a rich source of phenols and flavonoids.[56] The HPLC chromatogram of the ethanolic extract of *P. pashia* deciphers that the fruit has 4.24% (w/w) of lupeol. This study is a step to ensure the quality and safety of fruits of *P. pashia*, and HPLC quantification is an aid in the authentication and development of a monograph for *P. pashia* fruits.[56] This knowledge helps minimize adulteration, which mainly arises from improper knowledge, varied geographical conditions, plant morphology, associated problems of vernacular names, and microscopy. Further, it also ensures the reproducible quality of fruits.

The extraction of a crude herb with a particular solvent results in a solution containing different phyto-ingredients. The composition of these phytoconstituents in that solvent depends upon the nature of the herb and the polarity of the used solvent. As in the present study, hydroalcoholic and alcoholic extracts were studied and standardized. Further, the ash value deciphers the quality and purity of the herb.[57] The ash of an herb indirectly depicts the non-volatile inorganic components (metallic salts and silica) present in it, resulting from the controlled incineration of the herb, which varies within wide limits and is, therefore, an important criterion for the authentication of crude herbs.

Various physiochemical constants, such as extractive value, loss on drying, ash values, hemolytic index, foreign matter, foaming index, and swelling index, as well as loads of pesticide residues and heavy metals, were assessed. The values were found to be within the limits as prescribed by the WHO guidelines[58] for safety and associated side effects. As biotic and abiotic factors influence the chemical composition of the plant material,[59] it is necessary to check it before use for quality consistency, especially as globalization has synchronized the trade and availability of plant materials.

The chemical screening of the species has revealed the presence of saponins, triterpenes, carbohydrates, sterols, alkaloids, flavonoids, and tannins. Fruits of *P. pashia* are rich in phenolics and flavonoids and are used for biochemical actions such as antimutagenic, anticarcinogenic, and antioxidant effects, as well as can modify gene expression.[60,61] Certain phenolics have been reported for potential neuroprotective properties, aiming to be one of the greater challenges in new drug discovery today.[62] Additionally, flavonoids have been reported to possess multifaceted beneficial bioactive qualities for health, such as antiallergic, anticancer, and anti-inflammatory activities; lowering blood pressure and plasma lipids; and conferring cardioprotective and neuroprotective activities.[63]

HPLC studies revealed that the concentration of lupeol in the ethanolic extract of fruits of *P. pashia* is 4.24% (w/w). This wild berry fruit from the Himalayan region possesses various traditional medicinal properties.[63]

A recent effort to standardize the wild edible fruit of P. pashia exemplifies potential methodologies for future studies on other natural resources aimed at discovering new drug compounds. Moreover, the use of HPLC is a versatile, robust, and widely accepted technique for the phytochemical identification, analytical quantification, and purification of a mixture of herbs.[64] Such studies are necessary to prepare the monograph of any of the herbs.

SCOPE AND OPPORTUNITIES

P. pashia is a plant of choice for many health-related disorders and has different pharmacological properties, including anti-inflammatory, antioxidant, and hepatoprotective activities. Studies reveal that the hydroalcoholic extract of *P. pashia* has vasoconstrictive, bronchodilator, and spasmolytic properties through different mechanisms. The bronchodilator and spasmolytic activities are likely to be mediated through the blockade of Ca^{2+} ion channels, while vasoconstrictive activity is assumed due to the presence of serotonergic, α-muscarinic, adrenergic, and angiotensin II agonistic components. The Ca^{2+} ion channel blocking activity is to be attributed to the phytochemical constituents (i.e., anthraquinones, glycosides, flavonoids, and alkaloids) of *P. pashia* fruits.[55] Similar types of more detailed investigations are to be done for further authentication and therapeutic utilization of the *P. pashia* plant to ensure its quality and safety. *P. pashia* is a very less investigated species and requires detailed pharmacological studies to investigate and validate the therapeutic folk/traditional potential of *P. pashia* to treat cardiovascular, respiratory, and gastrointestinal ailments.

REFERENCES

1. Kala CP. 2007. Prioritization of cultivated and wild edibles by local people in the Uttaranchal hills of Indian Himalaya. *Indian Journal of Traditional Knowledge*. 6 (1): 239–244.
2. Matin A, Khan MA, Ashraf M, Qureshi RA. 2001. Traditional uses of herbs, shrubs, and tree of Shogran valley, Mansehra, Pakistan. *Pakistan Journal of Biological Sciences*. 4: 1101–1107.
3. Ahmad Z. 2007. *Country Report on Plant Genetic Resources for Food and Agriculture*. Pakistan Agricultural Research Council, Islamabad, Pakistan.
4. Thapa B, Walker DH, Sinclair FL. 1997. Indigenous knowledge of the feeding value of tree fodder. *Animal Feed Science and Technology*. 67: 97–114.
5. Tsering J, Gogoi BJ, Tag H. 2012. Ethnobotany and phytochemical analysis of *Pyrus pashia* leaves. *International Journal of Pharma Sciences and Research*. 3: 2721–2725.
6. Shinwari MI, Khan MA. 1998. Multiple dimensions of ethnobotany and its present status in Pakistan. *Hamdard Medicus*. 42: 5–10.
7. Maga JA. 1978. Simple phenol and phenolic compounds in food flavour. *Critical Reviews in Food Science and Nutrition*. 10: 323–372.
8. Negi VS, Maikhuri RK, Vashishtha DP. 2011. Traditional healthcare practices among the villages of Rawain valley, Uttarkashi, Uttarakhand, India. *Indian Journal of Traditional Knowledge*. 10 (3): 533–537.
9. Jambey T, Gogoi BJ, Tag H. 2012. Ethanobotany and phytochemical analysis of *Pyrus pashia* leaves. *IJPSR*. 3 (8): 2721–2725.
10. Zhen-Jie L, Zheng X, Chun-Ping W, Cai L, Li Y, Huang L, Ding ZT. 2016. A new phenolic compound with antioxidant activity from the branches and leaves of *Pyrus pashia*. *Journal of Natural Product Research*. 30: 1136–1143.
11. Sharma P, Agnihotry A, Sharma PP, Sharma L. 2013. Wild edibles of Murari Devi and surrounding areas in Mandi district of Himachal Pradesh, India. *International Journal*. 30 (5): 592–604.
12. Ambasta SP, Ramchandran K. 1986. *The Useful plants of India, Publications, and Information Directorate*. CSIR, New Delhi.
13. Sharma SK, Kumar N, Kumar H. 2009. *Ethnobotanical Studies on Trees, Shrubs and Climbers of Himalaya*. Satish Serial Publishing House.
14. Kumar M, Sheikh MA, Bussmann RW. 2011. Ethnomedicinal and ecological status of plants in Garhwal Himalaya, India. *Journal of Ethnobiology and Ethnomedicine*. 7 (1): 1–13.
15. Arya V, Gupta R, Gupta VK. 2011. Pharmacognostic and phytochemical investigations on *Pyrus pashia* Buch.-Ham.ex D. Don stem bark. *Journal of Chemical and Pharmaceutical Research*. 3 (3): 447–456.
16. Sawian JT, Jeeva S, Lyndem FG, Mishra BP, Laloo RC. 2007. Wild edible plants of Meghalaya, North-east India. *Natural Product Reseach*. 6 (5): 410–426.
17. Khan MA, Khan MA, Hussain M, Ghulam GM. 2010. An ethnobotanical inventory of Himalayan region Poonch valley Azad Kashmir (Pakistan). *Ethnobotany Research and Applications*. 8: 107–123.
18. Gairola S, Sharma J, Bedi YS. 2014. A cross-cultural analysis of Jammu, Kashmir and Ladakh (India) medicinal plant use. *Journal of Ethnopharmacology*. 155 (2): 925–986.
19. Abbasi AM, Khan MA, Ahmad M, Zafar M, Jahan S, Sultana S. 2010. Ethnopharmacological application of medicinal plants to cure skin diseases and in folk cosmetics among the tribal communities of North-West Frontier Province, Pakistan. *Journal of Ethnopharmacology*. 128 (2): 322–335.

20. Abbasi AM, Khan MA, Khan N, Shah MH. 2013. Ethnobotanical survey of medicinally important wild edible fruits species used by tribal communities of Lesser Himalayas-Pakistan. *Journal of Ethnopharmacology*. 148 (2): 528–536.
21. Gorsi MS, Miraj S. 2002. Ethnomedicinal survey of plants of Khanabad village and its allied areas, district Gilgit. *Asian Journal of Plant Sciences*. 1 (5): 604–615.
22. Arya KR. 2002. Traditional uses of some common plants in indigenous folklore of Dronagiri; A mythic hill of Uttaranchal. *Indian Journal of Traditional Knowledge*. 1 (1): 81–86.
23. Saklani S, Chandra S. 2012. Phytochemical screening of Garhwal Himalaya wild edible fruit *Ficus palmata*. *International Journal of Pharm Tech Research*. 4 (3): 1185–1191.
24. Rasineni GK, Siddavattam D, Reddy AR. 2008. Free radical quenching activity and polyphenols in three species of *Coleus*. *Journal of Medicinal Plants Research*. 2 (10): 285–291.
25. Guven K, Yucel E, Cetintas F. 2006. Antimicrobial activities of fruits of *Crataegus* and *Pyrus* species. *Pharmaceutical Biology*. 44 (2): 79–83.
26. Nassar MI, Mohamed TK, El-Toumy SA, Garra AH, El-Kashak WA, Brouard I, El Kousy SM. 2011. Phenolic metabolites from *Pyrus calleryana* and evaluation of its free radical scavenging activity. *Carbohydrate Research*, 346 (1): 64–67.
27. Imeh U, Khokhar S. 2002. Distribution of conjugated and free phenols in fruits: antioxidant activity and cultivar variations. *Journal of Agricultural and Food Chemistry*. 50: 6301–6306.
28. Bharali P, Tina M, Mahanta D, Kalita MC, Das AK. 2020. Phytoconstituent evaluation of *Pyrus pashia* Buch-Ham. ex D. Don-A potential ethnomedicinal plant from Arunachal Pradesh, India. *Pleione*. 13(2): 284–290.
29. Meyers KJ, Watkins CB, Pritts MP, Liu RH. 2003. Antioxidant and anti-proliferative activities of straw berries. *Journal of Agricultural and Food Chemistry*. 51: 6887–6892.
30. Chettri N, Sharma E, Lama S D. 2005. Non-timber forest produces utilization, distribution and status in a trekking corridor of Sikkim, India. *Lyonia*. 8: 89–101.
31. Khandelwal R, Paliwal S, Chauhan R, Siddiqui A. 2008. Phytochemical screening of hexane soluble fraction of *Pyrus pashia* fruits. *Oriental Journal of Chemistry*. 24: 773–774.
32. Lama YC, Ghimire SK, Aumeeruddy-Thomas A. 2001. *Medicinal Plants of Dolpo; Amchi's Knowledge and Conservation*. People and Plants Initiative and WWF Nepal Program Nepal.
33. Saklani S, Chandra S. 2012. Evolution of Garhwal Himalaya wild edible fruit *Pyrus pashia* Magapulp. *Journal of Pharmacy Research*. 5: 3030–3032.
34. Shui G, Leong LP. 2002. Separation and determination of organic acids and phenolic compounds in fruit juices and drinks by HPLC. *Journal of Chromatography A*. 977: 89–96.
35. Jiangsu New Medical College. 1986. *Dictionary of Chinese Traditional Medicine*. Shanghai People's Press, Shanghai, China.
36. Prakash O., Chauhan A. S., Kudachikar V. B.. 2021. *International Journal of Functional Nutrition*. 2: 9. doi:10.3892/ijfn.2021.19
37. Kala CP. 2000. *Medicinal plants of Indian Trans-Himalaya*. Bishen Singh Mahendra Pal Singh Dehradun, India.
38. Farooquee NA, Majila BS, Kala CP. 2004. Indigenous knowledge systems and sustainable management of natural resources in a high-altitude society in Kumaun Himalaya, India. *Journal of Human Ecology*. 16: 33–42.
39. Manandhar NP. 1994. An ethnobotanical survey of herbal drugs of Kaski District, Nepal. *Fitoterapia*. 65: 7–13.
40. Joshi AR, Edington JM. 1990. The use of medicinal plants by two village communities in the Central Development Region of Nepal. *Economic Botany*. 44: 71–83.
41. Shrestha PM, Dhillion SS. 2003. Medicinal plant diversity and use in the high lands of Dolakha district, Nepal. *Journal of Ethnopharmacology*. 86: 81–96.
42. Promila K, Dinesh Y. 2005. Indigenous animal healthcare practices of Kangra District, Himachal Pradesh. *Indian Journal of Traditional Knowledge*. 4 (2): 164–168.
43. Murad W, Ahmed A, Gilani SA and Khan MA. 2011. Indigenous knowledge and folk use of medicinal plants by the tribal communities of Hazar Nao Forest, Malak and District, North Pakistan. *Journal of Medicinal Plants Research*. 5 (7): 1072–1086.
44. Arzoo PM. 2016. Why is Pear so dear. *International Journal Research Ayurveda Phrma*. 7 (1): 108–112.
45. Thakur S, Sidhu MC. 2017. Medicinal plant remedies for dermatological problems. *Current Botany*. 8: 23–33.
46. Siddiqui SZ, Ali S, Rubab K. 2015. *Pyrus pashia*: a persuasive source of natural antioxidant. *Pakistan Journal of Pharmaceutical Sciences*. 28 (5): 1763–1772.
47. Saklani S, Chandra S. 2012. In-vitro antimicrobial activity nutritional profile of medicinal plant of Garhwal, Himalaya. *International Journal of Pharma Sciences and Research*. 3: 268–272.
48. Hussein FTK. 1983. *Medicinal plants in Libya*. Arab Encylopedia House, Beirut, Lebanon. pp. 7–822.
49. Meenakshi B, Rojini A, Chodhury MD. 2017. Hepatoprotective activity of aqueous extract of *Pyrus pashia* Buch-Ham ex d. don against CCl_4 induced liver damage. *International Journal of Pharmaceutical Sciences*. 8 (10): 4195–4200.
50. Pandey N, Singh A, Pant J. 2017. Anti-depressant activity of methanolic extract of *Pyrus pashia* leaves in Rats. *World Journal of pharmacy and Pharmaceutical Sciences*. 6 (10): 1175–1183.
51. Pandey N, Singh A, Pant J. 2017. In-vivo anti-inflammatory activity of methanolic extract of leaves part of *Pyrus pashia*. *World Journal of Pharmaceutical Research*. 6 (9): 621–628.
52. Chandra S, Saklani S, Kumar S. 2016. *In-vivo* anti-inflammatory activity of *Pyrus pashia* fruit. *World Journal of Pharmaceutical Sciences*. 4 (5): 273–276.
53. Chandra S, Ravindra, Malik SK. 2017. Evaluation of *Pyrus pashia* leaves extract as a disinfectant for Rainbow trout fertilized eggs. *International Journal of Current Microbiology and Applied Sciences*. 6 (1): 697–706.
54. Saini R, Verma G, Koushalya D. 2012. Comparative study of three wild fruits of Uttarakhand for antioxidant, anti-proliferative and polyphenolic composition. *Internationl Journal of Pharma and Biosciences*. 3 (4): 158–167.
55. Janbaz KH, Saqib F, Hawaz J. 2015. Scientific basis for used of *Pyrus pashia* Buch-Ham ex d.don fruit in GI, respiratory and cardiovascular ailments. *PLos One* 10(3): e0118605. doi:10.1371/journal.pone.0118605

56. Hemalatha S, Sharma P, Prasad SK. 2016. Quality control standardization of Wild Himalayan Pear: *Pyrus pashia*. *Pharmacognosy Journal*. 8 (4): 352–360.
57. Cho MH, Paik YS, Hahn TR. 2000. Enzymatic conversion of precarthamin to carthamin by a purified enzyme from the yellow petals of safflower. *Journal of Agricultural and Food Chemistry*. 48 (9): 3917–3921.
58. WHO. 2000. *Quality Control Methods for Medicinal Plant Materials*. WHO, Geneva.
59. Ncube B, Finnie JF, Staden JV. 2012. Review Quality from the field: the impact of environmental factors as quality determinants in medicinal plants. *South African Journal of Botany*. 82: 11–20.
60. Nakamura Y, Watanabe S, Miyake N, Kohno H, Osawa T. 2003. Dihydrochalcones: evaluation as novel radical scavenging antioxidants. *Journal of Agricultural and Food Chemistry*. 51 (11): 3309–3312.
61. Tapiero H, Tew KD, Ba GN, Mathe G. 2002. Polyphenols: do they play a role in the prevention of human pathologies? *Biomedicine and Pharmacotherapy*. 56 (4): 200–207.
62. Loers G, Yashunsky DV, Nifantiev NE, Schachner M. 2014. Neural cell activation by phenolic compounds from the Siberian Larch (Larixsibirica). *Journal of Natural Products*. 77 (7): 1554–15561.
63. Hwang SL, Shih PH, Yen GC. 2012. Neuroprotective effects of citrus flavonoids. *Journal of Agricultural and Food Chemistry*. 60 (4): 877–885.
64. Piana M, Zadra M, de Brum TF, Boligon AA, Gonçalves AF, da Cruz RC, de Freitas RB, Canto GS, Athayde ML. 2012. Analysis of rutin in the extract and gel of *Viola tricolor*. *Journal of Chromatographic Science*. 51 (5): 406–411.

24 *Pyrus pyrifolia* (Naspati/Wild Pear)

INTRODUCTION

Pears, genus *Pyrus* (family: Rosaceae), comprise two major types: the European (Western) and the Asian pears.[1] The European pears have a buttery, juicy texture that is rich in flavor and aroma, and Asian pears are characterized (Figure 24.1) by a crisp texture and sweet but sub-acid flavor. European pears are cultivars of *Pyrus communis*, whereas Asian cultivars are derived from *Pyrus pyrifolia*,[2] although the genus *Pyrus* has at least 22 species with over 5,000 subspecies or accessions.[3] Different terms, such as Chinese pear, Japanese pear, and Korean pear, are often used to reflect the geographic milieux from which differing accessions evolved, especially of *P. pyrifolia*. Based on evolutionary, geographical, and morphological characteristics, Asian pears are round-shaped (Figure 24.2), have crisp flesh, and contain high sugar content, especially fructose. The Western pear, especially *P. communis*, is gourd-shaped with smooth and soft flesh, few stone cells, flavor, and a stronger aroma.[4] A higher amount of arbutin, chlorogenic acid, and phenolics has been reported in the Asian pear cultivars than in the Western pears.[5,6]

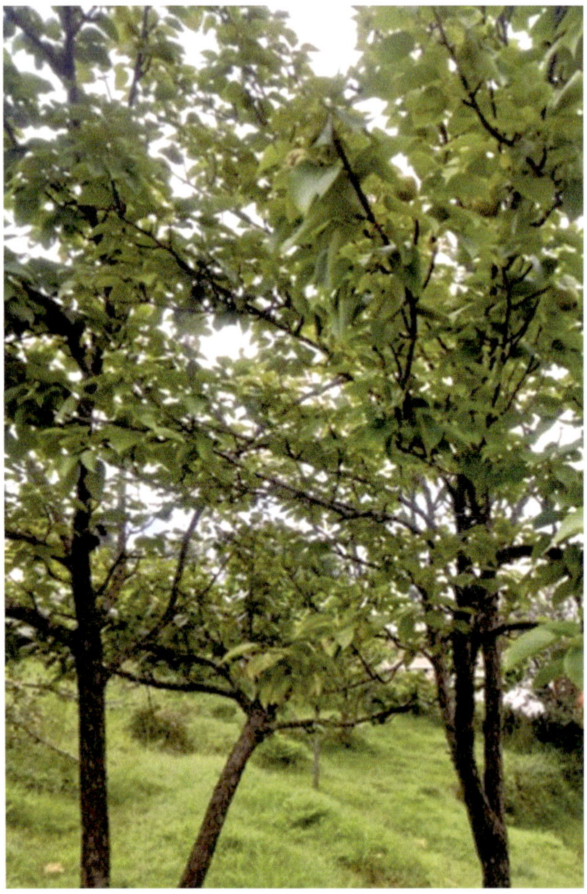

FIGURE 24.1 *Pyrus communis* trees.

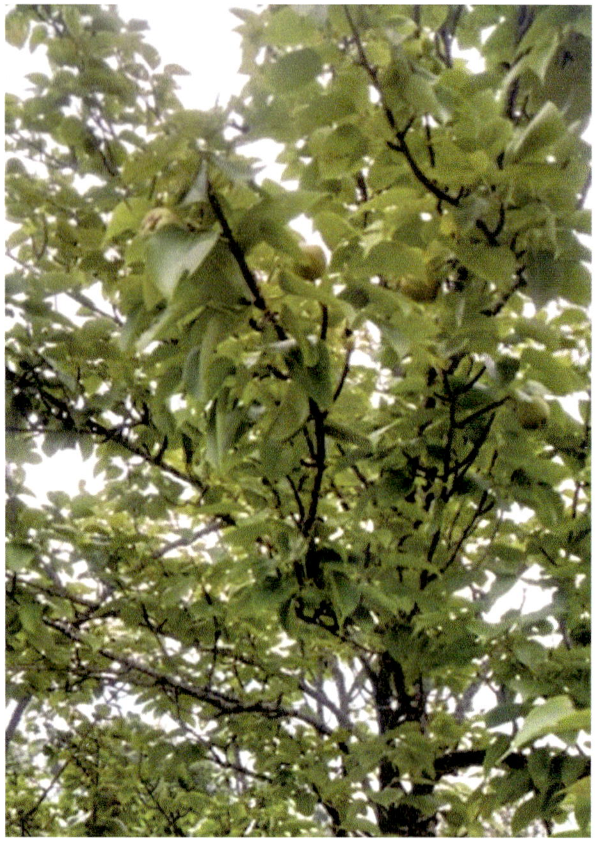

FIGURE 24.2 *P. communis* with fruits.

The Korean varieties are reported to have higher contents of sugar and potassium and are used for diverse medicinal applications, e.g., respiratory symptom relievers, fever management, inflammation treatment, alcohol hangovers, etc.[7,8] Traditionally in Korea, pears are used to aid in the digestion of meat, as a tenderizer in the cooking of beef, and as a dessert after meals. In addition, the traditional application of pears on alcohol hangovers has been confirmed by in vitro and in vivo studies that have revealed that eating *P. pyrifolia* stimulates the alcohol-metabolizing enzymes and eliminates the body burden of alcohol and aldehyde, respectively.[9] Further, clinical results have revealed the alleviation of hangover symptoms after eating pear fruits.[10]

Homer, an ancient Greek poet, described pears as the 'gifts of God'.[11] Pear cultivation has been in a semi-wild state for a long time, except in China and Japan. Its folk name in India is Bagu-goshaa or Naakh. Eating Bagu-goshaa (Naakh) fruits is recommended for maintaining a desirable acid balance in the body and normalizing elevated blood

DOI: 10.1201/9781003512868-26

glucose levels. Pear fruits are a good source of pectin, low in sucrose, and enriched in phenolics, the compounds known to boost body immunity.[2]

ETHNOPHARMACOLOGY

Humans have used *Pyrus* spp. as folk medicine and healthy food for thousands of years.[1] It is eaten either fresh or used in processed foods such as jams, jellies, purees, and juices.[3,12] In addition, pear fruits have been eaten in Asia to prevent constipation and cure coughs and the flu.[4] Its applications to treat gastric ulcers and inflammations have also been reported.[13–15]

Fresh pear juice is known for its therapeutic activity against *Escherichia coli*. The leaves of pears contain tannin, sorbitol, astragalin, isoquercitrin, ursolic acid, and arbutin.[16] Its barks contain friedelin, epifriedelanol, and β-sitosterol. The root's bark has phloridzin.[16] The plant extract is used to control the development of freckles and blemishes on the skin and prevents melanin formation, so it has application in skin lightening.[2]

Pear fruits are generally peeled before consumption due to concerns of pesticide and chemical contamination, presence of pectin and stone cells, and the skin's less desirable taste and texture.[17] The Chinese pharmaceutical encyclopedia has described the myriad uses of pears as a sweet and a little sour fruit that is cold and harmless; however, too much consumption of it makes people thin and weak and brings out diarrhea. It is used to treat fever, suppress cough, and quench thirst. Pear fruits in a slice form are used for relieving pain and preventing decomposition in burn wounds. These fruits provide benefits for defecation and urination, mollify chest tightness, dyspnea, and mental symptoms caused by hyperpyrexia, and are used to cool down the heart, moisturize lungs, remove sputum, and detoxify abscesses and alcohol poisoning. Pear flowers are used to cleanse dirt on a face, and during cold weather, the decoction of pear tree bark is beneficial for seasonal diseases. The leaves are enlisted to treat scrotal hernia, while pounded leaf extract is used against mushroom poisoning.[18]

Jun Heo, a Korean royal traditional physician (1546–1615 BC), described the usage of pears to treat chest tightness, irregular recurrent fever, and quenching thirst, particularly after drinking alcohol.[7] He also depicted the contraindications of pears, e.g., sword cuts or pregnancy, and described that too many pears make the stomach or intestines sick; however, cleaning with water boiled with pear barks provides benefits for scabies and tinea scores.[7] Zhang et al. have described that *P. pyrifolia* cv. Shingo has been used as a traditional medicine for alcohol hangovers in Korea and deciphered its richness in calcium, potassium, fiber, and water.[19]

PHYTOPHARMACOLOGY

P. pyrifolia has been reported to contain phenols and flavonoids (catechin, rutin, quercetin, and kaempferol), approximately 5 and 0.5 mmol/g of the dry weight of total fruit, respectively.[20] Its peel has 7- and 10-fold higher levels of total phenols (35 mmol/g) and flavonoids (9.5 mmol/g) than those in the flesh of western pears, respectively.[20] In human trials, the protective effects of the pears have been established against alcohol hangovers;[21] though protective mechanisms, yet, have not been established completely. Acetaldehyde, a main toxic metabolite of ethanol, is closely related to alcohol intoxification or hangover. Based on the results of in vitro studies by Lee et al., it has been concluded that the pear treatment stimulated anti-diuretic hormone or aldehyde dehydrogenase activities. The in vivo study results have revealed a decrease in alcohol levels in the blood after the pear treatment. This indicates that the pear treatment stimulated alcohol metabolism, reduced alcohol absorption, and sped up alcohol and aldehyde elimination through metabolic enhancement. Further, it was concluded that plenty of potassium, fructose, fiber, and water in Korean pear may have prevented alcohol-induced electrolyte imbalance, hypoglycemia, gastrointestinal disturbances, or dehydration to alleviate alcohol hangovers.[9]

Currently, there is an increasing trend to add functional materials to dairy products or functional peptides isolated from milk proteins. Park et al. studied the applications of crude enzymes obtained from *P. pyrifolia* on milk proteins and concluded that the peel of *P. pyrifolia* cv. Shingo can be used in the milk processing industry.[22]

Asian pear fruits are reported to contain arbutin and chlorogenic acid.[23]. Lin and Harnly have concluded that the phenolics in Asian pears are different from those in the European variety. A systematic study on the chemical constituents of *P. pyrifolia* fruits has been conducted, along with the isolation and structural elucidation of chemical constituents. The fruit peels of *P. pyrifolia* have much higher and more variable levels of phenolics than the pulp.[24]

Lee et al. have isolated seven phenylpropanoid malate derivatives from the peels of Asian pear[25] and reported eight phenolic compounds from the EtOAc with acidic pH.[26] The major components of pear fruits are water (approx. 80%), fiber (approx. 2%), and fructose and sugar (approx. 15%).[9] Polyphenols (flavonoids, phenolic acids), glucosides, and triterpenes are the major ingredients of pear fruits.[8,27] Phenolics are highest in the leaves, followed by seeds, peels, and pulps. Generally, phytonutrients are richer in peels than pulp.[28,29] The thick peel of pears has stone cells with lignified walls of abundant lignin and cellulose-containing pectin and is highly thickened.[30,31] The development of stone cells may be closely related to the transfer, synthesis, and deposition of lignin. For the monomeric compounds, arbutin, chlorogenic acid, oleanolic acid, epicatechin, ursolic acid, and rutin have been reported to be dominant in various pear cultivars, both in the flesh and in the peel.[6]

Arbutin is a well-known antibiotic[32] and skin-whitening compound of pears.[33,34] It degraded into hydroquinone, which is a skin-bleaching agent and is used in cosmetics as a melanin polymerization inhibitor, fragrance, and reducing agent. The in vitro and in vivo investigations have revealed that hydroquinone mediates immune function, though they have not yet been validated in humans.[34,35] Pear skins are one of the richest food sources of natural arbutin, especially those of *P. pyrifolia*,[36] and arbutin can be used as a potential pear-specific intake biomarker.[37]

Chlorogenic acid, the second most abundant (106.7–247.5 mg/100 g) phenolic compound in *P. pyrifolia* fruits, is present in both the flesh and peel,[38,39] and has been reported to have anti-inflammatory and antioxidant activities.[39] Chlorogenic acid reduces TNF-α, improves wound healing, and protects neurons.[40,41] It increases NOS and COX, resulting in the direct induction of endothelium-dependent vasodilation and endothelium-derived hyperpolarizing factor signaling pathways.[42] In addition, it is radioprotective, as it protects against DNA damage caused by radiation.[43]

Caffeic acid is a phenolic compound present in both the flesh and peel of the pear. It induces apoptosis, and reduces reactive oxygen species in the mitochondrial membrane, and has chemopreventive properties.[44]

Immature *P. pyrifolia* fresh fruits are reported to have flavonoids (182.5–368.9 mg/100 g)[33] (e.g., isorhamnetin, quercetin, etc.) and polymeric flavan-3-ols (epicatechin, proanthocyanidins, etc.).[45,46] These compounds are supposed to contribute to disease resistance of the plant, fruit quality, and color. Flavonoids are known for their biological properties, such as free radical scavenging, modulation of enzymatic activity, and inhibition of cellular proliferation. The potential applications of flavonoids include their use as antibiotic, anti-allergic, anticancer, anti-diarrheal, anti-inflammatory, and anti-ulcer agents in biological systems.[47] Epidemiological studies also acknowledge the role of flavonoids in human health.[48]

Malaxinic acid [4-(O-β-d-glucopyranosyl)-3-(3′-methyl-2′-butenyl)benzoic acid] is a major glucoside in *P. pyrifolia*.[49] In the immature fruits, malaxinic acid is 0.76–5.86 mg/100 gm (wt./wt.), although the amounts significantly decrease on maturity.[33] It has an antioxidative defense potential in blood circulation and inhibition of the growth of cancer cells (such as B16/BL6, HT1080, BAEC, and HeLa).[50,51] The isoprenyl side chain of malaxinic acid contributes to the inhibition of a 21–26 kDa protein response in cancer cell proliferation.[52] There is a need for more evidence related to the potential role of malaxinic acid as a cancer-preventive compound.

Eating pears has selectively stimulated the activities of microbial species in the gut region and induced reactions necessary for health benefits due to the presence of plenty of prebiotics in it.[53] The mixture of pear with carrot, sea buckthorn, and plum, containing inulin, confers the growth of *Lactobacillus*.[54] Additionally, pear fruits are rich in fiber and fructose, and this unique composition is responsible for their laxative properties.[37] Sugar alcohol, sorbitol, accounts for up to 90% of the total carbohydrate in pears, especially *P. pyrifolia*. In addition, malic, citric, ascorbic acids, and minerals (such as calcium, iron, potassium, and magnesium) in pears are likely to support blood pH and ionic homeostasis.[55]

PEARS AS ANTIDIABETIC FRUITS

The antihyperglycemic effects of pears and their consumption by diabetic patients are a matter of interest in treating the disease.[56–59] Further, the consumption of *P. pyrifolia* (pear) and *Malus domestica* (apple) has reduced the risk of type 2 diabetes mellitus by 18%.[59] The peel extract of *P. pyrifolia* significantly lowers fasting glucose levels compared to the control group, which is probably due to the inhibition of α-glucosidase.[60] Use of pears in humans may be an ideal herbal-nutrient option in the management of T2DM (type 2 diabetes mellitus).

ANTI-OBESITY ACTIVITY

Chemically, pear fruits are of low energy density (0.64 kcal/g) and rich in dietary fiber. These fruits are suitable for stomach satiety with less caloric intake, have reduced cortisol levels by 22% immediately after exercise, and promote fast recovery from strenuous exercises. Different investigations have supported the use of pears for obesity prevention and promoting exercise.[61]

ANTI-HYPERLIPIDEMIC EFFECTS

Velmurugan and Bhargava have reported that pear feeding in a dose-dependent manner significantly reduced the levels of total cholesterol, triglyceride, and low-density lipid concentration in hyperglycemic rats and increased levels of high-density lipid concentration.[56] It may be due to the catechin present in pears.

ANTI-MUTAGENIC AND ANTI-CARCINOGENIC EFFECTS

Pears have some anti-mutagenic and anticancer activities, which are supposedly due to polycyclic aromatic compounds.[62] The nitrite scavenging activity of Asian pears has been reported to be 80.7%–86.7%.[63,64] The pear fruits have comparably high nitrite scavenging properties than onions (50%) or kiwis (75.3%–81.8%).[8]

ANTI-INFLAMMATORY EFFECTS

Fruits such as apples, pears, red wine, and strawberries are part of the dietary chain to overcome noncommunicable diseases, as these fruits are a rich source of anthocyanin and flavanols, which have potent anti-inflammatory effects.[65] Arbutin exhibits anti-inflammatory effects on proinflammatory cytokines.[66] COVID-19 patients mostly have acute respiratory distress, resulting in lung damage, multi-organ failure, and finally death.[67] Hence, pears are a potential fruit to treat the cytokine storm.

RESPIRATORY PROTECTIVE EFFECTS

The intake of pears is strongly associated with a lower incidence of less diagnosed asthma, reduced bronchial hyper-reactivity, and fewer asthma symptoms. Many researchers have established an inverse correlation between pear consumption and asthma cases.[68] Further, the consumption of pears has significantly lowered the risk of chronic obstructive pulmonary disease in ex-smokers, with a hazard ratio of 0.70.[69] Studies using pears in in vitro reveal its bronchodilatory effects.[12] Lee et al. have reported that the sensitivity of the tracheal smooth muscle of mice can be treated with pectin of *P. pyrifolia*.[70] The mechanism of smoothing of tracheal muscle may be related to the unique combination of polyphenols and flavonoids.[12] The presence of quercetin and rutin in pears has a role in treating allergic diseases through the downregulation of mast cell activation.[71] The fresh pear juice reduced benzo(a)pyrene-induced lung cancer in A/J mice rather than heated juice,[72] concluding that heating fruit juice for preservation destroys the enzymes.

CARDIO-PROTECTIVE EFFECTS

Ingredients of the pear fruits, such as chlorogenic acid, improve ex vivo vessel function and protect endothelial cells against damage induced by hypochlorous acid, via induction of Hmox-1 and increased production of nitric oxide.[73] In vivo studies have confirmed the cardioprotective functions of pears via angiotensin-converting enzyme inhibition. However, the active compounds and process mechanisms are not fully deciphered. The hepatoprotective and alcohol detoxification properties of the pear fruits have been used as a traditional system to alleviate hangover symptoms.[7] The average scores of hangover severity have been noted to be significantly reduced in humans conditioned to the prior consumption of Korean pear juice before drinking alcohol.[10]

P. pyrifolia (Korean cultivar) enhances the growth of hepatocytes via the induced adenosine triphosphate synthesis in the cells.[74] Increased DNA synthesis has been reported in hepatic cells during the use of pear extracts. The pear peel extract has been reported for significant prevention in the levels of serum alanine aminotransferase and aspartate aminotransferase in mice.[75,76] The study has concluded that the use of Korean pears with alcohol may contribute to the prevention of liver damage from alcohol.

SKIN-WHITENING EFFECTS

Removing facial wrinkles and signs of a slowdown in the aging process are related to skin whitening, a cosmetic requirement, and pears are a natural source of abundant arbutin, a whitening compound.[8] Arbutin inhibits tyrosinase, an ingredient that generates melanin. Extracts of *P. pyrifolia* fruits have been reported to inhibit tyrosinase activity by 50% in mice. The use of the pear arbutin-enriched extract for the whitening effect has been reported much higher compared to arbutin itself.[77,78] Protocatechuic acid (PCA) is another phenolic compound in pear peels with skin-lightening and anti-melanogenic properties, which significantly suppresses melanogenesis through the inhibition of tyrosinase.[52]

SCOPE AND OPPORTUNITIES

The pear is a natural source of various therapeutic ingredients that can help to cure different body ailments. The ethnopharmacological and chemical information on pears may help researchers to explore more applications. Traditional applications of pears are still under investigation, and only a few have been confirmed with scientific evidence. Pears, an old and new fruit, have different therapeutic effects on various degenerative diseases and are used as a medicine or potential functional food for highly susceptible patients with underlying diseases to help prevent new communicable diseases like COVID-19 in the current era. Further studies on the molecular level to establish the role of pears for good health and a sound brain may help to find out new medicinal functions.

Pear extract with high amounts of cosmetic ingredients (e.g., arbutin and PCA) can treat facial problems like hyperpigmentation, and in the future, a new polyherbal formulation with a synergistic combination could be developed.

In recent years, the fruit processing industries have experienced rapid growth throughout the world, and fruit peels along with pulp are the major residues during processing. Though peels and pomace have a few major nutritional ingredients, they lack commercial applications. Due to the high industrial processing and domestic consumption of the edible parts of pears, a large volume of pear pomace is generated as residue, which may be utilized for animal feed or disposed of via compost manure, landfilling, and incineration. However, there is a scope to use pear peel residue as a source of nanocellulose.

REFERENCES

1. Yang M. 2018. *Detoxification of Pears. Daily Consumption of Korean Pears for Health*. Edited by Pear Research Institute, National Institute of Horticultural and Herbal Science: Rural Development Administration. pp. 55–67. Seoul, Republic of Korea.
2. Kaur R, Arya V. 2012. Ethnomedicinal and phytochemical perspectives of *Pyrus communis* Linn. *Journal of Pharmacognosy and Phytochemistry*. 1 (2): 14–19.
3. Wu J, Wang Y, Xu J, Korban S, Fei Z, Tao S, Ming R, Tai S, Khan AM, Postman JD, Gu C. 2018. Diversification and independent domestication of Asian and European pears. *Genome Biology*. 19 (1): 77.
4. Reiland H, Slavin J. 2015. Systematic review of pears and health. *Nutrition Today*. 50 (6): 301–305.
5. Sanchez ACG, Gil-Izquierdo A, Gil MI. 2003. Comparative study of six pear cultivars in terms of their phenolic and vitamin C contents and antioxidant capacity. *Journal of the Science of Food and Agriculture*. 83 (10): 995–1003.

6. Li X, Wang T, Zhou B, Gao W, Cao J, Huang L. 2014. Chemical composition and antioxidant and anti-inflammatory potential of peels and flesh from 10 different pear varieties (*Pyrus* spp.). *Food Chemistry*. 152: 531–8. https://doi.org/10.1016/j.foodchem.2013.12.010
7. Heo J. 2018. *Pyri Fructus / pear, part VII_Herbs 24 in DongUiBoGam (1613)*. Edited by Korea Institute of Oriental Medicine. https://mediclassics.kr/books/8/volume/21#content_756edition.
8. Min TS, Park MJ, Moon JH, Kim WS, Lee SH, Cho YD, Park SH. 2013. Bio-active substances and physiological activity of pears. *Journal of Applied Biological Chemisty*. 56 (2): 83–87. https://doi.org/10.3839/jabc.2013.014
9. Lee H, Isse T, Kawamoto T, Woo H, Kim AK, Park JY, Yang M. 2012. Effects and action mechanisms of Korean Pear (*Pyrus pyrifolia* cv. Shingo) on alcohol detoxification. *Phytotherapy Research*. 26: 1753–1758.
10. Lee H, Isse T, Kawamoto T, Baik HW, Park JY, Yang M. 2013. Effects of Korean pear (*Pyrus pyrifolia* cv. Shingo) juice on hangover severity following alcohol consumption. *Food and Chemical Toxicology*. 58: 101–106. https://doi.org/10.1016/j.fct.2013.04.007
11. Hedrick UP, Howe GH, Taylor OM, Francis EH, Turkey HB. 1921. The pears of New York. 29th Annual Report, New York Department of Agriculture. JB Lyon Co. Printers, Albany, New York.
12. James-Martin G, Williams G, Stonehouse W, O'Callaghan N, Noakes M. 2015. Health and Nutritional Properties of Pears (*Pyrus*): a Literature Review. https://australianpears.com.au/wp-content/uploads/2019/10/Pears-Health-Study-AP15010-Final-Report-Complete.pdf, as on 10th January 20222.
13. Choi J, Lee E, Kim J, Choi G, Jun S, Ham Y, Seo DC, Heo JS. 2006. Physiological activities according to cultivars and parts of Ulsan pear. *Journal of the Korean Society for Applied Biological Chemistry*. 49: 43–48.
14. Choi J, Lee S. 2013. Distribution of stone cell in Asian, Chinese, and European pear fruit and its morphological changes. *Journal of Applied Botany and Food Quality*. 86:185–189.
15. Jiang G, Yim S, Eun J. 2016. Physicochemical characteristics and antioxidant activities of new Asian pear cultivars. *Journal of Applied Biological Chemistry*. 59 (4): 337–343.
16. Nadkarni KM, Nadkarni AK. 2005. *Indian Materia Medica*, 3rd Edition. Popular Prakashan, Mumbai.
17. Chen YW, Hasanulbasori MA, Chait PF, Lee HV. 2019. *Pyrus pyrifolia* fruit peel as sustainable source for spherical and porous network based nanocellulose synthesis via one-pot hydrolysis system. *International Journal of Biological Macromolecules*. 123: 1305–1319
18. Li S. 2018. *Ben Cao Gang Mu (*1596). Edited by Korea Institute of Oriental Medicine. https://mediclassics.kr/books/190/volume/36
19. Zhang YB, Choi HJ, Han HS, Park JH, Kim S, Bae JH, Kim HK, Choi C. 2003. Polyphenolic compounds from Korean pear and their biological activities. *Food Science and Biotechnology*. 12: 262–267.
20. Hong SS. 2005. Determination of functional compounds and physiological activity in fruit of apple (*Malus* spp.) and pear (*Pyrus* spp.) Doctoral Dissertation, Department of Horticultural Science, Graduate School, Korea University, Seoul, South Korea.
21. Yang M, Park JY. 2010. Effects of Korean pears, *Pyrus pyrifolia* cv. Shingo, on alcohol detoxification. In *Functional Foods in the Prevention and Management of Metabolic Syndrome, The Proceeding of the 7th International Conference of Functional Food*, Dallas, TX. pp. 193–194.
22. Park MG, Kim HS, Nam IS, Kim WS. 2018. Application of crude enzymes obtained from *Pyrus pyrifolia* cv. Shingo on milk proteins. *Korean Journal of Agricultural Science*. 45 (4): 789–797.
23. Salta J, Martins A, Santos RS, Neng NR, Nogueira JMF, Justino J, Rauter AP. 2010. Phenolics composition and antioxidant activity of Rocha pear and other pear cultivars-A comparative study. *Journal of Functional Food*. 2: 153–157.
24. Lin LZ, Harnly JM. 2008. Phenolic compounds and chromatographic profiles of pear skins (Pyrus spp.). *Journal of Agricultural and Food Chemistry*. 56: 9094–9101.
25. Lee KH, Cho JY, Lee HJ, Park KY, Ma YK, Lee SH, Cho JA, Kim WS, Park KH, Moon JH. 2011. Phenylpropanoid malate derivatives from pear (*Pyrus pyrifolia* Nakai) fruit peel. *Journal of Agricultural and Food Chemistry*. 59: 10124–10128.
26. Lee KH, Cho JY, Lee HJ, Park KY, Ma YK, Lee SH, Cho JA, Kim WS, Park KH, Moon JH. 2011. Isolation and identification of phenolic compounds from an Asian Pear (*Pyrus pyrifolia* Nakai) fruit peel. *Food Science and Biotechnology*. 20 (6): 1539–1545.
27. Kolnia-Ostek J, Klopotowska D, Rutkowski KP, Skorupinska A, Kruczynska DE. 2020. Bioactive compounds and health-promoting properties of pears (*Pyrus communis* L.) fruits. *Molecules*. 25 (19): 4444.
28. Kolniak-Ostek J, Oszmiański J. 2015. Characterization of phenolic compounds in different anatomical pear (*Pyrus communis* L.) parts by ultra-performance liquid chromatography photodiode detector-quadrupole/time of flight-mass spectrometry (UPLC-PDA-Q/TOF-MS). *International Journal of Mass Spectrometry*. 392: 154–163.
29. Pascoalino LA, Reis FS, Prieto MA, Barreira JCM, Ferreira CFR, Barros L. 2021. Valorization of bio-residues from the processing of main Portuguese fruit crops: from discarded waste to health promoting compounds. *Molecules*. 26 (9): 2624.
30. Lee S, Cho J, Jeong HY, Jeong DE, Kim D, Cho S, Kim WS, Moon JH. 2015. Comparison of bioactive compound contents and *in-vitro* and *ex-vivo* antioxidative activities between peel and flesh of pear (*Pyrus pyrifolia* Nakai). *Food Science and Biotechnology*. 24 (1): 207–216.
31. Yan C, Yin M, Zhang N, Jin Q, Fang Z, Lin Y, Cai Y. 2014. Stone cell distribution and lignin structure in various pear varieties. *Scientia Horticulturae*. 174: 142–52.
32. Öztürk A, Demirsoy L, Demirsoy H, Asan A, Gül O. 2015. Phenolic compounds and chemical characteristics of pears (*Pyrus Communis* L.). *International Journal of Food Properties*. 18 (3): 536–546.
33. Cho J, Lee S, Kim EH, Yun HR, Hang YJ, Lee YG, Kim WS, Moon JH. 2015. Change in chemical constituents and free radical-scavenging activity during pear (*Pyrus pyrifolia*) cultivar fruit development. *Bioscience, Biotechnology, and Biochemistry*. 79 (2): 260–270.
34. Eun J, Eo J, Lee B. 2012. Functional compounds and biological activity of Asian pear. *Food Science and Industry*. 45 (1): 60–69.

35. Andersen FA, Bergfeld WF, Belsito DV, Hill RA, Klaassen CD, Liebler DC, Marks JG, Shank RC, Slaga TJ, Snyder PW. 2010. Final amended safety assessment of hydroquinone as used in cosmetics. *International Journal of Toxicology*. 29 (6_suppl): 274S–287S.
36. Deisinger PJ. 1996. Human exposure to naturally occurring hydroquinone. *Journal of Toxicology and Environmental Health, Part A*. 47 (1): 31–46.
37. Ulaszewska M, Vázquez-Manjarrez N, Garcia-Aloy M, Llorach R, Mattivi F, Dragsted LO, Praticò G, Manach C. 2018. Food intake biomarkers for apple, pear, and stone fruit. *Genes & Nutrition*. 13 (1): 29.
38. Kolniak-Ostek J. 2016. Chemical composition and antioxidant capacity of different anatomical parts of pear (*Pyrus communis* L.). *Food Chemistry*. 203: 491–497.
39. Wang Z, Barrow CJ, Dunshea FR, Suleria HAR. 2021. A comparative investigation on phenolic composition, characterization and antioxidant potentials of five different Australian grown pear varieties. *Antioxidants*. 10 (2): 151.
40. Hwang SJ, Kim Y, Park Y, Lee H, Kim K. 2014. Anti-inflammatory effects of chlorogenic acid in lipopolysaccharide-stimulated RAW 264.7 cells. *Inflammation Research*. 63 (1): 81–90.
41. Liang N, Kitts D. 2015. Role of chlorogenic acids in controlling oxidative and inflammatory stress conditions. *Nutrients*. 8: E16
42. Tom ENL, Girard-Thernier C, Demougeot C. 2016. The Janus face of chlorogenic acid on vascular reactivity: a study on rat isolated vessels. *Phytomedicine*. 23 (10): 1037–1042.
43. Mun G, Kim S, Choi E, Kim CS, Lee Y. 2018. Pharmacology of natural radioprotectors. *Archives of Pharmacal Research*. 41 (11): 1033–1050.
44. Jaganathan SK. 2012. Growth inhibition by caffeic acid, one of the phenolic constituents of honey, in HCT 15 colon cancer cells. *Scientific World Journal*. 2012 (1): 372345.
45. Fischer TC, Gosch C, Pfeiffer J, Halbwirth H, Halle C, Stich K, Forkmann G. 2007. Flavonoid genes of pear (*Pyrus communis*). *Trees*. 21 (5): 521–529.
46. Kolniak-Ostek J. 2016. Identification and quantification of polyphenolic compounds in ten pear cultivars by UPLC-PDA-Q/TOF-MS. *Journal of Food Composition and Analysis*. 49: 65–77.
47. Estrela JM, Mena S, Obrador E, Benlloch M, Castellano G, Salvador R, Dellinger RW. 2017. Polyphenolic phytochemicals in cancer prevention and therapy: bioavailability versus bio-efficacy. *Journal of Medicinal Chemistry*. 60 (23): 9413–9436.
48. Ross JA, Kasum CM. 2002. Dietary flavonoids: bioavailability, metabolic effects, and safety. *Annual Review of Nutrition*. 22 (1): 19–34.
49. Lee YG, Cho J, Park J, Lee S, Kim W, Park K, Moon JH. 2013. Large-scale isolation of highly pure malaxinic acid from immature pear (*Pyrus pyrifolia* Nakai) fruit. *Food Science and Biotechnology*. 22 (6): 1539–1545.
50. Lee HJ, Jeong HY, Jin MR, Lee HJ, Cho J, Moon J. 2017. Metabolism and antioxidant effect of malaxinic acid and its corresponding aglycone in rat blood plasma. *Free Radical Biology and Medicine*. 110: 399–407.
51. Truong XT, Park S, Lee Y, Jeong HY, Moon J, Jeon T. 2017. Protocatechuic acid from pear inhibits melanogenesis in melanoma cells. *International Journal of Molecular Sciences*. 18 (08): E1809.
52. Moon J, Cho J, Lee S, Kim W. 2017. Development and application of functional resource using pear. *Horticultural Science and Technology*. 35: 36–37.
53. Roberfroid M, Gibson GR, Hoyles L, McCartney AL, Rastall R, Rowland I, Wolvers D, Watzl B, Szajewska H, Stahl B, Guarner F. 2010. Prebiotic effects: metabolic and health benefits. *British Journal of Nutrition*. 104 (S2): S1–S63.
54. Ramnani P, Gaudier E, Bingham M, van Bruggen P, Tuohy KM, Gibson GR. 2010. Prebiotic effect of fruit and vegetable shots containing Jerusalem artichoke inulin: a human intervention study. *British Journal of Nutrition*. 104 (2): 233–240.
55. Brahem M, Renard CMGC, Eder S, Loonis M, Ouni R, Mars M, Le Bourvellec C. 2017. Characterization and quantification of fruit phenolic compounds of European and Tunisian pear cultivars. *Food Research International*. 95: 125–33.
56. Velmurugan C, Bhargava A. 2013. Anti-diabetic and hypolipidemic activitiy of fruits of *Pyrus Communis* L. in hyperglycemic rats. *Asian Journal of Pharmaceutical and Clinical Research*. 6 (5): 108–111.
57. Sarkar D, Ankolekar C, Pinto M, Shetty K. 2015. Dietary functional benefits of Bartlett and Starkrimson pears for potential management of hyperglycemia, hypertension and ulcer bacteria helicobacter pylori while supporting beneficial probiotic bacterial response. *Food Research International*. 69: 80–90.
58. Koch ER, Deo P. 2016. Nutritional supplements modulate fluorescent protein bound advanced glycation end products and digestive enzymes related to type 2 diabetes mellitus. *BMC Complementary and Alternative Medicine*. 16 (1): 338.
59. Guo X, Yang B, Tang J, Jiang J, Li D. 2017. Apple and pear consumption and type 2 diabetes mellitus risk: a meta-analysis of prospective cohort studies. *Food and Function*. 8 (3): 927–934.
60. Ci Z. 2018. Suppressive effect of polyphenols from immature pear fruits on blood glucose levels. *Journal of Food and Nutrition Research*. 6 (7): 445–449.
61. Nieman D, Gillitt N, Sha W, Meaney M, John C, Pappan K, Kinchen JM. 2015. Metabolomics-based analysis of banana and pear ingestion on exercise performance and recovery. *Journal of Proteome Research*. 14 (12): 5367–5377.
62. David RM, Gooderham NJ. 2018. Mechanistic evidence that benzo [a] pyrene promotes an inflammatory microenvironment that drives the metastatic potential of human mammary cells. *Archives of Toxicology*. 92: 3223–3239.
63. Heo B, Park Y, Park Y, Jung K, Cho J, Oh K, Chung US, Lee KD. 2009. Chemical composition and physiological activity of native pear c.v. 'Baekwoon'. *Korean Journal of Community Living Science*. 20: 549–558.
64. Kim D, Shin G, Lee Y, Lee JS, Cho J, Baik S, Lee OH. 2014. Assessment and comparison of the antioxidant activities and nitrite scavenging activity of commonly consumed beverages in Korea. *Food Chemistry*. 151: 58–64.
65. Cassidy A, Rogers G, Peterson J, Dwyer J, Lin H, Jacques P. 2015. Higher dietary anthocyanin and flavonol intakes are associated with anti-inflammatory effects in a population of US adults. *American Journal of Clinical Nutrition*. 102 (1): 172–181.
66. Migas P, Krauze-Baranowska M. 2015. The significance of arbutin and its derivatives in therapy and cosmetics. *Phytochemistry Letters*. 13: 35–40.

67. Ragab D, Salah Eldin H, Taeimah M, Khattab R, Salem R. 2020. The COVID-19 cytokine storm; what we know so far. *Frontiers in Immunology*. 11: 1446.
68. Hosseini B, Berthon BS, Wark P, Wood LG. 2017. Effects of fruit and vegetable consumption on risk of asthma, wheezing and immune responses: a systematic review and meta-analysis. *Nutrients*. 9 (4): 341.
69. Kaluza J, Larsson SC, Orsini N, Linden A, Wolk A. 2017. Fruit and vegetable consumption and risk of COPD: a prospective cohort study of men. *Thorax*. 72 (6): 500–509.
70. Lee J, Pak S, Lee S, Na C, Lim S, Song C, Bai YH, Jang CH. 2004. Asian pear pectin administration during presensitization inhibits allergic response to ovalbumin in BALB/c mice. *Journal of Alternative and Complementary Medicine*. 10 (3): 527–534.
71. Park H, Lee S, Son H, Park S, Kim M, Choi E, Singh TS, Ha JH, Lee MG, Kim JE, Hyun MC. 2008. Flavonoids inhibit histamine release and expression of proinflammatory cytokines in mast cells. *Archives of Pharmacal Research*. 31 (10): 1303–1311.
72. Yang M, Park C, Kim DJ, Jeong H. 2005. Antimutagenic and anti-carcinogegnic effects of Korean pears. *Cancer Prevention Research*. 10 (2): 124–127.
73. Jiang R, Hodgson JM, Mas E, Croft KD, Ward NC. 2016. Chlorogenic acid improves ex vivo vessel function and protects endothelial cells against HOCl-induced oxidative damage, via increased production of nitric oxide and induction of Hmox-1. *Journal of Nutritional Biochemistry*. 27: 53–60.
74. Yoon B, Kim K, Park S. 2006. Effects of pear extracts cultured under conventional and environment-friendly conditions on cell proliferation in rat hepatocytes. *Applied Biological Chemistry*. 49 (3): 233–237.
75. Ma JN, Xu HY, Ma CM. 2013. Chemical components and hepatoprotective effects of the extracts of apple-shaped pear peels on CCl_4-caused liver injury in mice. *International Conference on Biological, Medical and Chemical Engineering (Bmce 2013)*. p. 100–104.
76. Meng X, Li Y, Li S, Gan R, Li H. 2018. Natural products for prevention and treatment of chemical-induced liver injuries. *Comprehensive Reviews in Food Science and Food Safety*. 17 (2): 472–495.
77. Yim S, Nam S. 2015. Antioxidant and whitening activities of five unripe pear cultivars. *Journal of Applied Botany and Food Quality*. 88 (1): 186–91.
78. Park JJ, Hwang SJ, Kang YS, Jung J, Park S, Hong JE, Park Y, Lee HJ. 2019. Synthesis of arbutin–gold nanoparticle complexes and their enhanced performance for whitening. *Archives of Pharmacal Research*. 42 (11): 977–989.

25 *Quercus leucotrichophora* (Banj/Oak)

INTRODUCTION

Quercus leucotrichophora D. Don. (Hindi: Banj, Eng.: Oak), family: Fagaceae, is an evergreen tree, approximately 40 m in height, and is common in the Himalayan region at the range from 800 to 2,300 MSL.[1] The genus *Quercus* possesses immense medicinal properties and therapeutic applications.[2–5] It is a main source of fuel and fodder in the Himalayan region of India.[6] Barks, leaves, and seeds of the species are used to treat human ailments as well as for livestock.[7] Traditionally, gum of the species is used to treat gonorrhea and digestive disorders, especially in children.[8] The seeds act as a diuretic and astringent. Seeds are used to treat indigestion, diarrhea, and asthma in humans.[9] The stem bark of *Q. leucotrichophora* has quercetin, kaempferol,[10] and 23 volatile compounds, mainly monoterpenoids.[11] Fruits of *Q. leucotrichophora* have a higher amount of saturated fatty acid compared to unsaturated fatty acid.[11] Joshi and Juyal have reported that the plant *Q. leucotrichophora* is used in different folk healing systems but is still not deciphered for biological pathways to confirm its mechanism, activity, and medicinal properties.[12]

The *Quercus* genus, which often differs in its flowering and fruiting patterns, is comprised of around 450 species globally.[13] Depending on the locality, the *Q. leucotrichophora* seed ripens between November and March, but the ripe seeds may remain on the trees for several months.[14] *Q. leucotrichophora* bark is smooth and tan-brown at first but changes morphology to lightly furrowed and corky with age (Figure 25.1). The leaves are elongated ovals with

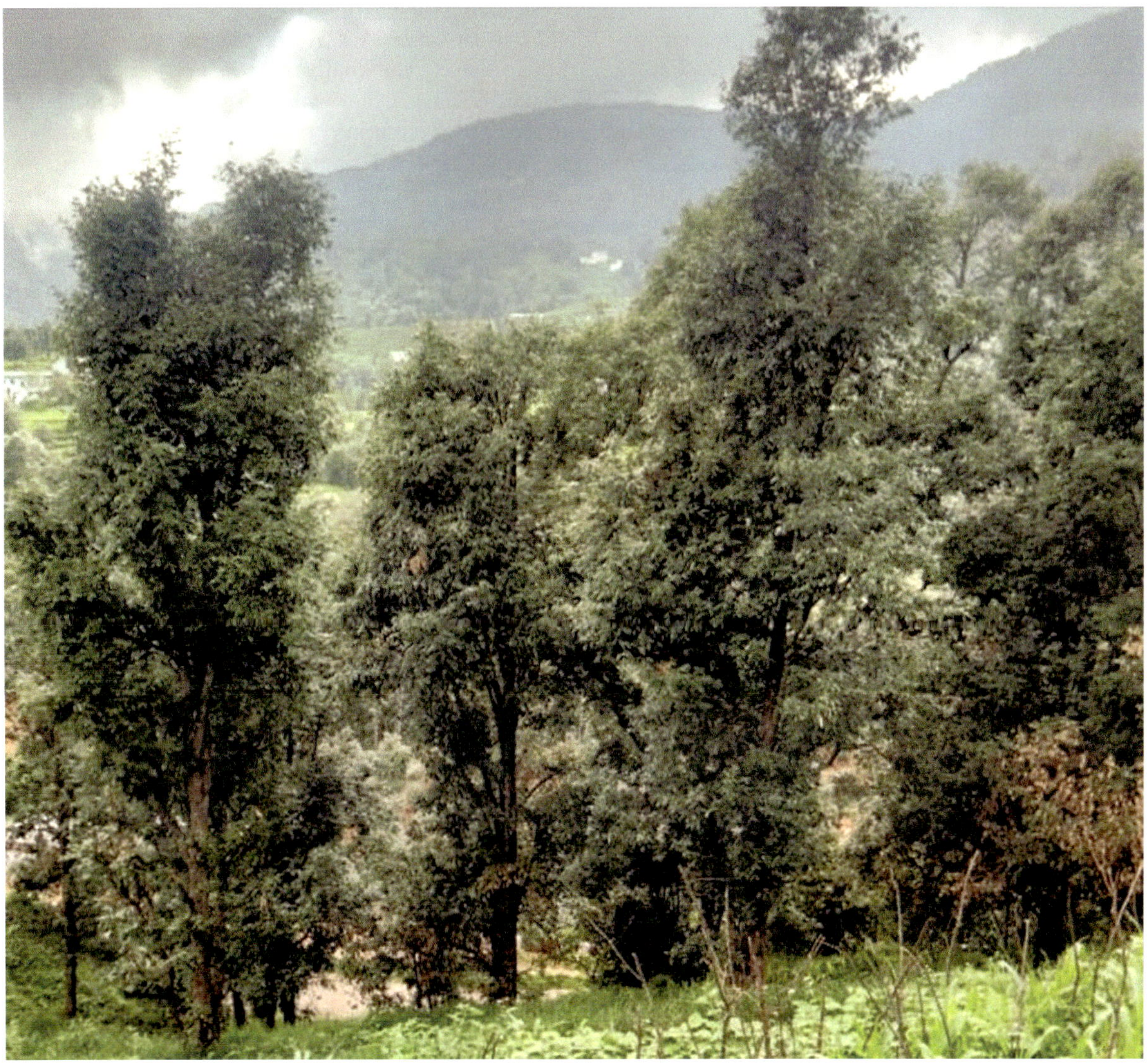

FIGURE 25.1 *Q. leucotrichophora* trees.

DOI: 10.1201/9781003512868-27

jagged teeth and are arranged alternately. Young leaves are pinkish purple in appearance and turn deep green on maturity at the upper surface, while the lower side becomes silvery grey due to the presence of white hairs (leucotrichophora=which has white hairs). The tiny, round female flower is borne at the base of leaves, and male inflorescence (catkins) develops at the tip of the branch. The fruits (acorns) are marble-sized, orange-tan colored.[14,15]

Joshi and Juyal[12] have surveyed the folklore efficacy of *Q. leucotrichophora* species and documented the ethnomedicinal information from tribal people of several areas and adjacent villagers of the Himalayan region. The concerned villages of the study areas were visited by the researchers for the identification of plant species with local medicine men to explore the traditional knowledge on the spot and authenticate the plant species. Saxena and Singh have reported that *Quercus* spp. is most effective in the strategy of soil and water conservation.[16] Due to the multifarious applications of the genus, all the species are overexploited for different purposes, but *Q. leucotrichophora* is the worst affected one among all.[16,17]

ETHNOMEDICINAL USES

For centuries, *Quercus* species have been in use as folk medicine to treat various diseases. Indigenous peoples on different continents have been using the genus to treat gastrointestinal disorders such as hemorrhoids and diarrhea, and as antiseptics. The bark of the *Q. leucotrichophora* is used to cure gastropathy and toothache, applied as an antiseptic and hemostatic, used to pacify inflammation, and as a healing agent in burn cases.[12,18] However, the resin of *Q. leucotrichophora* is used to cure diarrhea, asthma, dysentery, and gonorrhea.[12] *Q. infectoria* gallnut powder is used to restore uterine wall elasticity and treat aphthous ulcers.[19,20] The acorn (fruit) of the *Quercus* species is a rich source of nutrients (fat, proteins, and carbohydrates); hence, traditional application as food and as an ingredient in bread production or coffee powder is justified.[21] The acorns of the various species of *Quercus* are widely used in curing laryngopharyngitis diseases, obesity, diarrhea, stomach ulcers, and menorrhagia.[22,23] Pharmacological properties reported for the *Quercus* genus include anti-inflammatory, antimicrobial, hepatoprotective, neuro-generative, antioxidant, antidiabetic, anti-obesity, anticancer, gastrointestinal disorder, and skin disorder.[4,24–29] All these effects are due to the specific chemical composition, comprised mainly of tannins, flavonoids, and triterpenoids. Endo et al. have studied the anti-toxoplasma effect of the *Q. crispula* outer bark and isolated three pentacyclic triterpenoids, namely, ursolic acid acetate, oleanolic acid acetate, and 29-norlupane-3,20-dione, for therapeutic efficacy.[30] Authors have reported that these compounds have potent activities against the *Toxoplasma gondii* parasite.[30] Moreover, Lei et al. isolated new triterpenoids, identified as ursane, oleanane, and lupinane types, and reported them as anti-neuro-inflammatory compounds.[26] Different workers have described acorns as having strong antioxidant activity and being used to treat cancer, diabetes, and cardiovascular and inflammatory diseases.[31–33]

All parts of the *Quercus* species, including bark, leaves, and fruits, have been used for therapeutic properties in folk/traditional medicine in different civilizations and tribes to treat Parkinson's disease, asthma, gastritis, gonorrhea, pyrexia, and hepatic diseases,[34] including diarrhea, varicose veins, hemorrhoids, ulcers, and gastric and superficial injuries.[35] The bark of the genus is preferred as medicine and is used extensively as an energizer and an antiseptic. The decoctions prepared from the barks of *Q. robur* and *Q. petraea* are used in anti-inflammatory, antibacterial, and anti-hemorrhagic activities.[36] Patients with high levels of blood sugar[37] and sore throats are recommended to take the decoctions.[38] The leaves of *Q. virginiana* have antimicrobial properties and are used to treat gastrointestinal disorders.[39,40] The galls (Manjakani) of *Q. infectoria* are applied to restore the uterine wall elasticity and to treat inflammatory disorders,[20] while *Q. infectoria* galls (Manjakani) are used in Malay traditional medicine to treat wound infections after childbirth.[41] The practice is well-known since ancient times. Arabs, Persians, Indians, Chinese, and Malays have traditionally used Manjakani after childbirth as part of postpartum care to treat vaginal discharge and related postpartum infections.[41] In India, galls are used to treat toothache and gingivitis, and in Asia, they are widely used to treat infectious diseases, skin disorders, and inflammatory ailments of the body.[19] In the Kumaun and Garhwal regions of Uttarakhand, India, *Q. leucotrichophora* galls are used to treat urinary infections,[12] stomach pain,[42] gonorrhea, hemorrhages, asthma, dysentery, diarrhea,[43] urinary disorders,[44] and as diuretics.[45] In Korean folk medicine, they are used to treat diarrhea, skin diseases, and dysentery.[46]

Fruits (acorns) of *Quercus* are a rich source of energy, containing high amounts of amino acids, carbohydrates, lipids, sterols, and proteins. The Mesolithic era is known as the earliest period of acorn use as a foodstuff in Western Europe. In the North American WC, acorns make up more than half of the diet of native peoples.[47] *Q. humilis* fruits are mainly consumed raw, as an ingredient for making coffee, or in a roasted form.[21] In the northeast Iberian Peninsula, the fruit of *Q. ilex* is used raw, roasted, boiled (like coffee), or in the form of flour. The flour is mixed with cereal flour to make bread, while in Serbia, *Q. cerris* seeds are widely used for bread production.[48] The oil extracted from the acorn is used for cooking. It is nutritious and comparable to avocado, olive, cotton, and peanut oils for cooking purposes.[32]

Tribals from Tehri Garhwal, Uttarakhand, India, use *Q. leucotrichophora* (local name: Banj) gum resin to cure hemorrhages, gonorrhea, diarrhea, dysentery, and asthma.[49] The dry resin of *Q. leucotrichophora* is taken with water to cure stomach pain.[42] The people of Almora district, Uttarakhand, India, use the bark of the plant in the form of a gargle for tonsillitis (25 g bark in 100 mL hot water).[50] Tisane of leaves (about 10 mL) of *Q. leucotrichophora* is given thrice daily to treat dysentery and diarrhea.[51] According to the survey, fruits of *Q. leucotrichophora* are used as diuretics and astringents.[52] The natives of 'Haat Kali', a sacred grove in Kumaun Himalaya, Uttarakhand, India, use dried gum powder of the species with milk to cure general body weakness.[53]

PHYTOCHEMICALS

The genus *Quercus* contains various chemical classes of bioactive compounds such as phenolic acids, terpenoids, sterols, glycosides, flavonoids, tannins, and fatty acids. All the species of *Quercus* have flavonoids (particularly, flavan-3-ol), tannins, and phenolic acids (particularly, ellagic, gallic acids, and derivatives) in abundance.[32]

Semwal et al. have studied the methanolic extracts of leaves and bark of *Q. leucotrichophora* for their chemical composition with GC-MS and biological activities, and reported a total of 23 compounds from the bark and 62 compounds from the leaf extracts.[54] The major components identified in the bark extracts are epi-psi-taraxastanonol (14.20%), *cis*-vaccenic acid (13.10%), lupeol (17.91%), and linoleic acid (19.77%), while others have been reported in relatively small amounts. In leaf extract, the major components are simiarene (15.29%), linoleic acid (17.09%), D-quinic acid (9.29%), and flavone 4′-OH, 5-OH, 7-di-O-glucoside (15.26%), respectively. Antibacterial activity was evaluated for five bacterial strains, and it was observed that both extracts (bark and leaves, respectively) have activity against most of the tested bacterial strains.[54] Both extracts (bark and leaves) of *Q. leucotrichophora* have activity against all Gram-positive (*S. aureus*, *B. subtilis*, and *S. pyogenes*) and Gram-negative (*E. coli*, *P. aeruginosa*) bacterial strains. Methanolic extract of bark and leaves of the species, analyzed by GC-MS analysis, has revealed the presence of highly composite profiles of bioactive compounds, which are active against pathogenic microbes. The bark and leaves have pharmacological and industrial importance.

SCOPE AND OPPORTUNITIES

Quercus species have been used in different folk and traditional healing practices for a long time. The fruit, leaves, and bark of the species have been reported for a broad spectrum of biological effects, such as antidiabetic, anti-inflammatory, anticancer, antibacterial, and antioxidant. Phytochemical screening of the genus has deciphered the presence of gallic acid, ellagic acids and their derivatives, flavonoids, and tannins, ubiquitous in all the *Quercus* species. The anticancer, antidiabetic, and anti-inflammatory activities of the genus are due to triterpenoids, flavonoids, and phenolics, making the genus a promising candidate for the development of novel green medicines. In-depth research on *Q. leucotrichophora* species needs focusing attention from biochemists to assess its health effects and detailed chemical profile to evaluate the safety, efficacy, and side effects of its extracts.

Ethnobotanical information about the genus *Quercus* and its large applications for community healthcare programs has a clue to developing the new modern green medicines. The information is so potent that it has a long history without any side effects. Literature surveys and folklore reports on the application of *Quercus* reveal that its extracts have the potential to be anticancer, antimicrobial, and antioxidant, and can be applied in the pharmaceutical and nutraceutical industries to improve sensory quality. The high phenolic content, especially tannins, and their antioxidant properties have medicinal applications as herbal drugs. Pharmacological investigations have mostly been performed in vivo and in vitro, but clinical reports are scanty. Thus, clinical investigations are required to confirm in vitro and in vivo results for the rational application of the species, providing a clue for developing newer medicines to treat multidrug-resistant pathogens. Though *Quercus* products have been reported as generally safe, toxicological data are scanty. Large areas of *Quercus* forests, large amounts of annual forest waste (leaves and bark), waste resulting from wood processing, high availability, and their drought resistance property make *Quercus* species an important source of bioactive compounds. The present text describes the up-to-date information on traditional medicinal applications and phytopharmacology of *Q. leucotrichophora* to explore its therapeutic potential and develop modern green medicines in the future.

REFERENCES

1. Singh JS. 1992. *Forests of the Himalaya: Structure, Functioning and Impact of Man*. Gyanodaya Prakashan, India.
2. Hayouni EA, Abedrabba M, Bouix M, Hamdi M. 2007. The effects of solvents and extraction method on the phenolic contents and biological activities in vitro of Tunisian *Quercus coccifera* L. and *Juniperus phoenicea* L. fruit extracts. *Food Chemistry*. 105: 1126–1134.
3. Berahou A, Auhmani A, Fdil N, Benharref A, Jana M, Gadhi CA. 2007. Antibacterial activity of *Quercus ilex* bark's extracts. *Journal of Ethnopharmacology*. 112. 426–429.
4. Sanchez-Burgos JA, Ramírez-Mares MV, Larrosa MM, Gallegos-Infante JA, González-Laredo RF, Medina-Torres L, Rocha-Guzmán NE. 2013. Antioxidant, antimicrobial, anti-topoisomerase and gastroprotective effect of herbal infusions from four *Quercus* species. *Industrial Crops and Products*. 42: 57–62.
5. Jamil M, Ul Haq I, Mirza B, Qayyum M. 2012. Isolation of antibacterial compounds from *Quercus dilatata* L. through bioassay guided fractionation. *Annals of Clinical Microbiology and Antimicrobials*. 11: 1–11. https://doi.org/10.1186/1476-0711-11-11
6. Singh SP, Singh JS. 1986. Structure and function of the central Himalayan oak forests. *Proceedings: Plant Sciences*. 96: 159–189.

7. Al-Rousan WM, Ajo RY, Al-Ismail KM, Attlee A, Shaker RR, Osaili TM. 2013. Characterization of acorn fruit oils extracted from selected Mediterranean *Quercus* species. *Grasas Aceites*. 64: 554–560.
8. Soni PL, Sharma H, Gharia MM. 1993. Physicochemical properties of *Quercus leucotrichophora* (oak) starch. *Starch-Stärke*. 45: 127–130.
9. Chopra RN, Nayar SL, Chopra IC. 1986. *Glossary of Indian Medicinal Plants*. Council of Scientific & Industrial Research, New Delhi.
10. Sati SC, Sati N, Sati OP. 2011. Chemical investigation and screening of antimicrobial activity of stem bark of *Qurecus leucotrichophora*. *International Journal of Pharmacy and Pharmaceutical Science*. 3: 89–91.
11. Sati SC, Sati N, Sati OP, Biswas D, Chauhan BS. 2012. Analysis and antimicrobial activity of volatile constituents from *Quercus leucotrichophora* (Fagaceae) bark. *Natural Product Research*, formerly *Natural Produt Letters*. 26: 869–872.
12. Joshi AK, Juyal D. 2017. Traditional and ethnobotanical uses of *Quercus leucotrichophora* A. Camus (*Quercus oblongata* D. Don) in Kumaun and Garhwal regions of Uttarakhand, India; A review. *International Journal of Herbal Medicine*. 5: 6–8.
13. Tejerina D, Garcia TS, Vaca MC, Vasquez FM, Cava R. 2011. Acorns (*Quercus rotundifolia* Lam) and grass as natural sources of antioxidants and fatty acids in the "montanera" feeding of Iberian pig: intra- and inter-annual variations. *Food Chemistry*. 124: 997–1004.
14. Banj oak (*Quercus leucotrichophora*). https://www.feedipedia.org/node/108, as on 2nd September 2021.
15. Anonymous. 1998. *Quality Control Methods for Medicinal Plant Materials*. WHO, Geneva.
16. Saxena AK, Singh JS. 1982. A phytosociological analysis of woody species in forest communities of a part of Kumaun Himalaya. *Vegetatio*. 50: 3–22.
17. Pandey SK, Shukla RP. 2001. Regeneration strategy and plant diversity status in degraded sal forests. *Current Science*. 81: 95–102.
18. Khennouf S, Amira S, Arrar L, Baghiani A. 2010. Effect of some phenolic compounds and Q*uercus* tannins on lipid peroxidation. *World Applied Sciences Journal*. 8 (9): 1144–1149.
19. Sariozlu NY, Kivanc M. 2011. Gallnuts (*Quercus infectoria* Oliv, and *Rhus chinensis* Mill.) and their usage. In: *Health in Nuts and Seeds in Health and Disease Prevention*. Victor R. Preedy, Ronald Ross Watson, Vinood B. Patel (Eds.) Academic Press, Cambridge, MA. pp. 505–511. https://doi.org/10.1016/B978-0-12-375688-6.10060-X.
20. Hapidin H, Rozelan D, Abdullah H, Hanaffi WN, Soelaiman IN. 2015. *Quercus infectoria* gall extract enhanced the proliferation and activity of human fetal osteoblast cell line. *Malaysian Journal of Medical Sciences*. 22 (1): 12–22.
21. Garcıa-Gomez E, Perez-Badia R, Pereira J, Puri RK. 2017. The consumption of acorns (from *Quercus* spp.) in the central west of the Iberian Peninsula in the 20th century. *Economic Botany*. 71 (3): 256–268.
22. Moon HR, Chung MJ, Park JW, Cho SM, Choi DJ, Kim SM, Chun MH, KIM IB, Kim SO, Jang SJ, Park YI. 2013. Antiasthma effects through anti-inflammatory action of acorn (Q*uercus acutissimacarr*) *in- vitro* and *in-vivo*. *Journal of Food Biochemistry*. 37 (1): 108–118.
23. Kim H, Song MJ, Potter D. 2006. Medicinal effcacy of plants utilized as temple food in traditional Korean Buddhism. *Journal of Ethnopharmacology*. 104 (1–2): 32–46.
24. Gezici S, Sekeroglu N. 2019. Neuroprotective potential and phytochemical composition of acorn fruits. *Industrial Crops and Products*. 128: 13–17.
25. Huang J, Wang Y, Li C, Wang X, He X. 2016. Triterpenes isolated from acorns of *Quercus serrata* var. *brevipetiolata* exert anti-inflammatory activity. *Industrial Crops and Products*. 91: 302–309.
26. Lei Y, Huang Y, Wang Y, He X. 2018. Potential anti-neuro-inflammatory triterpenoids isolated from Chinese acorns (*Quercus serrata* var. *brevipetiolata*). *Journal of Functional Foods*. 50: 18–25.
27. Rocha-Guzman NE, Gallegos-Infante JA, GonzalezLaredo RF, Reynoso-Camacho R, Ramos-Gómez M, Garcia-Gasca T, Rodríguez-Muñoz ME, Guzmán-Maldonado SH, Medina-Torres L, Lujan-García BA. 2009. Antioxidant activity and genotoxic effect on HeLa cells of phenolic compounds from infusions of *Quercus resinosa* leaves. *Food Chemistry*. 115 (4): 1320–1325.
28. Medina-Torres A, Bisht M. 2018. Evaluation of in-vitro antioxidant potential and in-vivo hepato-protective activity of root extract of *Quercus oblongata* D. DON. *Journal of Drug Delivery and Therapeutics*. 8 (5): 152–161.
29. Xu J, Cao J., Yue J, Zhang X, Zhao Y. 2018. New triterpenoids from acorns of *Quercus liaotungensis* and their inhibitory activity against α -glucosidase, α -amylase and protein-tyrosine phosphatase 1B. *Journal of Functional Foods*. 41: 232–239.
30. Endo M, Shigetomi K, Mitsuhashi S, Igarashi M, Ubukata M. 2019. Isolation, structure determination and structure-activity relationship of anti-toxoplasma triterpenoids from *Quercus crispula* Blume outer bark. *Journal of Wood Science*. 65 (1): 1–11. https://doi.org/10.1186/s10086-019-1782-8
31. Karimi A, Moradi MT. 2015. Total phenolic compounds and in vitro antioxidant potential of crude methanol extract and the correspond fractions *of Quercus brantii* L. acorn. *Journals of Herbmed Pharmacology*. 4 (1): 35–39.
32. Vinha AF, Costa ASG, Barreira JCM, Pacheco R, Oliveira MBPP. 2016. Chemical and antioxidant profiles of acorn tissues from *Quercus* spp.: potential as new industrial raw materials. *Industrial Crops and Products*. 94: 143–151.
33. Silva JP, Gomes AC, Coutinho OP. 2008. Oxidative DNA damage protection and repair by polyphenolic compounds in PC12 cells. *European Journal of Pharmacology*. 601 (1–3): 50–60.
34. Uddin G, Rauf A. 2012. Phytochemical screening, antimicrobial and antioxidant activities of aerial parts of *Quercus robur* L. *Middle East Journal of Medicinal Plants Research*. 1 (1): 1–4.
35. Aslani A, Emami S, Ghannadi A, Ajdari M. 2009. Formulation and physicochemical evaluation of an herbal anti-hemorrhoid ointment from *Quercus*, black cumin and fenugreek for the treatment of internal anal hemorrhoids. *Journal of Pharmaceutical Sciences*. 14: 247–257.
36. Leporatti ML, Ivancheva S. 2003. Preliminary comparative analysis of medicinal plants used in the traditional medicine of Bulgaria and Italy. *Journal of Ethnopharmacology*. 87 (2–3): 123–142.

37. McCune LM, Johns T. 2007. Antioxidant activity relates to plant part, life form and growing condition in some diabetes remedies. *Journal of Ethnopharmacology*. 112 (3): 461–469.
38. Jamil M, Mirza B, Yasmeen A, Khan MA. 2012. Pharmacological activities of selected plant species and their phytochemical analysis. *Journal of Medicinal Plants Research*. 6 (37): 5013–5022.
39. McCutcheon AR, Ellis SM, Hancock REW, Towers GHN. 1992. Anti-biotic screening of medicinal plants of the British Columbian native peoples. *Journal of Ethnopharmacology*. 37 (3): 213–223.
40. Adonizio AL, Downum K, Bennett BC, Mathee K. 2006. Anti-quorum sensing activity of medicinal plants in southern Florida. *Journal of Ethnopharmacology*. 105 (3): 427–435.
41. Wunnoo S, Sermwittayawong D, Praparatana R, Voravuthikunchai SP, Jakkawanpitak C. 2024. Quercus infectoria Gall ethanolic extract accelerates wound healing through attenuating inflammation and oxidative Injuries in skin fibroblasts. *Antioxidants*. 13(9): 1094. https://doi.org/10.3390/antiox13091094
42. Uniyal B, Shiva V. 2005. Traditional knowledge on medicinal plants among rural women of the Garhwal Himalaya, Uttaranchal. *Indian Journal of Traditional Knowledge*. 4 (3): 259–266.
43. Chauhan PS, Bisht S, Ahmed S. 2017. Traditional and ethnobotanical uses of medicinal trees in district Tehri Garhwal (Western Himalayas). *International Journal of Ayurvedic and Herbal Medicine*. 7 (1): 2442–2448.
44. Rawat VS. 2016. Medicinal plants and sustainable livelihood in Pauri district of Garhwal Himalaya, Uttarakhand, India. *International Journal of Bioassays*. 5 (6): 4589–4592.
45. Ahmed E, Arshad M, Ahmad M, Saeed M, Ishaque M. 2004. Ethnopharmacological survey of some medicinally important plants of Galliyat areas of NWFP, Pakistan. *Asian Journal of Plant Sciences*. 3 (4): 410–415.
46. Kim JI, Kim HH, Kim S, Lee KT, Ham IH, Whang WK. 2008. Antioxidative compounds from *Quercus salicina* blume stem. *Archives of Pharmacal Research*. 31 (3): 274–278.
47. Bainbridge DA. 1986. Use of acorns for food in California: past, present, future. *Proceedings of the Symposium on Multiple Use Management of California's Hardwood Resources*, San Luis Obispo, CA, USA, November 1986. pp. 12–14.
48. Pinto D, Diaz Franco S, Silva AM, Cupara S, Koskovac M, Kojicic K, Soares S, Rodrigues F, Sut S, Dall'Acqua S, Oliveira MB. 2019. Chemical characterization and bioactive properties of a coffee-like beverage prepared from *Quercus cerris* kernels. *Food & Function*. 10 (4): 2050–2060.
49. Chauhan PS, Bisht S, Ahmad S. 2016. Traditional and ethnobotanical uses of medicinal trees in district Tehri Garhwal Western Himalayas. *Annals of Geriatric Education and Medical Sciences*. 1 (1): 14–19.
50. Kumari P, Joshi GC, Tewari LM. 2011. Diversity and status of ethno-medicinal plants of Almora district in Uttarakhand, India. *International Journal of Biodiversity and Conservation*. 3 (7): 298–326.
51. Sharma B, Sharma S, Bhardwaj SK, Ndungu CK, Dutt B. 2015. Ethnobotanical uses of common plant species growing along the National Highway 5 from Solan to Shimla in Himachal Pradesh. *World Journal of Pharmacy and Pharmaceutical Sciences*. 4 (2):1210–1218.
52. Gangwar KK, Gangwar RS. 2010. Ethnomedicinal plant diversity in Kumaun Himalaya of Uttarakhand, India. *Nature and Science*. 8 (5): 66–78.
53. Singh H, Agnihotri P, Dixit V, Pande PC, Husain T. 2015. An assessment of ethnomedicinal plant diversity in Haat Kali Sacred Grove in Kumaun Himalaya, Uttarakhand, India. *East Himalayan Society for Spermatophyte Taxonomy*. 9 (2): 456–464.
54. Semwal P, Painuli S, Badoni H, Bacheti RK. 2018. Screening of phyto-constituents and antibacterial activity of leaves and bark of *Quercus leucotrichophora* A. Camus from Uttarakhand Himalaya. *Clinical Phytoscience*. https://doi.org/10.1186/s40816-018-0090-y

26 *Rubus ellipticus* (Yellow Himalayan Raspberry)

INTRODUCTION

Rubus ellipticus Smith (family: Rosaceae) is native to tropical and subtropical India and is commonly called yellow Himalayan Raspberry, Hinsar, or Hisalu.[1] The species has been listed under the top ten wild edible medicinal plants[2] and under the world's 100 worst invasive plant species.[3] It grows along mountain valleys, hillsides, and roadsides, in thickets, slopes, and sparse forests at an altitude of 300–2,600 MSL.[4] The blooming season of the plant is March–April,[2] whereas the fruiting season is May–June, bearing golden yellow fruits.[5] The plant grows in regions with an annual rainfall of 2,000–6,500mm. It is weedy in wet forests and has vigorous growth in sunny open pastures and deep rainforests. The plant is very hard (Figure 26.1) and can adapt to environmental stress factors by its natural resistance mechanism.[6] The genus *Rubus* has over 750 species in 12 subgenera, and is very diverse, occurring on all continents except Antarctica.[2] *Rubus* species have ethnomedicinal and pharmacological applications.[7] The phytochemical, medicinal attributes, and health-promoting constituents of *Rubus* berries are universally acknowledged.[8] Its fruits (Figures 26.2 and 26.3) are edible, medicinally febrifuge, astringent, and have stomachic properties. The juice of fruits is used to treat sore throats, coughs, colic, and fever. The phloem (i.e., the inner bark) is used in Tibetan medicine for thermogenic potency. It has a sweet taste and sour flavor and is used as an anti-diuretic to make kidney tonic. Traditionally, it is used to treat weakening of the senses, polyuria, vaginal/seminal discharge, and micturition during sleep. In recent years, multiple resistances (chemical and drug type, respectively) of plant and human pathogenic microorganisms have been reported due

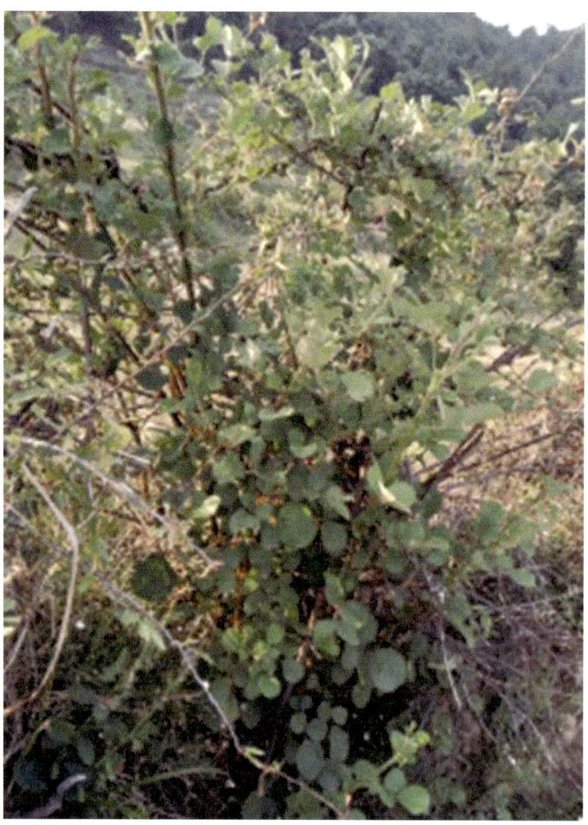

FIGURE 26.1 *R. ellipticus.*

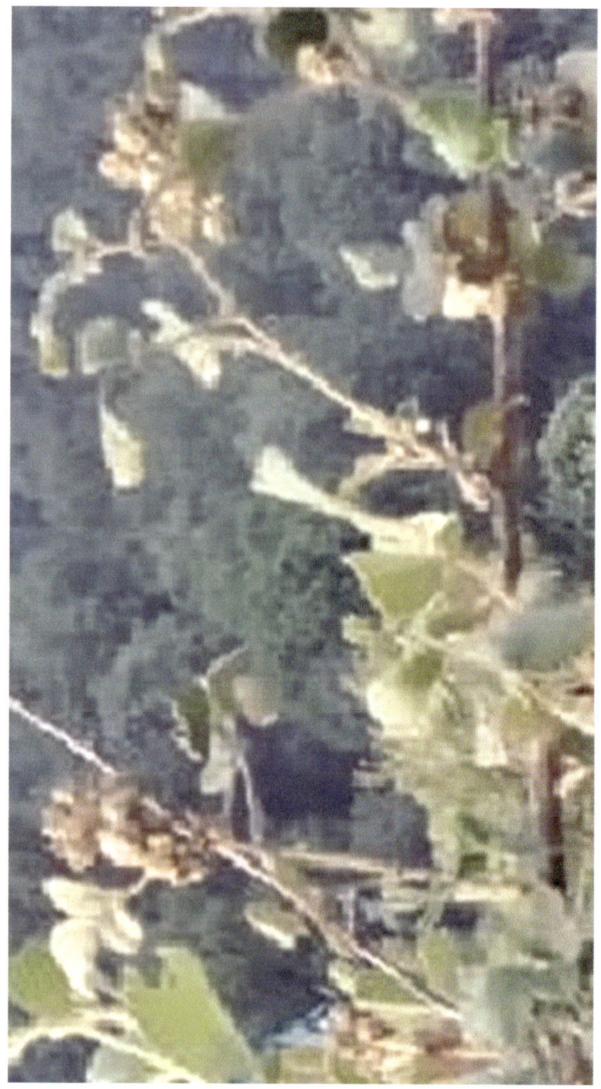

FIGURE 26.2 Immature fruits.

DOI: 10.1201/9781003512868-28

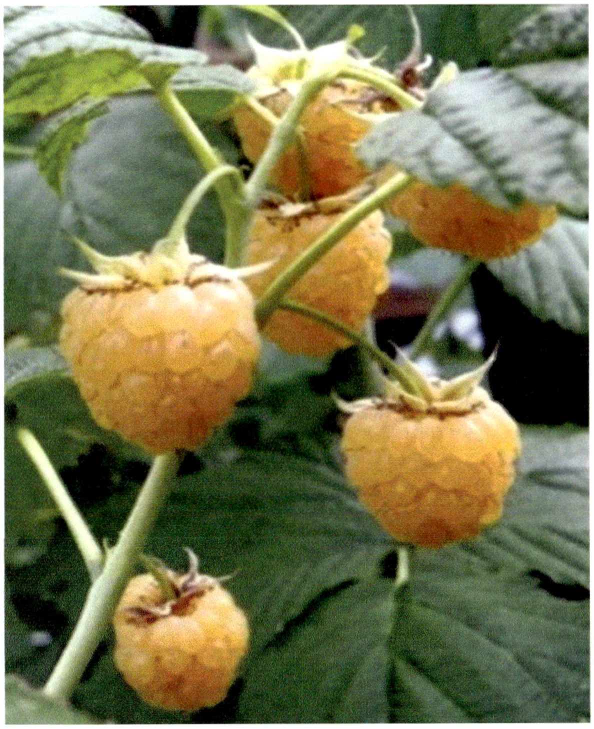

FIGURE 26.3 Ripened fruits.

to indiscriminate application of commercial antimicrobials (chemicals and drugs, respectively) to treat infectious diseases.[9]

The ethanolic extract of the root of the *R. ellipticus* has anti-inflammatory, antimicrobial, and antioxidant properties.[5] The fruits of *R. ellipticus* are rich in vitamins and sugars, highly delicious, and nutritious.[5] The plant is known for various therapeutic properties such as antipyretic, analgesic, anti-inflammatory, antiproliferative, antitumor, anticonvulsant, antioxidant, etc., and has immense ethnomedicinal applications because of its numerous bioactive compounds.[10,11] Current efforts are focused on developing new green medicines in the future using the unique chemicals of *R. ellipticus* and its nutritive values.

ETHNOMEDICINAL APPLICATIONS

The *R. ellipticus* is an excellent plant for cultivation as a hedge or boundary fence, practically with no cost of care except the cost of fruit picking. It is a source of additional income for farmers without any investment. Fruits have laxative action and are used in traditional medicine in Tibet to cure several body ailments. All plant parts have astringent properties and are used to reduce fevers, especially typhoid. The inner bark of the plant is applied as a kidney tonic and has an anti-diuretic function.[2] The juice from roots has antipyretic properties and is used to cure gastric problems, diarrhea, and dysentery. The root paste has wound-healing properties. Fruit juice is to reduce the temperature during fever and treats colic, sore throats, and colds.[2] The inner bark is used to treat patients with weakening senses in seminal or vaginal discharge.[2] In summer it is used to promote sweating.[7] Young shoots and roots of *R. ellipticus* are used to treat colic pain. A purplish-blue dye is produced from the fruits of *R. ellipticus*.[2] Traditionally, it is used for antifertility, wound healing, gastralgia, dysentery, antimicrobial, epilepsy, analgesic, ulcers, and diabetes mellitus.[13] The root bark decoction of the *R. ellipticus* is used twice a day to treat fever by the Naga tribe of Manipur.[14] The root bark is also used in the treatment of dysentery and diarrhea, as an emmenagogue, an abortifacient, and for healing fractured bones.[15] The root paste of the species is used as a poultice to treat bone fractures and applied on the forehead during severe headaches.[16] Ripe fruits have laxative properties and are used to treat constipation, and the paste of young fruits is taken in case of diarrhea, dysentery, and gastritis.[17] The root juice is used to treat urinary tract infections in the Tanahun district of Western Nepal.[18] The Lepcha tribe of Dzongu valley in North Sikkim, India, uses the species to cure different body ailments. The young shoot of *R. ellipticus* is chewed in raw form to relieve sudden stomach pain.[19]

PHYTOCHEMICAL SCREENING

Saklani et al. have reported the composition and nutraceutical values of fruits of *R. ellipticus*.[9] Fruits are reported to have crude protein (3.68%), carbohydrates (27.12%), crude fiber (2.35%), and ash content (1.30%). Minerals in *R. ellipticus* fruits have been reported as calcium, magnesium, potassium, and phosphorus, which are 0.95, 5.60, 1.82, and 0.20 mg/100 g, respectively. It is also revealed that the fruit contained a higher value of fat, protein, fiber, and minerals compared to apples. 200 g of *R. ellipticus* fruits contain enough nutrients required per day by a person.[9]

Phytochemical screening of *R. ellipticus* fruits depicts the presence of tannins, steroids, flavonoids, phenolic compounds, and carbohydrates.[22] Antioxidant properties of flavonoids and associated physiological functions are universally accepted for their therapeutic action in the prevention of coronary heart disease. Epidemiological studies have revealed the inverse relationship between the dietary intake of flavonoids and coronary heart disease.[23] Bidhani et al. reported that the fresh fruits of *R. ellipticus* have a total phenolic content of 3.95 mg GAE/100 g (±0.05), total flavonoids 4.99 (±0.15), total anthocyanin 0.58 (±0.02), vitamin C 4.46 (±0.53), and β-carotene 1.81(±0.02). Two phenolic acids, namely gallic acid and caffeic acid, have been reported in the highest amounts in fruits of the species. The fruits of *R. ellipticus* have been reported for the highest total phenolic acids compared to *Prunus armeniaca*, *Fragaria indica*, and *Pyracantha crenulata* fruits.[24]

Methanolic extract of fruits of *R. ellipticus* has relatively high antioxidant activity compared to other solvents, and it ranges from 45.97% to 84%.[25] Flavonoids and phenolics reported from the roots of the species are responsible for its antioxidant properties.[13] The overall antioxidant property of *R. ellipticus* is due to the phenolic compounds. Sharma et al. evaluated the total phenolic content and antioxidant properties of different leaf extracts of *R. ellipticus*. All the plant extracts have phenolic content except cold water; the methanolic extract has been deciphered for high phenolic content among all, and hexane had very little. Similarly, the free radical scavenging activity of the methanolic extract is higher compared to others. Free radicals have been implicated in many diseases, and superoxide radicals and singlet oxygen are highly harmful.[26] Ringmichon et al. reported that the root bark of *R. ellipticus* is grey to dark brown on the outer surface, while the inner surface is grey-light brown or slightly black to dark brown. It is fibrous and aromatic with a strong, bitter, and astringent taste. Histochemical analysis reveals the presence of starch, lipids, glucosides, proteins, tannins, mucilage, and saponins. The phelloderm of root bark is filled with tannin cells and starch grains.[14] Tannin-filled cells have a few prism-shaped calcium oxalate crystals. The roots of *R. ellipticus* have been reported for the presence of ursolic acid.[27] The leaves of *R. ellipticus* have been reported for elliptic acid,[28] tannins,[29] derivatives of kaempferol and quercetin, triterpenes, phenolic acids, vitamin C, minerals in the form of salts,[30] derivatives of ellagic acid,[31] methyl gallate, and methyl-brevifolin-carboxylate.[32] Bhakuni et al. have isolated 1-octacosanol from the roots of *R. ellipticus*.[12] *R. ellipticus* leaves have been reported for anticonvulsant activity against electrically induced convulsions.[33] The roots of *R. ellipticus* are reported for antiprotozoal activity against *Entamoeba histolytica* and hypoglycemic properties.[34] The Ayurvedic and Unani literature describes the antifertility activity of *R. ellipticus*. Saini et al. have reported potent free radical scavenging activity and lipid peroxidation inhibition activities in the *R. ellipticus* fruit extracts.[35]

HPLC analysis of *R. ellipticus* fruit extracts reveals the presence of a high quantity of ellagic acid and gallic acid in the fruit, which have antiproliferative activity against cervical cancer cells.[36] George et al. have reported the antipyretic, analgesic, and anti-inflammatory activities of *R. ellipticus* leaf methanol extract. Methanol extract from leaves of *R. ellipticus* (400 mg/kg) has a potent anti-inflammatory effect on carrageenan-induced inflammation.[37] *R. ellipticus* leaf methanolic extract has a potent peripheral analgesic effect in mice compared with paracetamol (100 mg/kg).[38] Sharma and Kumar have studied the protective effects of *R. ellipticus* fruits on the glucose tolerance and alloxan-induced diabetes, and reported a significant antidiabetic effect.[22] Oral administration of aqueous, ethanolic, and petroleum ether extracts from fruits of *R. ellipticus* (200 mg/kg) for 15 days significantly decrease the elevated blood glucose level to normal, and prove the traditional applications of *R. ellipticus* to cure type 2 diabetes mellitus.[22] The antidiabetic potential may be due to tannins, flavonoids, steroids, phenolic compounds, and carbohydrates. George et al. have investigated the wound-healing and antitumor properties of the species and reported that the *R. ellipticus* leaves methanol extract has significant antitumor and wound-healing properties.[6]

Sharma and Kumar have studied the therapeutic effects of *R. ellipticus* fruit extracts in acute acetaminophen-induced nephrotoxicity and reported that the ethanolic, aqueous, and petroleum ether extracts of *R. ellipticus* fruits have nephron-protective potential and improve histological derangements associated with acute-dose acetaminophen nephrotoxicity.[38]

COMPOSITION AND NUTRITIVE VALUE OF FRUITS

The *R. ellipticus* fruits have various amino acids, such as L-leucine, DL-valine, L-hydroxyproline, DL-2-aminobutyric acid, DL-isoleucine, DL-norleucine, DL-aspartic acid, L-glutamic acid, L-cysteine hydroxyl, DL-alanine, L-arginine, DL-methionine, L-cysteine-hydroxyl chloride, L-lysine monochloride, L-tyrosine, and DL-threonine.[39] Saklani et al. have concluded that, due to the high content of fiber, fats, minerals, and proteins, 200 g of *R. ellipticus* fruits are sufficient to fulfill the daily nutritional requirement of an individual.[39] Alkaloids have been reported to be absent in *R. ellipticus* fruits.[39]

Fruits of *R. ellipticus* are used as febrifuge, laxative, and carminative.[2] It is eaten during indigestion, as rich in fibrous, so helps in the digestive process.[2] Fruit juice is taken in case of sore throats, cold, and colic. The paste of young fruits is advised during gastritis, dysentery, and diarrhea.[2]

Children are given root juice decoction to get-rid-of stomach worms and for other gastric problems.[2] The juice is also given in case of kidney problems.[20] Juice from roots is given during fevers, diarrhea, and dysentery. Root paste is applied to aid in the fast healing of wounds.[2] The juice of the shoots is effective during colic pains,[7] and the decoction of young shoots is advised during stomachache.[20] Root bark decoction of *R. ellipticus* is advised during stomach ache.[20] Inner bark of the plant is used as anti-diuretic and kidney tonic.[2] Inner bark is helpful during vaginal discharge and the weakening of senses. Renal tonic is made from the inner bark is useful in the treatment of micturition during sleep.[2] Bark is used in cough, cold, and various blood disorders.[21]

Analytical reports reveal that fruits of *R. ellipticus* have the moisture of about 64.4%, crude fat 0.96% (±0.02), total nitrogen 0.58% (±0.07), vitamin C 1.05% (±0.03), soluble carbohydrates 27.12% (±0.12), K (1.82 mg/100 g, ±0.25), Ca (0.95 mg/100 g, ±0.10), total protein (3.68%, ±0.04), crude fiber (2.35%, ±0.05), ash (1.30%, ±0.05), P (0.2 mg/100 g, ±0.17), and Mg (5.60 mg/100 g, ±0.15).[39]

PHARMACOLOGY

The medicinal properties of the plant *R. ellipticus* are rich due to phytochemicals and minerals. Each part of the species is rich in one or more therapeutic ingredients, which are used either in the manufacturing of drugs or in ingredients used in various formulations such as decoctions, laxatives, and many more. The complete plant is astringent and is highly useful to lower the body temperature during typhoid, though it is used in normal fevers in folk.[2] The fruits of *R. ellipticus* are used in reducing oxidative stress and protecting the body against degenerative diseases, including cancer. Upon direct consumption, the property is cited due to its richness in antioxidants. The young roots and shoots of the plant are effective during colic pain, abdominal pain, stomachaches, etc. In Ayurveda and Unani, the antifertility property of the plant species has been reported.[2] The plant is also used for gastralgia, dysentery, diabetes mellitus, wound healing, ulcers, analgesia, epilepsy, and antimicrobials.[13]

SCOPE FOR VALUE-ADDITION AND FOOD SUPPLEMENTS

There are vast opportunities to utilize the delicious ingredients of *R. ellipticus* fruits in the food industry as a very good substrate. The antioxidant potential of fruits makes them useful for the development of various supplemented probiotic products and for producing a purplish-blue, food/pharma-grade dye. Currently, scientific intervention for the processing of the species is a lacking issue and is to be deciphered for the development of a wide range of food products. Owing to its composition, its berries can be utilized to develop numerous food products (jam, juice, jelly, candy, and squash) and pharma products with biotech interventions.

Currently, the phenolic compound of fruits, which has high nutritional value, can be used to modify the aroma of the food, its color, flavor, and taste. As *R. ellipticus* fruits are rich in phenolic contents, their utilization in food supplements has additional benefits. The juices of fruits have an attractive color and rich flavor and may be used for squash making.

R. ellipticus berries are seasonal and localized; so, their preservation can ensure yearlong availability and serve as a sustainable source of income for rural people. More focused research to attract food processors and industrialists to develop more value-added products with high nutritive and medicinal value is a need of the time.

There is a scope to develop an anti-inflammatory drug from *R. ellipticus* to treat various disorders and to investigate the mechanism/biological pathways behind these folk applications of the species. Moreover, with fruits like *R. ellipticus,* the gross pressure levied on a few fruit crops like guava, papaya, and mango will ease profoundly for different nutraceutical properties. As *R. ellipticus* is being hard crop grown in a wasteland of the mountainous region without much care or agronomic practices, its cultivation and utilization will prove cost-effective.

REFERENCES

1. Flynn T, Lorence DH. 1998. New naturalized plant records for the Hawaiian Islands. *Bishop Museum Occasional Papers. Honolulu*. 56: 5–6.
2. Pandey Y, Bhatt SS. 2016. Overview of Himalayan yellow raspberry (*Rubus ellipticus* Smith.): a nutraceutical plant. *Journal of Applied and Natural Science*. 8 (1): 494–499.
3. Lowe S, Browne M, Boudjelas S, De Poorter M. 2000. *100 of the World's Worst Invasive Alien Species: A Selection from the Global Invasive Species Database*. Vol. 12. Invasive Species Specialist Group, Auckland.
4. Wu K, Zhang J, Zhang G, Ding J. 2014. *Epiblema tetragonana* and *Epinotia ustulana* (*Lepidoptera: Tortricidae*), two potential biological control agents for the invasive plant, *Rubus ellipticus*. *Biological Control*. 77: 51–58.
5. Parmar C, Kaushal MK. 1982. *Rubus ellipticus. Wild Fruits*. Kalyani Publishers, New Delhi, India. pp. 84–87.
6. George BP, Parimelazhagan T, Saravanan S. 2013. Anti-inflammatory, analgesic, and antipyretic activities of *Rubus ellipticus* Smith. Leaf methanol extract. *International Journal of Pharmacy and Pharmaceutical Sciences*. 5 (2): 220–224.
7. Patel AV, Rojas-Vera J, Dacke CG. 2004. Therapeutic constituents and actions of *Rubus* species. *Current Medical Chemistry*. 11: 1501–1512.
8. Milivojevic J, Maksimovic V, Nikolic M, Bogdanovic J, Maletic R, Milatovic R. 2011. Chemical and antioxidant properties of cultivated and wild *Fragaria* and *Rubus* berries. *Journal of Food Quality*. 34 (1): 1–9.
9. Saklani S, Subhash C, Mishra AP. 2011. Evaluation of nutritional profile, medicinal value and quantitative estimation in different parts of *Pyrus pashia*, *Ficus palmate* and *Pyracantha crenulata*. *Asian Journal of Chemistry*. 2 (3): 350–354.
10. George BP, Parimelazhagan T, Kumar YT, Sajeesh T. 2015. Antitumor and wound healing properties of *Rubus ellipticus* Smith. *Journal of Acupuncture and Meridian Studies*. 8 (3): 134–141.
11. Badhani A, Rawat S, Bhatt ID, Rawal RS. 2015. Variation in chemical constituents and antioxidant activity in Yellow Himalayan (*Rubus ellipticus* Smith) and Hill Raspberry (*Rubus niveus* Thunb.). *Journal of Food Biochemistry*. 39 (6): 663–672.
12. Bhakuni RS, Shukla YN, Thakur RS. 1987. Chemical examination of the roots of *Rubus ellipticus*. *Indian Drugs*. 24: 272.
13. Vadivelan R, Bhadra S, Ravi AS, Singh K, Shanish A, Elango K, Suresh B. 2009. Evaluation of anti-inflammatory and membrane stabilizing property of ethanol root extract of *Rubus ellipticus* smith and albino rats. *Journal of Natural Remedies*. 9 (1): 74–78.
14. Ringmichon CL, Gopalkrishnan B, Dixit AP. 2013. Ethno-pharmacognostical studies on root bark of *Rubus ellipticus* Smith from Manipur. *Journal of Pharmacognosy and Phytochemestry*. 2 (2): 223–228.
15. Kirtikar KR, Basu BD. 2001. Indian medicinal plants. *Oriental Enterprises*. 5: 1487–1488.
16. Pradhan BK, Badola HK. 2008. Ethnomedicinal plant use by Lepcha tribe of Dzongu valley, bordering Khangchendzonga Biosphere Reserve, in North Sikkim, India. *Journal of Ethnobiology and Ethnomedicine*. 4: 22. https://doi.org/10.1186/1746-4269-4-22
17. Maity D, Pradhan N, Chauhan AS. 2004. Folk uses of some medicinal plants from North Sikkim. *Indian Journal of Traditional Knowledge*. 3: 66–71.
18. Uprety Y, Ram C, Asselin PH, Boon E. 2011. Plant biodiversity and ethnobotany inside the projected impact area of the Upper Seti Hydropower Project, Western Nepal. *Environment Sustainable Development*. 13: 463–492.

19. Pfoze NL, Kumar Y, Myrboh B. 2012. Survey and assessment of ethnomedicinal plants used in Senapati District of Manipur State, Northeast India. *Phytopharmacology*. 2: 285–311.
20. Hazarika TK, Pongener M. 2018. Potential wild edible fruits of Nagaland, North-east India and its significance in the livelihood and nutritional security of rural, indigenous people. *Genetic Resources and Crop Evolution*. 65 (1): 199–215.
21. Wangchuk P, Yeshi K, Jamphel K. 2017. Pharmacological, ethnopharmacological, and botanical evaluation of subtropical medicinal plants of Lower Kheng region in Bhutan. *Integrative Medicine research*. 6 (4): 372–387.
22. Sharma US, Kumar A. 2011. Anti-diabetic effect of *Rubus ellipticus* fruit extracts an alloxan induced diabetic rats. *Journal of Diabetology*. 2 (4): 11–15.
23. Hertog MG, Hollman PC, Katan MB, Kromhout D. 1993. Dietary antioxidant flavonoids and risk of coronary heart disease. *Lancet*. 342: 1007–1011.
24. Bidhani A, Sakalani S, Mishra AP. 2011. Variation in biochemical and antioxidant activity of some wild edible fruit of Uttarakhand. *Report and Opinion*. 3: pp. 25–29.
25. Ahmad M, Masood S, Sultana S, Hadda TB, Bader A, Zafar M. 2015. Antioxidant and nutraceutical value of wild medicinal *Rubus* berry. *Pakistan Journal of Pharmaceutical Science*. 28 (1): 241–247.
26. Sharma M, Neerajani G, Kumar A, Basak D. 2014. Evaluation of total phenolic content and antioxidant properties of different leaf extract of *Rubus ellipticus*. *Ethiopian International Journal of Multidisciplinary Research*. 2 (2): 14–17.
27. Talapatra SK, Shrestha KM, Talapatra B. 1989. Chemical investigation of some medicinal plants of Nepal: part II. *Indian Journal of Chemistry*. 28: 880–881.
28. Dutta SGL, Ganguly KN. 1997. Isolation and structure elucidation of new pentacyclic triterpene acid from the Leaves of *Rubus ellipticus*. *Natural Product Sciences*. 32: 108–110.
29. Okuda T, Yoshida T, Hatano T, Iwasaki M, Kubo M, Orime T, Yoshizaki M, Naruhashi N. 1992. Hydrolysable tannins as chemotaxonomic markers in the Rosaceae. *Phytochemistry*. 31: 3091–3096.
30. Gudej J, Rychlinska I. 1996. Flavonoid compounds from the leaves of *Rubus idaeus* L. *Herbal Journal of Poland*. 42: 257–261.
31. Gudej J. 2003. Kaempferol and quercetin glycosides from *Rubus idaeus* L. leaves. *Acta Poloniae Pharmaceutica*. 60: 313–316.
32. Gudej J, Tomczyk M, Urban E, Tomczykowa M. 1998. Analysis of chemical composition of *Rubus saxatilis* L. leaves. *Herbal Journal of Poland*. 44: 340–344.
33. Rana AC, Santana DD, Saluja AK. 1990. Pharmacological screening of the alcohlic extract of the leaves of *Rubus ellepticus*. *Indian Journal of Pharmaceutical Science*. 52: 174–177.
34. Abraham Z, Bhakuni DS, Garg HS, Geol AK, Mehrotra BN, Patniak GK. 1986. Screening of Indian plants for biological activity. *Indian Journal of Experimental Biology*. 24: 48–68.
35. Saini R, Dangwal K, Singh H, Garg V. 2012. Antioxidant and Anti-proliferative activities of phenolics isolated from fruits of Himalayan Yellow Raspberry (*Rubus ellipticus*). *Journal Food Science and Technology*. 5: 22–23.
36. You BR, Moon HJ, Han YH, Park WH. 2010. Gallic acid inhibits the growth of HeLa cervical cancer cells via apoptosis and or necrosis. *Journal of Food Science and Technology*. 48: 1334–1340.
37. George BP, Parimalazhagan T, Kumar YT, Sajees T. 2013. Antitumor and wound healing properties of *Rubus Ellipticus* Smith. *Journal of Acupuncture and Meridian Studies*. 5 (3): 100–106.
38. Sharma US, Kumar A. 2010. Therapeutic efficacy of *Rubus ellipticus* (smith) fruits extracts in acute acetaminophen induced nephrotoxicity in rats. *Pharmacologyonline*. 3: 514–526.
39. Saklani S, Chandra S, Badoni PP, Dogra S. 2012. Antimicrobial activity, nutritional profile and phytochemical screening of wild edible fruit of *Rubus ellipticus*. *International Journal of Medicinal and Aromatic Plants*. 2 (2): 269–274.

27 *Rubus occidentalis* (Black Raspberry)

INTRODUCTION

The genus *Rubus*, the family Rosaceae, is ubiquitous, especially in the temperate parts of the northern hemisphere. The genus comprises around 700 species, and a few are cultivated as industrial plants for fruits. The fruit is eaten either alone in fresh form or as a value-added product, e.g., jams, jellies, and pastry fillings.[1]

Soon after the Ice Age, *Rubus* species were a source of medicine and food for native peoples. Genus *Rubus* is an example of the earliest historical knowledge of medicinal use.[2] Asian medicinal traditions (the Ayurvedic tradition of India and the traditional Chinese medicine) and folk traditions throughout the world have also used *Rubus* for multiple medicinal purposes. In modern times, *Rubus* species are grown for vitamin-rich fruits and delicious taste. In ancient times it was used either as a whole plant or in parts, as branches, flowers, leaves, roots, and stems were used in plasters or oil, decoctions, wine extractions, condensates, and infusions.[3] Decoctions of branches are used to stop dyeing hair, cure diarrhea, act as an antivenom for snakebites, and prevent vaginal discharge. Leaves are chewed as a plasterer to constrain shingles and strengthen gums, headscarves, hemorrhoids, and prolapsed eyes. Flowers triturated with oil are used to reduce eye inflammations and cool skin rashes, and infusions with wine-aided or water are used for stomach ailments. Romans and Greeks were using leaves for female applications, whereas the Chinese used them to treat male disorders. Medicinal properties of the genus *Rubus* continue in Renaissance and modern therapeutic practices, as leaf infusions are recommended as a gargle for throat cankers and sore mouth and a wash for wounds. Barks rich in tannins were and are used as a tonic for diarrhea. The root extract has cathartic and emetic properties.[3] Current molecular studies have acknowledged *Rubus* fruits for their high phenolics, anthocyanins, ellagic acid, and antioxidants. Fruit extracts have anticarcinogenic properties and are used as colorants,[4] antivirals, cosmetic moisturizing agents, and antiallergenic compounds.[3] All species of the genus are used for their health-healing properties in different ways.

R. occidentalis Linn. (Eng.: Black Raspberry) is an important folklore medicinal plant of the genus *Rubus*. It can be found specifically along roadsides, in disturbed areas, and in woodlands. Commercial cultivation is preferred in sunny and dry sites with adequate rain, as fruits do not develop properly in water scarcity. Furthermore, too much shade is not good for better fruiting of the *R. occidentalis* plant. It is a heat-tolerant plant that prefers moist, partially sunny sites with highly organic soil.[5] The propagation of black raspberries depends on various biotic and abiotic factors and may affect rooting, including the cutting position, cutting type, and the presence of auxin.[6] Currently, photostable auxin, indole butyric acid, and auxins are commonly used to promote the rooting of the species.[6]

R. occidentalis plant has flowers arranged in terminal panicles, and its fruits are in clusters, small, and their dark purple color is attractive. These small fruits have excellent nutritional properties, as they contain more than twice the anthocyanins compared to the red raspberry fruits.[6]

The vegetative propagation of species in the genus *Rubus* is via root and stem cuttings, as well as tissue culture.[6] Black raspberry, yellow raspberry, blackberry, and red raspberry produce a few buds from roots. In black raspberries, the use of woody stems and herbaceous cuttings is a viable alternative for vegetative propagation.[6] The cutting technology is an inexpensive and rapid method of asexual propagation and allows the retention of the original characteristics of plants, an objective of agricultural interest preferred to avoid species mixing.[6]

ETHNOPHARMACOLOGY

The *Rubus* species have been associated with several health-healing benefits, such as antirheumatic, analgesic, antibacterial, anti-inflammatory, anticancer, and hypoglycemic properties.[7–9] Radiocarbon dating has revealed that soon after the Ice Age, *Rubus* species were a main source of medicine and food for native peoples.[10] Radiocarbon dating results have deciphered that raspberries were harvested by the ancient Greeks in 370 BCE (before the Christian Era).[11] Pompey had introduced raspberries from Turkey to Rome in 65 BCE.[12]

Ayurvedic medicine has a similitude to ancient Greek medicine, as both systems are based on humor.[3] *Rubus* is used as an astringent and diuretic in Indian traditional medicines. Leaves of raspberry have been combined with many other herbs to produce an astringent juice (Kashay) in Ayurveda.[3] The decoction of *R. occidentalis* produces clarity, causes a rigid mouth, stimulates a feeling of heaviness, contracts the tongue, and diminishes saliva. The infusion of *Rubus* leaves in the Ayurvedic system is used as an aid in childbirth, menopause, and stomach problems.[3]

Extracts of *Rubus* species have been used in traditional medicines to treat wounds, burn inflammation, and microbial infections.[1]

PHYTOCHEMISTRY

Phytochemical screening of plants and its results are the basis to support or deny the traditional therapeutic applications of plants. The genus *Rubus* is characterized to

DOI: 10.1201/9781003512868-29

accumulate and synthesize triterpenoids, ellagitannins, anthocyanins, and flavonoids, and each chemical class is known for its unique therapeutic properties.[1] Information on the pharmacological activities of compounds isolated from *R. occidentalis* and their structures supports their applications in the traditional healing system.[1]

R. occidentalis has different structural conjugates of phenolic acids and tannins. Phenolic compounds are an important part of the human food chain and comprise the largest groups of secondary metabolites of plants.[13] Plant-derived phenolics have health-healing and health-promoting properties, mainly as an antioxidant. Soft fruits, such as raspberry, are a rich source of phenolics.[1]

Black raspberry has delicious fruits that are consumed either fresh or in processed forms such as juices, liquors, and jams. Phenolic compounds present in berry extracts have a strong capacity to scavenge free oxygen radical species and to inhibit oxidation, as well as the growth of pathogenic bacteria.[14] The major phenolics in *Rubus* berries are represented by hydrolyzable tannins (gallotannins and ellagitannins), with anthocyanins, a black pigment of the fruit. Flavan-3-ols, hydroxycinnamic acids, flavonols, and proanthocyanidins are the minor chemical classes present in fruits.[15,16] Anthocyanins of *R. occidentalis* are of pharmaceutical interest to researchers for healthcare purposes globally.

Hydrolyzable tannins consist of a polyol core (e.g., quinic acid or glucose) esterified with either gallic acid(s) (gallotannins) or hexahydroxydiphenic acid(s) (ellagitannins). Ellagitannins are present in the highest concentration in fruits of *R. occidentalis*. The flavonoid content estimated by high performance liquid chromatography (HPLC) has been reported in higher quantity in blackberry leaves than in black raspberry leaves.[17]

Anthocyanins, a naturally occurring phenolic group of compounds, impart color to flowers and fruits and also have therapeutic properties. *R. occidentalis* contains a high quantity of anthocyanins and is used either in diet or in some therapeutic applications. Different *Rubus* species have different anthocyanin compositions. *R. occidentalis* has a distinct spectrum of anthocyanins.[18] The major components of *R. occidentalis* anthocyanin are cyanidin and cyanidin-3-sophoroside, with traces of cyanidin-3-glucoside, cyanidin-3-(2-G-glucosylrutinoside), pelargonidin, cyanidin-3-rutinoside, etc., and their glycosides.[18]

The *Rubus* species are reported to contain triterpenoids. Terpenoids are in abundance in the plant kingdom and possess different types of biological properties. Ursane-type triterpene has been identified in the *Rubus* species along with β-sitosterol and β-sitosterol-3-β-D-glucose.[18]

PHARMACOLOGICAL PROPERTIES

The *R. occidentalis* plant is known for its antinociceptive, antioxidant, and anti-inflammatory properties.[19,20] These properties of *R. occidentalis* are attributed to ellagic acid, anthocyanins, and other phenolic compounds. The bioactivity of different compounds has been reported to be dependent on the maturity stage of fruits.[19,21,22] In a study on premature black raspberry fruits, a high content of phenolics, flavonoids, and vitamin C has been reported, implying the potential of the premature black raspberry fruits to be used as a medicine or functional food.[21]

Berries are the richest dietary source of anthocyanins, and black raspberries have the highest anthocyanin content among all.[23] Studies have revealed that black raspberry anthocyanins have potent chemoprotective properties.[4,24,25] The geographical source of fruit may affect its chemoprotective efficacy, as biotic and abiotic factors are known to affect the anthocyanin quantity and antioxidant properties of *R. occidentalis* fruits.[26,27]

In herbals, pharmacological studies are generally focused on the bioactive fractions of either a plant part as an extract or a crude drug. However, several investigations have a successful history of focusing on the bioactivity of specific isolated compound(s), even bioassay-guided fractionation after detecting bioactivity in the plant part.[1]

Folklore utilization of *R. occidentalis* is mainly for inflammatory diseases, and its use has been proven highly potent. The genus *Rubus* overall is used as medicine, food, and as a dye for clothing. *R. occidentalis* has a high capacity to quench free oxygen radicals,[28] and its fruits have high antioxidant activity compared to other red raspberries.[29] Wang and Jiao have investigated the antioxidant activities of *R. occidentalis* against hydrogen peroxide, superoxide radicals, singlet oxygen, and hydroxyl radicals. Anti-inflammatory properties of *R. occidentalis* are used to treat several pathologies in traditional medicine all over the world.[30] Triterpenoids and tannins have been reported as the responsible compounds of *R. occidentalis* for their antioxidant activities and anti-inflammatory properties. Some of these compounds have been isolated by the bioassay-guided fractionation method, which was previously detected in part of the plants for the same activity.[31,32]

Rubus species have been deciphered to suppress tumor development. The use of R. occidentalis fruits is an effective non-invasive treatment that reduces the severity and incidence of cancer.. Ellagitannins and triterpenoids have been reported as responsible compounds for the antineoplastic activity of the genus. Paivarinta et al. have reported that natural ellagitannins are a chemopreventive agent for intestinal tumorigenesis.[33] Some of these compounds have been isolated and studied by bioassay-guided fractionation and have been proven useful in treating cancer.[33]

Carcinogenesis is a multistage, micro-evolutionary process, and the tumor is derived from single abnormal cells. Carcinogenesis can be divided into three major stages: initiation, promotion, and progression. The initiation is a result of DNA damage, and cells so initiated transform into malignancy on promotion and progression. Promotion accounts for a major portion of the lengthy latent period of carcinogenesis and is partly reversible. The final stage of cancer is the progression to a malignant neoplasm. The conventional treatments, such as radiological, chemotherapy, and surgical, are not fully satisfactory, as prevention of disease or at least stopping it at its inception is important, and the application of black raspberry may be beneficial.[33] Mallery et al. have also reported that *R. occidentalis* fruits may be used in preventing oral cancer.[34]

R. occidentalis fruits have been reported to inhibit oral cavity tumors in hamsters, which were fed with 5% and 10% freeze-dried black raspberries (LBR) in the diet for 2 weeks before treatment for a known carcinogen and for 10 weeks thereafter. A significant difference has been reported in the number of tumors between the 5% LBR and control groups. Studies on tumors in the 10% berry-treated animals have revealed that dietary black raspberries inhibit tumor formation in the oral cavity.[35]

SCOPE AND OPPORTUNITIES

Fruits of *R. occidentalis* have a unique phenolic composition dominated by ellagitannins and anthocyanins. Due to this polyphenolic combination, *R. occidentalis* fruits have a high antioxidant capacity and have been reported to reduce cancer, the rate of proliferation, and inflammation at a molecular level. Fruits of *R. occidentalis* have been proven to be effective at the initiation and progression stages of tumor development by reducing the growth rate of premalignant cells, affecting carcinogen metabolism, reducing tissue inflammation, promoting apoptosis, and inhibiting angiogenesis in different types of cancers. The results of different in vivo and in vitro investigations have concluded that *R. occidentalis* is a promising herb for checking cancer at an early stage, but results have not been completely translated into clinical trials.

Rubus berries are a highly potent source of phenolic compounds. Phenolic compounds were previously considered anti-nutrients; however, interest in food phenolics has grown significantly due to their antioxidant properties, capacity to neutralize free radicals, and effectiveness in metal chelation. The possible role of phenolics of *R. occidentalis* in human health, such as being friendly for cardiovascular health and reducing the risk of cancer and other pathologies, has been reported.

Currently, *R. occidentalis* used for medicines is either from cultivated plants or wild sources. A worldwide survey on the production of *Rubus* spp. conducted in 2005 revealed that there were an estimated 20,035 ha. of berries planted and commercially cultivated worldwide, recording a 45% increase since 1995.[36]

Wu et al. (2006) investigated the bioavailability of *R. occidentalis* anthocyanins in the gastrointestinal tract and suggested that anthocyanins are stable in the intestine.[37] Tian et al. have examined human absorption and metabolism of anthocyanins of *R. occidentalis* in male volunteers and reported the intact excretion of anthocyanins, which are converted into methylated derivatives in human urine.[38] There is still a knowledge gap to illustrate the bioavailability of phenolics from the genus *Rubus* fruits in the human gastrointestinal tract. Detailed investigations on the anthocyanins inside the human intestine may lead to a new mode of drug delivery.

Currently, there is no specification for the minimum anthocyanin concentration of a black raspberry dietary supplement even in the USA. Most people are unable to distinguish black raspberries, red raspberries, and blackberries, usually in modified physical form. Lee and Finn have developed an HPLC analytical method for individual anthocyanins using HPLC/DAD/MS (diode array detector mass spectrometry),[39] and results were expressed as mg of cyanidin-3-glucoside in different samples having black raspberry fruits.[39] The anthocyanin profile for identifying food and dietary supplements prepared from black raspberry fruits may help in checking the adulteration and shelf life of the product, an important parameter for global business.[40,41]

REFERENCES

1. Rocabado GO, Bedoya LM, Abad MJ, Bermejo P. 2008. *Rubus* – a Review of its phytochemical and pharmacological profile. *Natural Product Communications*. 3 (3): 423–436.
2. Jin C, Yin-Chun S, Gui-Qin C, Wen-Dun W. 1999. Ethnobotanical studies on wild edible fruits in southern Yunnan: folk names, nutritional value and uses. *Economic Botany*. 53 (1): 2–14. https://doi.org/10.1007/BF02860785
3. Humme KE. 2010. *Rubus* pharmacology: antiquity to the present. *Horticultural Science*. 45(11):1587–91
4. Seeram NP. 2008. Berry fruits for cancer prevention: current status and future prospects. *Journal of Agricultural and Food Chemistry*. 56: 630–635.
5. N C State Extension Plant Toolbox. *Rubus occidentalis*. https://plants.ces.ncsu.edu/plants/rubus-occidentalis/, as on 25th January 2022.
6. Villa F, Stumm DR, da Silva DF, Menegusso FJ, Ritter G, Kohler TR. 2018. Rooting of black raspberry with plant growth regulator. Ciencia Rural, Santa Maria. 48 (3): e20161023
7. But MT. 1997. *International Collation of Traditional and Folk Medicine*. World Scientific. New Jersey.
8. Moerman DE. 1998. *Native American Ethnobotany*. Timber Press, Portland.
9. Heywood VH. 1978. *Flowering Plants of the World*. University Press, Oxford.
10. Connolly TJ. 1999. Newberry Crater: a ten-thousand-year record of human occupation and environmental change in the basin-plateau borderlands. Anthropological Papers No. 121. University of Utah, Salt Lake City, UT.
11. Handley D, Pritts M. (Eds.) 1989. *Bramble Production Guide*. Northeast Regional Agr Eng Serv. NRAES-35, Ithaca, NY.
12. Trager J. 1995. *The Food Chronology: A Food Lover's Compendium of Events and Anecdotes from Prehistory to the Present*. Henry Holt and Co., New York.
13. Krondatyuk TP, Pezzuto JM. 2004. Natural product polyphenols of relevance to human health. *Pharmaceutical Biology*. 42: 46–63.
14. Kähkönen MP, Hopia AI, Heinonen M. 2001. Berry phenolics and their antioxidant activity. *Journal of Agricultural and Food Chemistry*. 49: 4076–4082.

15. Moyer RA, Hummer KE, Fim CE, Frei B, Wrolstad RE. 2002. Anthocyanins, phenolics and antioxidant capacity in diverse small fruits: *Vaccinium*, *Rubus* and *Ribes*. *Journal of Agricultural and Food Chemistry*. 50: 519–525.
16. Maatta-Riihinen KR, Kamal-Eldin A, Torronen AT. 2004. Identification and quantification of phenolic compounds in berries of *Fragaria* and *Rubus* species (Family Rosaceae). *Journal of Agricultural and Food Chemistry*, 52: 6178–6187.
17. Marinova D, Ribarova F. 2007. HPLC determination of carotenoids in Bulgarian berries. *Journal of Food Composition and Analysis*. 20: 370–374.
18. Dugo P, Mondello L, Errante G, Zappia G, Dugo G. 2001. Identification of anthocyanins in berries by narrow-base high-performance liquid chromatography with electrospay ionization detection. *Journal of Agricultural and Food Chemistry*. 49: 3987–3992.
19. Johnson JL, Bomser JA, Scheerens JC, Giusti MM. 2011. Effect of black raspberry (*Rubus occidentalis* L.) extract variation conditioned by cultivar, production site, and fruit maturity stage on colon cancer cell proliferation. *Journal of Agricultural and Food Chemistry*. 59 (5): 1638–1645.
20. Dai J, Patel JD, Mumper RJ. 2007. Characterization of blackberry extract and its antiproliferative and anti-inflammatory properties. *Journal of Medicinal Food*. 10 (2): 258–265.
21. Shin D, Chae K, Choi H, Lee S, Gim S, Kwon G, Lee HT, Song YC, Kim KJ, Kong HS, Kwon JW. 2018. Bioactive and pharmacokinetic characteristics of pre-matured black raspberry, *Rubus occidentalis*. *Italian Journal of Food Science*. 30 (3): 428–439.
22. Bhandary B, Lee HY, Back HI, Park SH, Kim MG, Kwon JW, Song JY, Lee HK, Kim HR, Chae SW, Chae HJ. 2012. Immature *Rubus coreanus* shows a free radical-scavenging effect and inhibits cholesterol synthesis and secretion in liver cells. *Indian Journal of Pharmaceutical Sciences*. 74 (3): 211–216.
23. Tian Q, Giusti M, Stoner G, Schwartz S. 2006. Characterization of a new anthocyanin in black raspberries (*Rubus occidentalis*) by liquid chromatography electrospray ionization tandem mass spectrometry. *Food Chemistry*. 94: 465–468.
24. Stoner G, Wang L, Zikri N, Chen T, Hecht S, Huang C, Sardo C, Lechner J. 2007. Cancer prevention with freeze-dried berries and berry components. *Seminars in Cancer Biology*. 17: 403–410.
25. Wang L, Stoner G. 2008. Anthocyanins and their role in cancer prevention. *Cancer Letters*. 269: 281–290.
26. Ozgen M, Wyzgoski F, Tulio A, Gazula A, Miller A, Scheerens J, Reese R, Wright S. 2008. Antioxidant capacity and phenolic antioxidants of Midwestern black raspberries grown for direct markets are influenced by production site. *HortScience*. 43: 2039–2047.
27. Wyzgoski F, Paudel L, Rinaldi P, Reese R, Ozgen M, Tulio A, Miller A, Scheerens J, Hardy J. 2010. Modelling relationships among active components in black raspberry (*Rubus occidentalis* L.) fruit extracts using high-resolution 1 H nuclear magnetic resonance (NMR) spectroscopy and multivariate statistical analysis. *Journal of Agricultural and Food Chemistry*. 58: 3407–3414.
28. Wada L, Ou B. 2002. Antioxidant activity and phenolic content of Oregon caneberries. *Journal of Agricultural and Food Chemistry*. 50: 3495–3500.
29. Pantelidis GE, Vasilakakis M, Manganaris GA, Diamantidis GR. 2007. Antioxidant capacity, phenol, anthocyanin and ascorbic acid contents in raspberries, blackberries, red currants, gooseberries and cornelian cherries. *Food Chemistry*. 102: 777–783.
30. Wang SY, Jiao H. 2000. Scavenging capacity of berry crops on superoxide radicals, hydrogen peroxide, hydroxyl radicals and singlet oxygen. *Journal of Agricultural and Food Chemistry*. 48: 5677–5684.
31. Choi J, Lee KT, Ha J, Yun SY, Ko CD, Jung HJ, Park HJ. 2003. Antinociceptive and anti-inflammatory effects of niga-ichigoside F1 and 23-hydroxytormentic acid obtained from *Rubus coreanus*. *Biological & Pharmaceutical Bulletin*. 26: 1436–1441.
32. Nam JH, Jung HJ, Choi J, Lee KT, Park HJ. 2006. The anti-gastropathic and anti-rheumatic effect of niga-ichigoside F1 and 23-hydroxytormentic acid isolated from the unripe fruits of *Rubus coreanus* in a rat model. *Biological & Pharmaceutical Bulletin*. 29: 967–970.
33. Paivarinta E, Pajari AM, Torronen R, Mutanen M. 2006. Ellagic acid and natural sources of ellagitannins as possible chemo-preventive agents against intestinal tumorigenesis in the Min mouse. *Nutrition and Cancer*. 54: 79–83.
34. Mallery SR, Zwick JC, Pei P, Tong M, Larsen PE, Shumway BS, Lu B, Fields HW, Mumper RJ, Stoner GD. 2008. Topical application of a bioadhesive black raspberry gel modulates gene expression and reduces cyclooxygenase 2 protein in human premalignant oral lesions. *Cancer Research*. 68: 4945–4957.
35. Casto BC, Kresty LA, Kraly CL. 2002. Chemoprevention of oral cancer by black raspberries. *Anticancer Research*. 22: 4005–4015.
36. Strik BC, Clark JR, Finn CE, Banados MP. 2007. Worldwide blackberry production. *Horttechnology*. 17: 205–213.
37. Wu X, Pittman HE, Prior RL. 2006. Fate of anthocyanins and antioxidant capacity in contents of the gastrointestinal tract of weanling pigs following black raspberry consumption. *Journal of Agricultural and Food Chemistry*. 54: 583–589.
38. Tian Q, Giusti MM, Stoner GD, Schwartz SJ. 2006. Urinary excretion of black raspberry (*Rubus occidentalis*) anthocyanins and their metabolites. *Journal of Agricultural and Food Chemistry*. 54: 1467–1472.
39. Lee J, Finn CE. 2007. Anthocyanins and other polyphenolics in American elderberry (*Sambucus canadensis*) and European elderberry (*S. nigra*) cultivars. *Journal of the Science of Food and Agriculture*. 87: 2665–2675.
40. Sanzini E, Badea M, Santos AD, Restani P, Sievers H. 2011. Quality control of plant food supplements. *Food Function*. 2: 740–746.
41. Lee J. 2014. Marketplace analysis demonstrates quality control standards needed for black raspberry dietary supplements. *Plant Foods for Human Nutrition*. 69: 161–167.

28 *Solanum nigrum* (Black Nightshade)

INTRODUCTION

The plant *Solanum nigrum* Linn. (Family: Solanaceae) is commonly called black nightshade in English and makoi in Hindi. It is an annual herb, erect, divaricately branched, unarmed, and suffrutescent. Its fruits are purplish-black or reddish berries. These species are semi-cultivated in a few African countries and Indonesia and are largely utilized as vegetables. It is a volunteer crop that occurs as a weed in cultivated fields, near buildings, in weedy plant communities, along fences, under trees and roads, on wasteland, and in shaded areas, including on fertile land to be used as vegetables or in home gardens.[1]

S. nigrum has diverse therapeutic and biological control-based potentials. During the last few decades, both aqueous and organic solvent-based extracts of *S. nigrum* have been prepared to recover from infections, internal and external wounds, inflammations, and cancer, as well as to control many body ailments like hepatic, gastric, cardiovascular, and enzymatic complications, and cytotoxicity. The plant has been reported effective in reducing aging and is an ideal low-cost source of phytomedicines.[2]

ETHNOPHARMACOLOGY

The leaves and berries of *S. nigrum* are mainly used for medicinal purposes, besides the other parts of the species. The leaves are applied as a poultice for gouty joints (swollen and painful), rheumatic pains, and skin diseases, are used to treat tuberculosis, and are reported to produce diaphoresis. Additional applications of leaves have been reported to treat nervous disorders, nausea, and dropsy. The decoction of the flowers and berries is useful in erysipelas, pulmonary tuberculosis, bronchitis, and cough. The juice of berries is used as an antidiarrheal and for treating hydrophobia, ophthalmopathy, anasarca, and heart diseases. The use of berries has been reported as cathartic, diuretic, and tonic. Seeds are used to cure giddiness and dry throat and treat skin diseases and inflammations. The roots are useful in hepatitis, retinopathy, and ophthalmopathy. The whole plant is used as an expectorant, antiseptic, cardiotonic, anti-inflammatory, laxative, diuretic, digestive, sedative, and diaphoretic to treat asthma, swelling, and cough. The plant is also effective in curing dropsy, cardiopathy, leprosy, hemorrhoids, nephropathy, general debility, and ophthalmopathy. Decoction of the plant species is used to depress the CNS and enhance the biological activities in the spinal cord.[1,3–10]

Additionally, folk applications of its fruits have been described to treat cataracts, blindness, and optical bacterial infection, and to stop kids' bedwetting.[8,11] Roots of *S. nigrum* are described as being used to relieve cough, increase feminine fertility, and treat other respiratory infections.[12,13] The whole plant application has been described as a remedy for complications of oncogenic origin, dermal infections, burns, and snake venom.[11,14–16]

Different chemical classes have been identified for the therapeutic action of *S. nigrum*. Leaves of the species are rich in minerals (phosphorus, iron, and calcium), fat, protein, and carbohydrates.[17] *S. nigrum* is traditionally used to treat liver diseases.[18] The aerial parts of *S. nigrum* are used to suppress ulcers due to excess acid in the stomach and aspirin-induced ulceration.[19]

PHYTOPHARMACOLOGY

Bioactive compounds of herbal origin in food are subject to modifications during cooking and inside the gastrointestinal tract. In addition, the bio-accessibility and bioavailability of active ingredients from herbal sources are further dependent on the intestinal barrier, metabolism, and retention in the body before excretion. Mostly, bioactive molecules ingested orally have low bioavailability,[20] which hinders their potential effects on human health, an important factor focused on during in vivo and in vitro evaluations of herbals.

A literature survey on *S. nigrum* reveals that it consists of antinutrient factors (tannins), phytosterols, reducing sugars,[21] glycosides,[22] glycoproteins,[23] proteins, carbohydrates, alkaloids,[22] saponins,[24] linoleic acid,[25] steroidal glycosides, and steroid alkaloids,[24] along with protein (30.26%) (mainly proline and glycine) and carbohydrates (69.74%).[26] The concentration of solasodine is found less in mature plants, but its concentration is higher in unripe fruits.[25,27] Ascorbic acid has been reported in fruits of the species.[28] There may be many more unidentified compounds in fruits, as FTIR data reveal the presence of functional groups with different peaks, such as anhydrides, alkyl, carboxylic acid, ether, and alcoholic groups.[29]

Phytochemical investigations have revealed that *S. nigrum* contains alkaloids,[22] steroids,[24] steroidal saponins,[30] and glycoproteins,[26] and it exhibits antitumor activity.[31] *S. nigrum* has been reported to contain osmotin, a protein.[32] A new glycoprotein (150 kDa) has been isolated from *S. nigrum*, which consists of carbohydrate (69.74%) and protein moiety (30.26%), and it has more than 50% hydrophobic amino acids such as glycine and proline.[33] Small unripe fruits of *S. nigrum* have a high concentration of solasodine, but both the concentration and the absolute amount per fruit decrease with fruit maturation.[25] The berries of *S. nigrum* collected from New Zealand have four steroidal alkaloidal glycosides, namely, α-solanigrine, β-solanigrine,

DOI: 10.1201/9781003512868-30

solasonine, and solamargine. The berries of *S. nigrum* have been found to contain tigogenin by mixed melting point analysis and IR spectroscopy.[34] *S. nigrum* fruits and roots have been reported for the presence of ascorbic acid, and the concentration of ascorbic acid is higher in fruits compared to roots.[35] Seeds of the *S. nigrum* have a high lipid content, while mineral and protein contents are also present in considerable amounts. The seed oil of *S. nigrum* is an important natural source of linoleic acid.[23]

Steroidal glycosides of *S. nigrum* are utilized for different steroidal drugs, sexual hormones, corticosteroids, and oral contraceptives,[36–38] and are used to cure several dermal and ophthalmic disorders and hydrophobia.[36] Alkaloids, flavonoids, steroidal lactones, and glycosides of *S. nigrum* are considered pharmacologically potential ingredients for antidysentery, antiseptic, and diuretic applications.[39] The exceptional medicinal importance of *S. nigrum* is due to its anticancer, antioxidant, cytotoxic, antiulcerogenic, and antimicrobial potential (against *Aspergillus niger*, *Klebsiella pneumonia*, *Aspergillus fumigatus*, *Bacillus subtilis*, *Candida albicans*, *Escherichia coli*, *Salmonella typhiurium*, *Micrococcus luteus*, and *Vibrio cholera*). The role of other ingredients of *S. nigrum*, such as the minerals phosphorus, iron, calcium, and vitamins A and C found in leaves of *S. nigrum*, has additional applications for the plant.[40]

Phenolics are characterized by a structure of a hydroxy group (-OH) linked to an aromatic ring and are classified into non-flavonoids and flavonoids.[41] During gastrointestinal digestion, phenolics are highly unstable, resulting in low bioavailability.[42,43] *S. nigrum* has major phenolic compounds, namely 5-caffeoylquinic acid, 3-caffeoylquinic acid, 4,5-dicaffeoylquinic acid, 3,4-dicaffeoylquinic acid, and myricetin.[44] The healing properties of the *Solanum* genus are attributed to these phenolics, which exhibit antidiabetic, anti-inflammatory, antioxidant, anti-obesity, and cardioprotective.[42,43]

The genus *Solanum* (Family: Solanaceae) is known for its antiproliferative effects and alkaloid content. Alkaloids are grouped based on their origin, chemical characteristics, biosynthetic pathways, or their structure, such as pseudoalkaloids, true alkaloids, and proto-alkaloids.[45] The health-promoting effects attributed to alkaloids from *S. nigrum* are antidiabetic and antioxidant and are considered potential drugs for treating neurodegenerative disorders (e.g., Huntington's disease, Parkinson's disease, epilepsy, schizophrenia, and Alzheimer's disease).[7,46,47] Solanine and other steroidal glycoalkaloids (e.g., solasodine, α-solamargine, β-solamargine, β-2-solasonine, solasonine, solamargine, and 12-β, 27-dihydroxy solasodine) are the main ingredients of *S. nigrum*.[48–50]

Saponins, consisting of sapogenin (aglycone) linked to one or more N, O, P, R, and S oligosaccharide units,[51] are grouped according to their structure as steroidal or triterpenoid saponins.[52,53] Saponins have foaming properties in aqueous solutions, so they are poorly absorbed in the intestine and exert a hemolytic effect. These compounds have a bitter taste and astringency,[52] and they have proven potential anti-obesogenic effects and anti-insulin resistance.[54] Saponins from *Solanum* species are used for their antiviral, anti-inflammatory, antitumor, antioxidant, hypoglycemic, hypolipidemic, and antimycotic properties.[55,56]

Carotenoids, the lipophilic isoprenoids, are classified as acyclic or cyclic according to the absence or presence of a ring at the end of their structure.[57,58] The most common carotenoids reported in blood plasma are β-carotene, lutein, and lycopene.[59] Several health benefits have been attributed to carotenoids, such as protecting the skin from UV damage, improving brain functions during childhood,[60,61] immunomodulation, improving eye,[62] heart health,[63] and cancer prevention.[64] Carotenoids are provitamin A compounds, a key vitamin for protecting against diseases, reproduction, growth, and good vision.[7]

There are many more structural changes in therapeutic ingredients after ingestion, which start at the processing point, from mashing or cutting to baking or boiling, even at low temperatures, that can help release these compounds and finally affect the degree of their bio-accessibility. Cooking in water can reduce the content of hydrophilic compounds, but oil cooking can cause synergy and increase the bio-accessibility of lipophilic compounds. High temperatures result in the breakdown of cell walls and could increase phytochemicals' bio-accessibility, but the stability of thermosensitive compounds is overruled due to degradation.[65] The future course of phytochemicals after ingestion from the oral route depends on the gastrointestinal tract's physiological data of digestion, digestive enzymes, dilution, pH, electrolytes, and time of digestion.[66] In the gastrointestinal tract, it can be degraded and transformed into another compound, e.g., one that is highly pH sensitive, such as anthocyanins, etc. Glycosides can also break into aglycone (genin) and glycone (sugar). Enzymes like lactase, hydrolase, etc., can hydrolyze the sugar moieties from glycosylated bioactive molecules.[20] Cooking may result in the breakdown of cell walls, release bioactive molecules, and increase their bio-accessibility, but these compounds may be more susceptible to degradation.[67] Common household processes such as making the paste and drying significantly increased total flavonoid, phenolic, lycopene, and total antioxidant properties. Thermal processing has been reported to disrupt cell walls and cell membranes, releasing lycopene from the insoluble portion of the botanical matrix.[68] Synergic interactions among different molecules have been reported to increase bio-accessibility, e.g., red cabbage, on co-digestion with different vegetables, enhancing the bio-accessibility of total anthocyanins by 10%–15%. On the contrary, when samples were carotenoid-rich, like tomatoes, the carotenoid bio-accessibility is reported to decrease by 42%–56%. This example of phyto-molecular interaction reveals that a few combinations exert synergy and others antagonize bio-accessibility.[69] Anthocyanins are highly sensitive to pH changes in the intestinal tract, which influence bio-accessibility and bioactivity.[70]

Studies in white and purple potatoes after boiling reveal that the bio-accessibility of polyphenols increased in the in vitro digestion but reduced in the intestinal phase, and boiled undigested samples have been reported for a lower content of polyphenols. The pharmacological and biological activities of S. nigrum are attributed to bioactive compounds that enhance its significance in pharmaceuticals, as mentioned below.

ANTIBACTERIAL ACTIVITY

Different extracts of roots, seeds, and leaves of *S. nigrum* have been reported to have potent antifungal and antibacterial activity. The sensitivity of microorganisms to the used extract depends on the nature of the solvent used for extraction and the type of tested microorganisms.[71,72] The methanol extracts of the seeds and leaves of *S. nigrum* have potent activity against *Staphylococcus aureus, E. coli, Pseudomonas aeruginosa, Shigella flexneri, Yersinia aldovae, Trichophyton rubrum*, Saccharomyces, *Aspergillus parasiticus, Candida albicans*, and *Fusarium solani*.[73] The ethanolic extract of roots has antifungal properties against *A. brassicicola*.[74] Different extracts of *S. nigrum* prepared from seeds, roots, and leaves using ethanol and ethyl acetate, respectively, have been studied for their antifungal activity against a few fungal strains (*Aspergillus niger, Trichoderma viride, Penicillium notatum*, and *Fusarium oxysporum*). The extracts from seeds have been reported for antifungal properties.[75]

ANTI-HCV ACTIVITY

Hepatitis C virus (HCV) is a serious global health problem, and Javed et al. have reported that chloroform and methanol extracts of seeds of *S. nigrum* have potential antiviral activity against HCV.[76] Both extracts have been reported to inhibit HCV by 37% to 50% at nontoxic doses. The seed's chloroform extract of *S. nigrum* reduces the function of the HCV protease in a dose-dependent manner.[76]

The water extract of *S. nigrum* has been reported as hepatoprotective against liver damage by CCl_4 (carbon tetrachloride) in rats. The hepatoprotective effect of *S. nigrum* is suggested due to the free radical scavenging and antioxidant effects of the ingredients of the plant and subsequent detoxification by enzymes. Oral administration of *S. nigrum* significantly reduces thioacetamide-induced hepatic fibrosis by reducing TGF-1 secretion. Methanol extracts of *S. nigrum* have also been reported as hepatoprotective against liver injury induced by injection of CCl_4 in rats. The berries' ethanolic extract of *S. nigrum* has potent hepatoprotective properties.[77]

S. nigrum fruits have glycoprotein (150 kDa) with scavenging activity against DPPH, OH, and O free radicals, and its properties are similar to those of ascorbic acid in the DPPH assay. It concludes that *S. nigrum* glycoprotein functions as a natural antioxidant.[78,79]

SCOPE AND OPPORTUNITIES

S. nigrum is a potent and preferential plant to restore Cd-contaminated soils. Studies in a post-culture experiment reveal that *S. nigrum* can accumulate cadmium (Cd) up to 103.8 and 124.6 mg/kg in stem and leaves, respectively, without phototoxic symptoms and reduction in growth.[80] The *S. nigrum* plant has been reported to purify Cd-contaminated soils[81] from multi-metal-contaminated soils.[82]

Bioactive compounds from the genus *Solanum* have different mechanisms of action to prevent or reduce the intensity of diseases and their complications, but the transformation mechanism during digestion and absorption for effective and safe phytopharmaceuticals is not clear. Aerial parts, fruits, and roots of *S. nigrum* have been reported beneficial to humans if consumed as part of their daily diet. Traditionally, *S. nigrum* is used to cure hepatotoxicity, cancer, and ulcers, along with immense applications in abdominal problems, central nervous system and brain functioning, and body pain. Noting the high concern for the useful benefits of the plant species, detailed clinical investigations for different applications may lead to the new modern green medicines standardized for the dose.

REFERENCES

1. Saleem TSM, Chetty CM, Ramkanth S, Alagusundaram M, Gnanaprakash K, Thiruvengada Rajan VS, Angalaparameswari S. 2009. *Solanum nigrum* Linn. – a Review. *Pharmacognosy Reviews*. 3 (6): 342–345.
2. Vaved A, Aslam S, Qayyum Z, Fatima A, Sadiq A, Kubra KT. 2022. Changing trends of *Solanum nigrum* based pharmacognosy. Haya: *The Saudi Journal of Life* Sciences. 7 (2): 29–33.
3. Dancey JE, Chen HX. 2006. Strategies for optimizing combinations of molecularly targeted anticancer agents. *Nature Reviews Drug Discovery*. 5: 649–659.
4. Cowan MM. 1999. Plant products as antimicrobial agents. *Clinical Microbiology Reviews*. 564–582.
5. Lin HM, Tseng HC, Wang CJ. 2008. Hepatoprotective effects of solanum nigrum Linn extract against CCl_4 – induced oxidative damage in rats. *Chemico-Biological Interactions*. 171: 283–293.
6. Kaunda JS, Zhang Y-J. 2019. The genus *Solanum*: an ethnopharmacological, phytochemical and biological properties review. *Natural Products and Bioprospecting*. 9: 77–137.
7. Contreras-Angulo L, Emus-Medina A, Gutierrez-Grijalva E, Ambriz-Perez D, Elizalde-Romero C, Heredia JB. 2020. Pharmacological potential of *Solanum* Genus. In: *Solanum: An Overview. Plant Science Research and Practices*. Souza AV (Ed.) Nova Science, New York. Vol. 1. pp. 199.
8. Moshi MJ, Otieno DF, Mbabazi PK, Weisheit A. 2009. The ethnomedicine of the Haya people of Bugabo ward, Kagera Region, North-western Tanzania. *Journal of Ethnobiology and Ethnomedicine*. 5: 24. https://doi.org/10.1186/1746-4269-5-24
9. Muthu, C, Ayyanar M, Raja N, Ignacimuthu S. 2006. Medicinal plants used by traditional healers in Kancheepuram district of Tamil Nadu, India. *Journal of Et hnobiology and Ethnomedicine*. 2: 43.

10. Kala CP. 2005. Ethnomedicinal botany of the Apatani in the Eastern Himalayan region of India. *Journal of Ethnobi ology and Ethnomedicine*. 1: 11.
11. Boulos L. 1983. *Medicinal Plants of North Africa*. Algonac, Michigan.
12. Parveen UB, Roy S, Kumar A. 2007. Traditional uses of medicinal plants among the rural communities of Churu district in Thar Desert, India. *Journal of Ethnopharmacology*. 113: 387–399.
13. Sikdar M, Dutta U. 2008. Traditional phytotherapy among the Nath people of Assam. *Ethno-Medicine*. 2: 39–45.
14. Chifundera K. 1998. Livestock diseases and the traditional medicine in the Bushi area, Kivu province, Democratic Republic of Congo. *African Study Monographs*. 19: 13–33.
15. Javed A, Usman M, Haider SM, Zafar B, Iftikhar K. 2019. Potential of indigenous plants for skin healing and care. *American Scientific Research Journal for Engineering, Technology, and Sciences*. 51(1):192–211.
16. Javed A, Kabeer A. 2018. Implication of flora for skin wound healing and regeneration from Pakistan. *IJCR*. 10 (6): 639383–639388.
17. Jainu M, Srinivasulu C, Devi S. 2006. Antiulcerogenic and ulcer healing effects of *S. nigrum* L. on experimental ulcer models: possible mechanism for the inhibition of acid formation. *Journal of Ethnopharmacology*. 104: 156–163.
18. Ikeda T, Tsumagari H, Nohara T. 1992. Steroidal oligoglycosides from *Solanum nigrum* growing in Azerbaijan. *Biologicheskie Nauki*. 3: 15–18.
19. Albouchi F, Attia M, Hanana M, Hamrouni L. 2018. Ethnobotanical notes and phytopharmacologiques on *Solanum nigrum* Linn. (Family: Solanaceae). *American Journal of Phytomedicine and Clinical Therapeutics*. 6 (1): 5. doi:10.21767/2321-2748.100341
20. Velderrain-Rodríguez GR, Palafox-Carlos H, Wall-Medrano A, AyalaZavala JF, Chen CY, Robles-Sanchez M, Astiazaran-García H, Alvarez-Parrilla E, González-Aguilar GA. 2014. Phenolic compounds: their journey after intake. *Food Function*. 5: 189–197. https://doi.org/10.1039/C3FO60361J
21. Akubugwo IE, Obasi AN, Ginika SC. 2007. Nutritional potential of the leaves and seeds of black nightshade-*Solanum nigrum* L. Var virginicum from Afikpo-Nigeria. *Pakistan Journal of Nutrition*. 6 (4): 323–326.
22. An L, Tang JT, Liu X M, Gao NN. 2006. Review about mechanisms of anti-cancer of *Solanum nigrum*. *China Journal of Chinese Materia Medica*. 31: 1225–1226.
23. Dhellot JR, Matouba E, Maloumbi MG, Nzikou, JM, Dzondo MG, Linder M, Parmentier M, Desobry S. 2006. Extraction and nutritional properties of *Solanum nigrum* L seed oil. *African Journal of Biotechnology*. 5 (10): 987–991.
24. Ji YB, Gao SY, Ji C F, Zou X. 2008. Induction of apoptosis in HepG2 cells by solanine and Bcl-2 protein. *Journal of Ethnopharmacology*. 115: 194–202.
25. Elsadig A, Alia ES, Anzari A, James, G. 1997. Changes in the steroidal alkaloid solasodine during development of *Solanum nigrum* and *Solanum incanum*. *Phytochemistry*. 46(3): 489–494.
26. Heo KS, Lee SJ, Ko JH, Lim K, Lim KT. 2004. Glycoprotein isolated from *Solanum nigrum* L. inhibits the DNA-binding activities of NF-κB and AP-1, and increases the production of nitric oxide in TPA-stimulated MCF-7 cells. *Toxicology in-vitro*. 18 (6): 755–763.
27. Daniell H, Lee SB, Grevich J, Saski C, Quesada-Vargas T, Guda C, Jansen RK. 2006. Complete chloroplast genome sequences of *Solanum bulbocastanum*, *Solanum lycopersicum* and comparative analyses with other Solanaceae genomes. *Theoretical and Applied Genetics*. 112 (8): 1503
28. Chauhan R, Ruby KM, Shori A, Dwivedi J. 2012. *Solanum nigrum* with dynamic therapeutic role: a review. *International Journal of Pharmaceutical Sciences Review and Research*. 15 (1): 65–71.
29. Zia U, Sheraz A, Nazish V, Sajjad H, Saima G, Sabir K, Shabhum S. 2012. Nutritional potential and antioxidant activity of *Solanum nigrum* and *Oenothera speciose* from Northern area of Pakistan. *International Journal of Biological and Pharmaceutical Research*. 3: 974–979.
30. Zhou X, He X, Wang G, Gao H, Zhou G, Ye W, Yao X. 2006. Steroidal saponins from *Solanum nigrum*. *Journal of Natural Products*. 69: 1158–1163.
31. Lina W, Fang H, Hsieha C. 2008. Inhibitory effect of *Solanum nigrum* on thioacetamide-induced liver fibrosis in mice. *Journal of Ethnopharmacology*. 119: 117–121.
32. Kirti PB, Jami SK, Anuradha TS, Guruprasad L. 2007. Molecular, biochemical and structural characterization of osmotin-like protein from black nightshade (*Solanum nigrum*). *Journal of Plant Physiology*. 164: 238–252.
33. Lee SJ, Lim KT. 2006. 150 kDa glycoprotein isolated from *Solanum nigrum* Linne stimulates caspase-3 activation and reduces inducible nitric oxide production in HCT-116 cells. *Toxicology in Vitro*. 20: 1088–1097.
34. Varsheny IP, Sharma SC. 1965.Saponins and sapogenins -XXIX: the sapogenin of *Solanum nigrum* L. berries. *Phytochemistry*. 4: 967–968.
35. Kapoor BBS, Khatri JS, Bhumika Ranga P. 2004. Herbal plants of Hanuman Garh District; New source of ascorbic acid. *Journal of Phytological Research*. 17(1): 111–112.
36. Rajathi M, Modilal D, Anandan R, Sindhuand R, Logeshwari MN. 2015. Screening of *Solanum nigrum* for its phytochemical and antimicrobial activity against respiratory tract pathogens. *International Journal of Pure and Applied Zoology*. 3(3): 210–215.
37. Kumari M. 2014. *Solanum nigrum*: a wild plant effective against breast cancer and prostate cancer. *International Journal of Green and Herbal Chemistry*. 3 (1): 4–31.
38. Desai S, Tatke P, Gabhe SY. 2015. Quantification of diosgenin in extracts and formulations containing *Solanum nigrum*. *International Journal of Pharma Sciences and Research*. 6 (2): 676–681.
39. Kiran K R, Rani M, Pal A. 2009. Reclaiming degraded land in India through the cultivation of medicinal plants. *Botany Research International*. 2: 174–181.
40. Ikeda T, Tsumagari H, Nohara T. 2000. Steroidal oligoglycosides from *Solanum nigrum*. *Chemical and Pharmaceutical Bulletin*. 48: 1062–1064.
41. Laura A, Moreno-Escamilla JO, Rodrigo-Garcia J, Alvarez-Parrilla E. 2019. *Phenolic Compounds. Postharvest Physiology and Biochemistry of Fruits and Vegetables*. Elsevier, Queretaro. pp. 253–271.
42. Plazas M, Andujar I, Vilanova S, Hurtado M, Gramazio P, Herraiz FJ, Prohens J. 2013. Breeding for chlorogenic acid content in eggplant: interest and prospects. *Notulae Botanicae Horti Agrobotanici Cluj-Napoca*. 41: 26–35. https://doi.org/10.15835/nbha4119036

43. Gurbuz N, Uluişik S, Frary A, Frary A, Doganlar S. 2018. Health benefits and bioactive compounds of eggplant. *Food Chemistry*. 268: 602–610. https://doi.org/10.1016/j.foodchem.2018.06.093
44. Moyo SM, Serem JC, Bester MJ, Mavumengwana V, Kayitesi E. 2020. The impact of boiling and *in-vitro* human digestion of *Solanum nigrum* complex (Black nightshade) on phenolic compounds bioactivity and bioaccessibility. *Food Research International*. 137: 109720. https://doi.org/10.1016/j.foodres.2020.109720
45. Gutierrez-Grijalva EP, López-Martínez LX, Contreras-Angulo LA, ElizaldeRomero CA, Heredia JB. 2020. Plant alkaloids: structures and bioactive properties. In: *Plant-derived Bioactives: Chemistry and Mode of Action*. Swamy MK (Ed.) Springer Singapore, Singapore. pp. 85–117.
46. Jayakumar K, Murugan K. 2016. *Solanum* alkaloids and their pharmaceutical roles: a review. *Journal of Analytical & Pharmaceutical Research*. 3: 00075. https://doi.org/10.15406/japlr.2016.03.00075
47. Hussain G, Rasul A, Anwar H, Aziz N, Razzaq A, Wei W, Ali M, Li J, Li X. 2018. Role of plant derived alkaloids and their mechanism in neurodegenerative disorders. *International Journal of Biological Sciences*. 14: 341–357. https://doi.org/10.7150/ijbs.23247
48. Atanu F, Ebiloma U, Ajayi E. 2011. A review of the pharmacological aspects of *Solanum nigrum* Linn. *Biotechnology and Molecular Biology Reviews*. 6: 1–7.
49. Gu X-Y, Shen X-F, Wang L, Wu Z-W, Li F, Chen B, Zhang GL, Wang MK. 2018. Bioactive steroidal alkaloids from the fruits of *Solanum nigrum*. *Phytochemistry*. 147:125–131. https://doi.org/10.1016/j.phytochem.2017.12.020
50. Keerthana SD, Philip A, Abdul R, M RK, Syed SA, Syed A, Bharath DR 2022. Ethnopharmacology of *Solanum nigrum*: A review. *World Journal of Current Med and Pharm Research*. 4(4): 48–52. https://www.wjcmpr.com/index.php/journal/article/view/223https://doi.org/10.20959/wjpps201712-10538
51. Jeepipalli SPK, Du B, Sabitaliyevich UY, Xu B. 2020. New insights into potential nutritional effects of dietary saponins in protecting against the development of obesity. *Food Chemistry*. 318: 126474. https://doi.org/10.1016/j.foodchem.2020.126474
52. Mohan VR, Tresina PS, Daffodil ED. 2016. Antinutritional factors in legume seeds: characteristics and determination. In: *Encyclopedia of Food and Health*. Caballero B, Finglas PM, Toldra F (Eds.) Academic Press, Oxford. pp. 211–220.
53. Navarro del Hierro J, Herrera T, Fornari T, Reglero G, Martin D. 2018. The gastrointestinal behavior of saponins and its significance for their bioavailability and bioactivities. *Journal of Functional Foods*. 40: 484–497. https://doi.org/10.1016/j.jff.2017.11.032
54. Luo Z, Xu W, Zhang Y, Di L, Shan J. 2020. A review of saponin intervention in metabolic syndrome suggests further study on intestinal microbiota. *Pharmacological Research*. 160: 105088. https://doi.org/10.1016/j.phrs.2020.105088
55. Chen F-F, Zhou J, Zhang Y-W, Chen Y-P, Wang Y-R, Zhao Y-F, Liu W, Huang XF. 2021. Five new steroidal saponins from the seeds of *Solanum melongena* L. *Phytochemistry Letters*. 41: 21–26. https://doi.org/10.1016/j.phytol.2020.10.008
56. Perez Colmenares A, Rojas LB, Mitaine-Offer A-C, Pouységu L, Quideau S, Miyamoto T, Tanaka C, Paululat T, Usubillaga A, Lacaille-Dubois MA. 2013. Steroidal saponins from the fruits of *Solanum torvum*. *Phytochemistry*. 86: 137–143. https://doi.org/10.1016/j.phytochem.2012.10.010
57. Milani A, Basirnejad M, Shahbazi S, Bolhassani A. 2017. Carotenoids: biochemistry, pharmacology, and treatment. *British Journal of Pharmacology*. 174: 1290–1324. https://doi.org/10.1111/bph.13625
58. Rodriguez-Concepcion M, Avalos J, Bonet ML, Boronat A, Gomez-Gomez L, Hornero-Mendez D, Limon MC, Meléndez-Martínez AJ, Olmedilla-Alonso B, Palou A, Ribot J. 2018. A global perspective on carotenoids: metabolism, biotechnology, and benefits for nutrition and health. *Progress in Lipid Research*. 70: 62–93. https://doi.org/10.1016/j.plipres.2018.04.004
59. Zimmer JP, Hammond Jr BR. 2007. Possible influences of lutein and zeaxanthin on the developing retina. *Clinical Ophthalmology*. 1: 25–35.
60. Walk AM, Khan NA, Barnett SM, Raine LB, Kramer AF, Cohen NJ, Moulton CJ, Renzi-Hammond LM, Hammond BR, Hillman CH. 2017. From neuro-pigments to neural efficiency: the relationship between retinal carotenoids and behavioral and neuroelectric indices of cognitive control in childhood. *International Journal of Psychophysiology*. 118: 1–8. https://doi.org/10.1016/j.ijpsycho.2017.05.005
61. Cheng HM, Koutsidis G, Lodge JK, Ashor AW, Siervo M, Lara J. 2019. Lycopene and tomato and risk of cardiovascular diseases: a systematic review and meta-analysis of epidemiological evidence. *Critical Reviews in Food Science and Nutrition*. 59: 141–158. https://doi.org/10.1080/10408398.2017.1362630
62. Chew EY, Clemons TE, SanGiovanni JP, Danis RP, Ferris FL, Elman MJ, Antoszyk AN, Ruby AJ, Orth D, Bressler SB, Fish GE. 2014. Secondary analyses of the effects of lutein/zeaxanthin on age-related macular degeneration progression: AREDS2 report No. 3. *JAMA Ophthalmology*. 132: 142–149. https://doi.org/10.1001/jamaophthalmol.2013.7376
63. Palmer AC, West KP, Dalmiya N, Schultink W. 2012. The use and interpretation of serum retinol distributions in evaluating the public health impact of vitamin A programmes. *Public Health Nutrition*. 15: 1201–1215. https://doi.org/10.1017/S1368980012000560
64. Wan L, Tan H-L, Thomas-Ahner JM, Pearl DK, Erdman JW, Moran NE, Clinton SK. 2014. Dietary tomato and lycopene impact androgen signaling-and carcinogenesisrelated gene expression during early TRAMP prostate carcinogenesis. *Cancer Prevention Research*. 7: 1228–1239. https://doi.org/10.1158/1940-6207.CAPR-14-0182
65. Navajas-Porras B, Perez-Burillo S, Valverde Moya Á, Hinojosa-Nogueira D, Pastoriza S, Rufián Henares J. 2020. Effect of cooking methods on the antioxidant capacity of plant foods submitted to in vitro digestion–fermentation. *Antioxidants*. 9: 1312. https://doi.org/10.3390/antiox9121312
66. Brodkorb A, Egger L, Alminger M, Alvito P, Assunçao R, Ballance S, Boutrou R, Carrière F, Clemente A. 2019. INFOGEST static in vitro simulation of gastrointestinal food digestion. *Nature Protocols*. 14: 991–1014.
67. Rodriguez-Jimenez JR, Amaya-Guerra CA, Baez-Gonzalez JG, AguileraGonzalez C, Urias-Orona V, Nino-Medina G. 2018. Physicochemical, functional, and nutraceutical properties of eggplant flours obtained by different drying methods. *Molecules*. 23: 3210.

68. Kamiloglu S, Demirci M, Selen S, Toydemir G, Boyacioglu D, Capanoglu E. 2014. Home processing of tomatoes (*Solanum lycopersicum*): effects on in vitro bioaccessibility of total lycopene, phenolics, flavonoids, and antioxidant capacity. *Journal of the Science of Food and Agriculture.* 94: 2225–2233.
69. Phan MAT, Bucknall MP, Arcot J. 2019. Co-ingestion of red cabbage with cherry tomato enhances digestive bioaccessibility of anthocyanins but decreases carotenoid bioaccessibility after simulated in vitro gastro-intestinal digestion. *Food Chemistry.* 298: 125040. https://doi.org/10.1016/j.foodchem.2019.125040
70. Condurache NN, Aprodu I, Craciunescu O, Tatia R, Parfene G, Barbu V, Enachi E, Râpeanu G, Bahrim GE, Oancea A, Stănciuc N. 2019. Probing the functionality of bioactives from eggplant peel extracts through extraction and microencapsulation in different polymers and whey protein hydrolysates. *Food and Bioprocess Technology.* 12: 1316–1329.
71. Avat T, Mohammad MK. 2013. Chemical composition analysis of the essential oil of *Solanumn nigrum* L. by HS/SPME method and calculation of the biochemical coefficients of the components. *Arabian Journal of Chemistry.* 10(2): S2372–2375. https://doi.org/10.1016/j.arabjc.2013.08.015
72. Kavishankar GB, Lakshmidevi N, Mahadeva MS. 2011. Phytochemical analysis and antimicrobial properties of selected medicinal plants against bacteria associated with diabetic patients. *International Journal of Pharmaceutical and Biology Sciences.* 2: 509–518.
73. Britto AJD, Gracelin DHS, Kumar PR. 2011. Antimicrobial activity of a few medicinal plants against gram negative bacteria. *International Journal of Applied Biology and Pharmaceutical Technology.* 2: 457–461.
74. Muto M, Mulabagal V, Huang HC. 2010. *Japan Toxicity of Black Nightshade (Solanum nigrum) Extracts on Alternaria Brassicicola, Causal Agent of Black Leaf Spot of Chinese Cabbage* (*Brassica pekinensis*). Department of International Agricultural Development, Tokyo University of Agriculture, Sakuragaoka, Setagaya-ku, Tokyo.
75. Sridhar TM, Josthna P, Naidu CV. 2011. Antifungal activity phytochemical analysis of *Solanum nigrum* (L.) an important antiulcer medicinal plant. *Journal of Ecobiotechnology.* 3: 11–15.
76. Javed T, Usman AA, Sana R. 2011. In-vitro antiviral activity of solanum nigrum against Hepatitis C Virus. *Virology Journal.* 8: 26.
77. Subash KR, Ramesh KS, Binoy V. 2011. Study of Hepatoprotective activity of Solanum nigrum and Cichorium intybus. *International Journal of Pharmacology.* 7: 504–509.
78. Kung SH, Sei JL, Lim KT. 2004. Cytotoxic effect of glycoprotein isolated from *Solanum nigrum* L. through the inhibition of hydroxyl radical-induced DNA-binding activities of NF-kappa B in HT-29 cells. *Environmental Toxicology and Pharmacology.* 17: 45–54.
79. Jin BJ, Ben O. 2010. Lunasin peptide purified from solanum nigrum L. protects DNA from oxidative damage by suppressing the generation of hydroxyl radical via blocking fenton reaction. *Cancer Letters.* 293: 58–64.
80. Wei SH, Zhou QX, Koval PV. 2006. Flowering stage characteristics of cadmium hyperaccumulator *Solanum nigrum* L. and their significance to phytoremediation. *Science of Total Environment.* 369: 441–446.
81. Ji PH, Sun TH, Song YF, Ackland ML. 2011. Strategies for enhancing the phytoremediation of cadmium-contaminated agricultural soils by *Solanum nigrum* L. *Environmental Pollution.* 159: 762–768.
82. Liang C, Shenglian L, Jueliang C, Yong W. 2012. Diversity of endophytic bacterial populations associated with Cd-hyperaccumulator plant *Solanum nigrum* L. grown in mine tailings. *Applied Soil Ecology.* 62: 24–30.

29 *Syzygium cumini* (Jamun)

INTRODUCTION

Syzygium cumini (Linn.) Skeels (Hindi: Jamun) is an evergreen tropical and subtropical indigenous plant (Figure 29.1, fam.: Myrtaceae) of the Indian subcontinent, and frequently occurs in Bangladesh, Ceylon, India, Myanmar, and Pakistan. The *S. cumini* plant attains about 100 feet in height and is a rapidly growing species that starts fruiting in summer.[1,2] Other common names of the species are Black Plum, Java Plum, Jambul, Indian Blackberry, Jamun Jamblang, etc. The species fruits once a year, and the berries turn black from purple on maturity (Figure 29.2), taste bittersweet, and are available in India from May to July. Though it is a tropical and subtropical plant, it occurs in the lower ranges of the Himalayas up to an altitude of 1300 meters above MSL. Different parts of the species, such as bark, leaves, and seeds, are used in herbal healthcare throughout India. The fruits are highly effective in the treatment of type 2 diabetes mellitus and are used for their antifungal, antibacterial, nitric oxide scavenging, antioxidant, radioprotective, and anti-HIV properties. During the ancient era, seeds, bark, flowers, and leaves were used for healing purposes. Namasivayam et al. (2008) have reported using the bark of the species to treat dysentery, which is rich in tannins and carbohydrates.[3] Chaudhari et al. (1990) have reported Jamun seeds as antioxidants and anti-inflammatories in diabetic rats.[4] The whole family Myrtaceae is known to be rich in volatile oils, which have medicinal properties,[5] and the fruits are edible.[6]

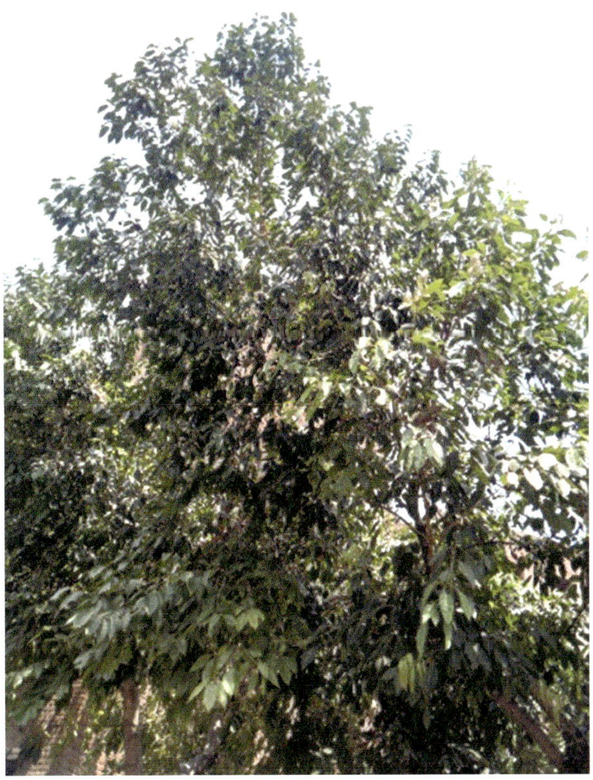

FIGURE 29.1 *S. cumini* tree.

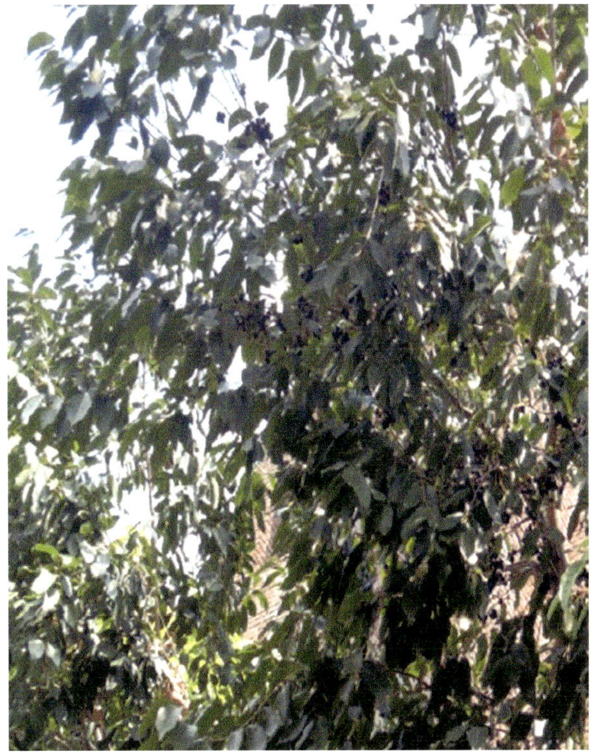

FIGURE 29.2 *S. cumini* branches with fruits.

ETHNOBOTANY

The Jamun plant has its religious importance globally. In Buddhism, it is venerated and planted near Hindu temples as a sacred tree to Lord Krishna.[1,7] The plant is commercially cultivated for fruit production, as an ornamental, and for timber. The fruits of the species are fleshy, luscious, and dark-purple or nearly black berries with a single large seed.[8,9] The purple berries have a very sweet flavor and turn slightly astringent on the edges as the fruit gains maturity. The dark violet-colored ripe fruits resemble the fruit of the olive tree in both shape and weight, and have an astringent taste,[10] and are used globally to treat diabetes, dysentery, cough, ringworm, and inflammation.[6,11] In Unani medicine, different plant parts of the tree are used to enrich the blood, as a liver tonic to strengthen teeth and gums, and as a lotion to treat ringworm infection of the head.[12] In the early studies (1960–1970), preliminary reports on the antidiabetic

DOI: 10.1201/9781003512868-31

activity of different parts of Jamun in diabetic animals are available.[12] In Madagascar, Jamun seeds are used to cure the slow, debilitating impacts of diabetes.[13] In Tamil Nadu, India, villagers used the seed extract to treat *Candida albicans* infections, resulting in ulcers (in the genitourinary tract, throat, and mouth), as well as cough, cold, and fever.[14]

Jamun fruits are also eaten raw and can be made into sauces, jams, and tarts. Good-quality Jamun juice is excellent for different household Indian drinks. Jamun fruits have been reported for a few adverse effects when consumed in excess or during body ailments, as they lower blood sugar. Therefore, they should be avoided for 1 week before and a minimum of 2 weeks after surgery, as they affect the healing. Eating Jamun fruits on an empty stomach and after drinking milk may produce an adverse effect. Pregnant women and breastfeeding mothers are not advised to eat Jamun fruits. Excess eating of Jamun fruits may cause sputum accumulation in the lungs, cough, fever, and body aches.[2,15]

The Ayurvedic Pharmacopeia of India deciphers the antidiabetic effect of Jamun, which states that the seed powder of Jamun is effective in controlling high blood sugar levels. Jamun has been in practice to control blood sugar levels for more than 130 years in Western countries; however, clinical results are mixed, as a few patients have shown control of blood sugar levels after Jamun therapy, whereas others did not show any improvement.[16]

Charak Samhita describes the use of seeds, leaves, and fruits as decoctions for diarrhea and bark as an astringent. Sushruta has described the use of Jamun fruits to treat vaginal discharges, menstrual disorders, obesity, and as a cold infusion for intrinsic hemorrhage.[17] The juice of the bark is prescribed for chronic diarrhea, menorrhagia, and dysentery. Decoction of the bark is an effective gargle and mouthwash to treat a relaxed throat, spongy gums, stomatitis, and other diseases of the oral cavity. The bark is used for coloring fishnets, curing inflammation of the skin, and for dyeing and tanning purposes.[18] Diarrhea with blood is treated by ingestion of juice of Jamun, Amra, and Amalaka leaves mixed with goat milk and honey. Leaf juice of *S. cumini* is mixed with milk every morning and used orally to treat diabetes. The stomach pain is treated using the fresh leaf juice of *S. cumini* orally.[19] The syrup of ripe fruits is a very pleasant drink, and syrup or vinegar prepared from ripe fruits is used to treat spleen enlargement and is useful as an astringent in chronic diarrhea. Hot water extract from dried fruits is used to treat stomach ulcers and to reduce acidity and diabetes.[20–22] The Jamun fruit syrup is very effective in curing diarrhea, and it is a carminative, diuretic, and stomachache remedy, and has cooling and digestive properties.[23] Jamun fruits are a good source of Vitamin C and Vitamin E.[24, 25] Fruits are used in making jellies, vinegar, jam, squash, and ice cream for their attractive purple color.[18]

PHYTOPHARMACOLOGY

The plant of *S. cumini* is a rich source of glucoside, anthocyanins, kaempferol, ellagic acid, myricetin, and isoquercetin. Seeds of *S. cumini* have jambosine (an alkaloid) and a glycoside (jambolin or antimellin), which inhibit the diastatic conversion of starch into sugar. The seed extract has been reported to reduce blood pressure by 34.6% and is attributed to the ellagic acid content in the species.[1]

The leaves of Jamun are rich in tannin,[1] quercetin, myricetin, myricetin-3-O-4-acetyl-L-rhamnopyranoside,[26] triterpenoids,[27] esterase, galloyl carboxylase,[28] and acylated flavonol glycosides.[5] The tender leaves juice of Jamun with mango (*Mangifera indica*) leaves and myrobalan (*Terminalia chebula*) are mixed and prescribed orally with goat's milk and honey to treat dysentery with bloody discharge. Further, the juice of tender leaves alone or in combination with cardamom or cinnamon is given in goat's milk to treat diarrhea in children.[29] The ash of the leaves of *S. cumini* is used for strengthening the gums and teeth.[30]

Sagrawat et al. have reported that the leaves of *S. cumini* have crategolic (maslinic) acid, β-sitosterol, n-hentriacontane, mycaminose, betulinic acid, n-octacosanol, hepatcosane, n-nonacosane, n-dotricontanol, n-triacontanol, myricitrin, myricetin, and quercetin. These chemicals have been widely used in pharmacology to cure various diseases.[12] Eshwarappa et al. have reported the leaf gall extract of the species has antioxidant properties and is used to treat various metabolic disorders such as arthritis, cancer, diabetes mellitus, liver disorder, etc. Further, it was narrated that the aqueous and methanolic extract of *S. cumini* leaf has flavonoids, phenolics, phytosterols, tannin, triterpenoids, saponins, and alkaloids.[31]

Kumar et al. have investigated the antimicrobial properties of leaves of *S. cumini* and reported that ethyl acetate extract of leaves has maximum antimicrobial activity at a concentration of 200 mg/mL.[32] Jagetia et al. concluded that dichloromethane extract of *S. cumini* leaf has radioprotective effects in various concentrations (1.56, 3.125, 6.25, 12.5, 25, 50, and 100 μg/mL) and reduces the radiation-induced DNA damage.[33]

The stem bark of *S. cumini* is rich in friedelin, betulinic acid, epifriedelanol, ß-sitosterol, fatty acid ester of epifriedelanol, eugenin,[34] quercetin, ß-sitosterol, ellagic acid, gallic acid, myricetin, kaempferol,[35] bergenins,[36] tannins, and flavonoids.[37] The gallotannins and ellagitannins have been attributed to the astringent property of stem bark. The bark is digestive, sweet, acrid, and astringent to the bowels and is used to treat asthma, sore throat, bronchitis, biliousness, thirst, ulcers, and dysentery. The bark is considered a good blood purifier.[30]

An application of different extracts with different concentrations of different solvents (n-hexane, alcohol, and aqueous alcohol) from different plant parts of *S. cumini* (bark of stem and roots, fruits, and leaves) as an antifungal against *Ascochyta rabiei* has been reported by Jabeen and Javaid (2010),[34–38]who reported that all aqueous extracts have significant antifungal activity.[38] Ivan has reported the presence of betulinic acid in the bark of the species.[39] Yogeswari and Sriram have reported that betulinic acid has selective cytotoxicity against many specific tumors. ß-sitosterol in the bark of the plant has been attributed to reducing blood cholesterol and has an anti-inflammatory property.[40] Pandey and Khan reported that ethanolic extract of *S. cumini* bark has anti-inflammatory activity against serotonin, histamine, and prostaglandin.[41]

The flowers of *S. cumini* are rich in quercetin, isoquercetin, kaempferol, myricetin, quercetin-3-D-galactoside, myricetin-3-L-arabinoside, oleanolic acid, dihydromyricetin, acetyl oleanolic acid, eugenol-triterpenoid A, and eugenol-triterpenoid B.[42] Ramya et al. have reported that the flowers of *S. cumini* contain galactoside, oleanolic acid, erategolic acid (maslinic acid), dihydromyricetin, kaempferol, quercetin3-D-acetyl oleanolic acid, flavonoids-isoquercitrin, quercetin, myricetin-3-L-arabinoside, eugenol-triterpenoid A, and eugenol-triterpenoid B.[43] Sagrawat et al. have narrated that the flower of *S. cumini* contains isoquercetin, quercetin, oleanolic acid, ellagic acids, myricetin, and kaempferol.[12]

The roots of *S. cumini* are rich in flavonoid glycosides[27] and iso-rhamnetin-3-O-rutinoside.[44] Fruits of *S. cumini* are rich in fructose, glucose, raffinose,[45] citric acid, malic acid,[46] anthocyanins, gallic acid,[47] petunidin-3-gentiobioside, delphinidin-3-gentiobioside, malvidin-3-laminaribioside,[48] petunidin, malvidin, and cyanidin diglycoside.[49] The sourness of fruits is attributed to the presence of gallic acid.[48] The fruit contains 83.70%–85.80% moisture, 0.70%–0.13 % protein, 0.15%–0.30 % fat, 0.30%–0.90% crude fiber, 14.00% carbohydrate, 0.32%–0.40% ash, and minerals (calcium, magnesium, phosphorus, iron, sodium, potassium, copper, and sulfur), vitamin A, thiamine, riboflavin, niacin, ascorbic acid, and folic acid.[50] One of the varieties found in Brazil has been reported to contain malvidin-3-glucoside and petunidin-3-glucoside.[51] The peel powder of the species is used as a colorant for foods and pharmaceuticals.[52]

The fruit of Jamun is astringent, acrid, sweet, cooling, antidiabetic, useful in biliousness, diuretic, stomachic, removes bad smells from the mouth,[29] and has a very long history of health healing applications for various body ailments. Currently, it has a large market to treat chronic diarrhea and other enteric disorders.[52] Vinegar prepared from ripe fruit juice is a stomachic and carminative, used as a diuretic, and useful to treat spleen enlargement and chronic diarrhea.[30] The fruit of *S. cumini* is purple due to the presence of cyaniding diglycosides.[53] S. *cumini* seeds have potent therapeutic properties and are extensively used as antidiabetic, hypolipidemic, anti-inflammatory, neuroprotective, and radioprotective.[54]

Raza et al. reported that fruit extract reduces elevated blood glucose levels and regulates insulin levels in hyperglycemic animals. Experimental data were recorded that fruit extract has attenuated serum glucose levels to 5.35% and 12.29% in normal and hyperglycemic animals, respectively, and insulin levels were improved by 2.82% and 6.19%, respectively. The seed extract of *S. cumini* was noted to reduce glucose by 7.04% and 14.36% and increase insulin levels by 3.56% and 7.24% in normal and diabetic animals, respectively.[55] The research concluded that both the seed and fruit have a potent role in managing type 2 diabetes mellitus.[55] Chauhan and Intelli have reported the different therapeutic biochemicals in the *S. cumini* fruits.[56]

The essential oils extracted from the freshly collected different plant parts of *S. cumini*[57] have been deciphered for the presence of ß-pinene, limonene, α-pinene, camphene, α-copaene, terpinolene, cis-ocimene, trans-ocimene, γ-terpinene, myrcene, bornyl acetate, α-humulene, ß-caryophyllene, γ-cadinene, δ-cadinene,[10] ß-myrcene, α-terpineol, trans-ocimene, cis-ocimene, dihydrocarvyl acetate, terpinyl valerate, geranyl butyrate,[58] α-terpineol, α-humulene, α-muurolol, ß-caryophyllene, ß-selinene, cis-farnesol, calacorene, α-santalol, lauric, palmitic, myristic, stearic, oleic, malvalic, linoleic, vernolic, and sterculic acids.[59,60]

PHARMACOLOGICAL PROPERTIES OF *S. CUMINI*

Seeds, fruits, and bark of the species *S. cumini* possess promising properties against diabetes mellitus, and it has been supported by several molecular and clinical investigations.[61–64] Tisane prepared from leaves of *S. cumini* has been reported to have an antihyperglycemic impact.[65] The bark of the stem induces insulin secretion in treated animals,[66] and a significant decrease in blood glucose levels has been observed with the stem bark by oral glucose tolerance test.[67]

The seed powder extracted in water has also been reported to reduce blood sugar levels in diabetic rabbits,[68] and the aqueous seed extract at a dose of 1 g/kg b.wt. in diabetic animals has been reported to reduce the elevated blood glucose levels to the normal range.[69]

Ahmad Raza et al. evaluated the potential of both *S. cumini* seed and fruit extracts against type 2 diabetes mellitus and reported that both the fruit and seed extracts reduce the blood glucose level significantly and regulate the insulin levels in diabetic animals.[70] Karnic has described that the *S. cumini* ethanolic extract decreased the blood sugar level by 20% after 1 hour of excessive glucose in experimental animals.[71] Dhawan and Singh have reported the antiviral properties of the species.[72,73]

SCOPE AND OPPORTUNITIES

Traditionally, *S. cumini* is widely used to treat type 2 diabetes mellitus and related complications. The unique chemical composition of the secondary metabolites of the species confers most of the characteristics of the plant. Mostly, pharmacological investigations are focused on seeds for antihyperglycemic properties, but the therapeutic potential of the other parts of the plant is to be explored in detail. Additionally, synergistic combinations with other plant species to treat type 2 diabetes mellitus are also lacking. Based on current molecular evidence, the role of plant species in various treatments and health ailments suggests that further phytochemical and clinical research may lead to a new vista of modern green medicine.

Further, the mechanism of action of *S. cumini* to normalize the elevated blood glucose levels and reduce low-density lipids is not accurately known. As diabetes triggers, there is an increased availability of free radicals, and *S. cumini* has the potential to quench or reduce these free radicals and improve the functioning of β-cells in the pancreas, resulting in the reduction of sugar levels. *S. cumini* also stimulates the activity of enzymes like glutathione S-transferase, and catalase glutathione peroxidase and increases the synthesis of glutathione. Further, *S. cumini* depletes lipid peroxidation, resulting in reduced cholesterol levels in the blood. *S. cumini* reduces the α-amylase activity, which is unregulated in diabetics.[74]

Traditional applications and modern molecular knowledge reveal that the *S. cumini* plant has the potential to treat diabetes and related complications and has antineoplastic activities. Molecular studies have revealed that *S. cumini* is selective in its action in breast cancer cells. The effect of *S. cumini* and its phytochemicals is still to be investigated as a chemopreventive agent in different models of carcinogens, including chemical, radiation, and viral models. Raw *S. cumini* and its value-added products may offer greater health benefits to the urban population.

REFERENCES

1. Morton J. 1987. Jambolan. In: *Fruits of Warm Climates*. Morton JF (Ed.) pp. 375–378. Miami, FL, Winterville, N.C.: J.F. Morton, Distributed by Creative Resources Systems in English.
2. Jagetia GC. 2017. Phytochemical composition and pleotropic pharmacological properties of Jamun, *Syzygium cumini* Skeels. *Journal of Exploratory Research in Pharmacology*. 2 (2):54–66.
3. Namasivayam R, Ramachandrani B, Deecaraman M. 2008. Effect of aqueous extract of *Syzygium cumini* pulp on antioxidant defense system in streptozotocin induced diabetic rats. *International Journal of Post-Harvest* Technology. 7: 137–145.
4. Chaudhuri N, Pal A, Gomes S. 1990. Anti-inflammatory and related action of *Syzygium cumini* seed extract. *Phytotherapy Research*. 4 (2): 5–10.
5. Mahmoud II, Marzouk MS, Moharram FA, El-Gindi MR, Hassan AM. 2001. Acylated flavonol glycosides from Eugenia jambolana leaves. *Phytochemistry*. 58: 1239–1244.
6. Reynertson KA, Basile MJ, Kennelly EJ. 2005. Antioxidant potential of seven myrtaceous fruits. *Ethnobotany Research and Applications*. 3: 25–35.
7. Ayyanar M, Subash-Babu P. 2012. Syzygium cumini (L.) Skeels: a review of its phytochemical constituents and traditional uses. *Asian Pac J Trop Biomed*. 2(3): 240–246. doi: 10.1016/S2221-1691(12)60050-1
8. Gamble JS. 1935. *The Flora of the Presidency of Madras*. Adlard & Son LTD, London.
9. Hooker JD. 1879. *The Flora of British India*. Nabu Press, London. pp. 499.
10. Craveiro AA, Andrade CHS, Matos FJA, Alencer JW, Machado MIL. 1983. Essential oil of *Eugenia jambolana*. *Journal of Natural Products*. 46: 591–592.
11. Jain SK. 1991. *Dictionary of Indian Folk Medicine and Ethnobotany*. Deep Publications Paschim Vihar, New Delhi.
12. Sagrawat H, Mann AS, Kharya MD. 2006. Pharmacological potential of *Eugenia jambolana:* a review. *Pharmacogenesis Magazice*. 2: 96–104.
13. Ratsimamanga U. 1998. Native plants for our global village. *TWAS News Letters*. 10: 13–15.
14. Chandrasekaran M, Venkatesalu V. 2004. Antibacterial and antifungal activity of *Syzygium jambolanum* seeds. *Journal of Ethnopharmacology*. 91: 105–108.
15. Thomson. 2000. *PDR for Herbal Medicines*, 2nd Edition. Medical Economics, Montvale. pp. 429–430.
16. Helmstädter A. 2008. *Syzygium cumini* (L.) SKEELS (Myrtaceae) against diabetes –125 years of research. *Pharmazie*. 63 (2): 91–110.
17. . Nair AG, Subramanian S. 1962. Chemical examination of flowers of *Eugenia-jambolana*. *Journal of Scientific & Industrial Research*. 21 (9): 457–458.
18. Kirtikar KR, Basu BD. 1975. *Indian Medicinal Plants*. Periodical Experts, New Delhi. Vol-II. pp. 1052–1053.
19. Bhandary MJ, Chandrashekar KR, Kaveriappa KM. 1995. Medical ethnobotany of the siddis of Uttara Kannada district, Karnataka, India. *Journal of Ethnopharmacology*. 47 (3): 149–158.
20. Katiyar D, Singh V, Ali M. 2016. Recent advances in pharmacological potential of *Syzygium cumini*: a review. *Advances in Applied Science Research*. 7: 1–2.
21. Jain SR, Sharma SN. 1967. Hypoglycemic drugs of Indian indigenous origin. *Planta Medica*. 15 (04): 439–442.
22. Singh N, Gupta M. 2007. Effects of ethanolic extract of *Syzygium cumini* (Linn) seed powder on pancreatic islets of alloxan diabetic rats. *Indian Journal of Experimental Biology*. 45: 861–867.
23. Sharma IP, Kanta C, Semwal SC, Goswami N. 2017. Wild fruits of Uttarakhand (India): Ethnobotanical and medicinal uses. *Int J Complement Alt Med*. 8(3): 00260. doi: 10.15406/ijcam.2017.08.00260.
24. Carr AC, Frei BA. 1999. Toward a new recommended dietary allowance for vitamin C based on antioxidant and health effects in humans. *American Journal of Clinical Nutrition*. 69 (6): 1086–1107.
25. Simon JA, Hudes ES. 2000. Serum ascorbic acid and gallbladder disease prevalence among US adults: the Third National Health and Nutrition Examination Survey (NHANES III). *Archives of Internal Medicine*. 160 (7): 931–936.
26. Timbola AK, Szpoganicz B, Branco A, Monache FD, Pizzolatti MG. 2002. A new flavonoid from leaves of *Eugenia jambolana*. Fitoterapia. 73: 174–176.
27. Gupta GS, Sharma DP. 1974. Triterpenoid and other constituents of *Eugenia jambolana* leaves. *Phytochemistry*. 13: 2013–2014.

28. Bhatia IS, Sharma SK, Bajaj KL. 1974. Esterase and galloyl carboxylase from *Eugenia jambolana* leaves. *Indian Journal of Experimental Biology*. 12: 550–552.
29. Nadkarni KM. 1976. *Indian Materia Medica*. Popular Prakashan Ltd, Bombay.
30. Kiritikar KR, Basu BD. 1987. *Indian Medicinal Plants*. International Book Distributors, Dehradun. pp. 1052–1054.
31. Eshwarappa RSB, Iyer RS, Subbaramaiah SR, Austin-Richard S, Dhananjaya BL. 2014. Antioxidant activity of *S. cumini* leaf galls extracts. *Bioimpacts*. 4: 101–107.
32. Kumar D, Arora S, Alam M. 2014. Pharmacognostical standardization and anti-microbial activity of leaves of *Syzygium cumini* (Linn.) from various regions of North India. *International Research Journal of Pharmacy*. 5 (2): 62–65.
33. Jagetia GC, Shetty PC, Vidyasagar MS. 2008. Treatment of mice with leaf extract of Jamun (Syzygium cumini Linn. Skeels) protects against radiation-induced damage in the intestinal mucosa of mice exposed to different doses of γ-radiation. *Pharmacologyonline* . 1: 169–195.
34. Sengupta P, Das PB. 1965. Terpenoids and related compounds. Part IV. triterpenoids the stembark of *Eugenia jambolana* Lam. *Indian Chemical Society*. 42: 255–258.
35. Bhargava KK, Dayal R, Seshadri TR. 1974. Chemical components of *Eugenia jambolana* stem bark. *Current* Sciene. 43: 645–646.
36. Kopanski L, Schnelle G. 1988. Isolation of bergenin from barks of *Syzygium cumini*. *Planta Medica*. 54 (6): 572.
37. Bhatia IS, Bajaj KL. 1975. Chemical constituents of the seeds and bark of *Syzygium cumini*. *Planta Medica*. 28: 347–352.
38. Jabeen K, Javaid A. 2010. Antifungal activity of *Syzygium cumini* against *Ascochyta rabiei*, the cause of chickpea blight. *Natural Product Research*. 24 (12): 1158–1167.
39. Ivan AR. 2006. *Medicinal Plant of World: Chemical Constituents, Traditional Uses and Modern Medicinal Uses*. Human Press, Totowa, NJ. pp. 283–289.
40. Yogeswari P, Sriram D. 2005. Betulinic acid and its derivatives; A review on their biological properties. *Current Medicinal Chemistry*. 12 (6): 657–666.
41. Pandey M, Khan A. 2002. Hypoglycemic effect of defatted seeds and water-soluble fibre from the seeds of *Syzygium Cumini* (Linn.) Skeels in alloxan diabetic rats. *Indian Journal of Experimental Biology*. 40 (10): 1178–1182.
42. Subramanian SS, Nair RAG. 1972. Flavonoids of the flowers of *Eugenia jambolana*. *Current Science*. 41: 703–704.
43. Ramya S, Neethirajan K, Jayakumararaj R. 2012. Profile of bioactive compounds in *Syzygium cumini* – a review. *Journal of Pharmacy Research*. 5 (8): 4548–4553.
44. Vaishnava MM, Gupta KR. 1990. Isorhamnetin-3-O-rutinoside from *Syzygium cumini* Lam. *Journal of the Indian Chemical Society*. 67: 785–786.
45. Srivastava HC. 1953. Paper chromatography of fruit juices. *Journal of Scientific and Industrial Research*. 12B: 363–365.
46. Lewih YS, Dwarakanath CT, Johar DS. 1956. Acids and sugars in *Eugenia jambolana*. *Journal of Scientific and Industrial Research*. 15C: 280–281.
47. Jain MC, Seshadri TR. 1975. Anthocyanins of *Eugenia jambolana* fruits. *Indian Journal of Chemistry*. 3: 20–23.
48. Venkateswarlu G. 1952. On the nature of the coloring matter of the jambul fruit (*Eugenia jambolana*). *Journal of the Indian Chemical Society*. 29: 434–437.
49. Sharma JN, Sheshadri TR. 1955. Survey of anthocyanins from Indian sources Part II. *Journal of Scientific and Industrial Research*. 14: 211–214.
50. Noomrio MH, Dahot MU. 1996. Nutritive value of *Eugenia jambosa* fruit. *Journal of Islamic World Academy of Sciences*. 9 (1): 9–12.
51. Silva VGd, Nogueira GF, Soares CT, Oliveira R Ad. 2023. Anthocyanin-rich Jamun (*Syzygium cumini* L.) pulp transported on protein-coated ionic gelation microparticles of calcium alginate: Production and morphological characteristics. *Polysaccharides*. 4: 33–50. https://doi.org/10.3390/polysaccharides4010002.
52. Veigas JM, Narayan MS, Laxman PM, Neelwarne B. 2007. Chemical nature stability and bioefficacies of anthocyanins from fruit peel of *Syzygium cumini* Skeels. *Food Chemistry*. 105: 619–627.
53. 1982. *The Wealth of India*. CSIR, New Delhi. Vol-X. pp. 100–104.
54. Anjali V, Sindhu G, Girish C. 2017. A review on pharmacology and phytochemistry of *syzygium cumini*. *Indian Journal of Pharmaceutical and Biological Research*. 5 (4):24–28.
55. Raza A, Butt MS, Iahtisham-UL-Haq, Ansar H, Suleria R. 2017. Jamun seed and fruit extracts attenuate hyperglycemia in diabetic rats. *Asian Pacific Journal of Tropical Biomedicine*. 7(8):750–754. https://doi.org/10.1016/j.apjtb.2017.07.006
56. Chauhan A, Intelli. 2015. *Syzygium cumini* (Jamun): Potential benefits in hyperglycemia. *SOJ Pharmacy & Pharmaceutical Sciences*. 2 (3): 1–3.
57. Kumar A, Naqvi AA, Kahol AP, Tandon S. 2004. Composition of leaf oil of *Syzygium cumini* L, from north India. *Indian Perfum*. 48: 439–441.
58. Vijayanand P, Rao LJM, Narasimham P. 2001. Volatile flavor components of Jamun fruit (*Syzygium cumini*). *Flavour and Fragrance Journal*. 16: 47–49.
59. Daulatabad CMJD, Mirajkar AM, Hosamani KM, Mulla GMM. 1988. Epoxy and cyclo-propenoid fatty acids in *Syzygium cuminii* seed oil. *Journal of the Science of Food and Agriculture*. 43: 91–94.
60. Gupta RD, Agrawal SK. 1970. Chemical examination of the unsaponifiable matter of the seed fat of *Syzygium cumini*. *Scientific Culture*. 36: 298.
61. Sigogneau-Jagodzinski M, Bibal-Prot P, Chanez M, Boiteau P. 1967. Contribution to the study of the action of a principle extracted from the myrtle of Madagascar (*Eugenia jambolana*, Myrtaceae) on blood sugar of the normal rat. *Comptes Rendus Hebdomadaires des Seances de L'academie des sciences. Serie D: Sciences Naturelles*. 264: 1223–1226.
62. Lal BN, Choudhuri KD. 1968. Observations on *Momordica charantia* Linn, and *Eugenia jambolana* Lam. as oral antidiabetic remedies. *Indian Journal of Medical Research* 2: 161.
63. Shrotri DS, Kelkar M, Deshmukh VK, Aiman R. 1963. Investigations of the hypoglycemic properties of *Vinca rosea*, *Cassia auriculata* and *Eugenia jambolana*. *Indian Journal of Medical Research*. 51: 464–467.
64. Bose SN, Sepha GC. 1956. Clinical observations on the antidiabetic properties of *Pterocarpus marsupium* and *Eugenia jambolana*. *Journal of the Indian Medical Association*. 27: 388–391.

65. Teixeira CC, Knijnik J, Pereira MV, Fuchs FD. 1989. The effect of tea prepared from leaves of "jambolao" (*Syzygium cumini*) on the blood glucose levels of normal rats an exploratory study. *Proceedings of the Brazilian-Sino Symposium on Chemistry and Pharmacology of Natural Products*, Rio de Janeiro Brazil. pp. 191.
66. Schossler DRC, Mazzanti CM, Almeida da Luzi SC, Filappi A, Prestes D, Ferreria da Silveira A, Cecim M. 2004. *Syzygium cumini* and the regeneration of insulin positive cells from the pancreatic duct. *Brazilian Journal of Veterinary Research and Animal Science*. 41: 236–239.
67. Villasenor IM, Lamadrid MRA. 2006. Comparative anti-hyperglycemic potentials of medicinal plants. *Journal of Ethnopharmacology*. 104: 129–131.
68. Brahmachari HD, Augusti KT. 1961. Hypoglycemic agents from Indian indigenous plants. *Journal of Pharmacy and Pharmacology*. 13: 381–182.
69. Kedar P, Chakrabarti CH. 1983. Effects of Jambolan seed treatment on blood sugar, lipids and urea in streptozotocin induced diabetes in rabbits. *Indian Journal of Physiology and Pharmacology*. 27 (2): 135–140.
70. Raza A, Masood SB, Iahtisham-Ul-Haq, Suleria HAR. 2017. *Syzygium cumini* seed and fruit extract attenuate hyperglycemia in diabetic rats. *Asian Pacific Journal of Tropical Biomedicine*. 7 (8): 750–754.
71. Karnic CR. 1991. A clinical trial of a composite herbal drug in treatment of diabetic mellitus (madhumeha). *Aryavaidyan*. 5: 36–46.
72. Dhawan BN, Patnaik GK, Rastogi RP, Singh KK, Tandon JS. 1977. Screening of Indian plants for biological activity: part VI. *Indian Journal of Experimental Biology*. 15 (3): 208–219.
73. Singh R. 1971. In-activation of potato virus X by plant extracts/ In-attivazione del virus X della Patata da parte di estratti di piante. *Phytopathologia Mediterranea*. 10 (2): 211–213.
74. Gajera HP, Gevariya SN, Hirpara DG, Patel SV, Golakiya BA. 2017. Antidiabetic and antioxidant functionality associated with phenolic constituents from fruit parts of indigenous black jamun (*Syzygium cumini* L.) landraces. *Journal of Food Science and Technology*. 54 (10): 3180–3191.

30 *Terminalia chebula* (Haritaki/Harad)

INTRODUCTION

Terminalia chebula Retz. (fam.: Combretaceae) is commonly known as Harad (Hindi), Chebulic myrobalan (English), and Haritaki (Sanskrit).[1] The tree is tall, about 17–26 m in height, with a round crown and spreading branches. The *T. chebula* plant has dark brown stem bark with some longitudinal cracks, and flowers are dull white to yellow and monoecious with a strong unpleasant odor. The flowering season for the species is May–June, and fruiting is from July to December. Fruits are about 1–2 inches in size, with five lines (ribs) on the outer skin. Unripe fruits are green and yellowish-grey at the ripened stage (Figures 30.1 and 30.2). November–January is the time of fruit formation, and it is harvested from January to April.[2] The fruit of the species has diverse health potential and has been used as a household remedy and treatment of various body ailments since antiquity.[3,4] It is a popular traditional medicinal plant, chiefly used in Ayurveda, Unani, Siddha, and overall, in homeopathy. Its wide applications in homeopathy and other folk/traditional systems are due to its wide spectrum of pharmacological properties associated with bioactive compounds present in the plant.[5] *T. chebula* fruits are a common folk medicine in Asia and Africa. It is an important ingredient of the most common Ayurvedic preparation, the 'Triphala', together with *Emblica officinalis* (amalaki) and *Terminalia bellerica* (bibhitaki). Triphala is described in the Ayurvedic texts as a therapeutic formulation used to balance the rejuvenating effects on constitutional elements (three senses of humor: vata, pitta, and kapha).[6] *T. chebula* fruits have different classes of chemicals, such as alkaloids, anthocyanins, flavonoids, polyphenols, glycosides, and terpenes. These ingredients are mainly responsible for the pharmacological properties of the fruit of *T. chebula*.[7] Extracts from the roots, flowers, leaves, and seeds of *T. chebula* have antibacterial activity against severe bacterial strains. The plant has been reported to have properties like antiviral, antioxidant, antifungal, cardioprotective, antineoplastic, antidiabetic, immune-modulatory, etc.[8] The genus *Terminalia* has 250 species and is widely distributed in tropical areas of the world.[9] The health benefits and information on the phytopharmacology of the plant still have many unanswered questions, although no fatal cases have been reported from its traditional applications. In Ayurveda, *T. chebula* is listed first because of its extraordinary therapeutic properties and has been described for the seven varieties of fruits, namely, Rohini, Putana, Vijaya, Abhaya, Amrita, Chetaki, and Jivanti.[10,11]

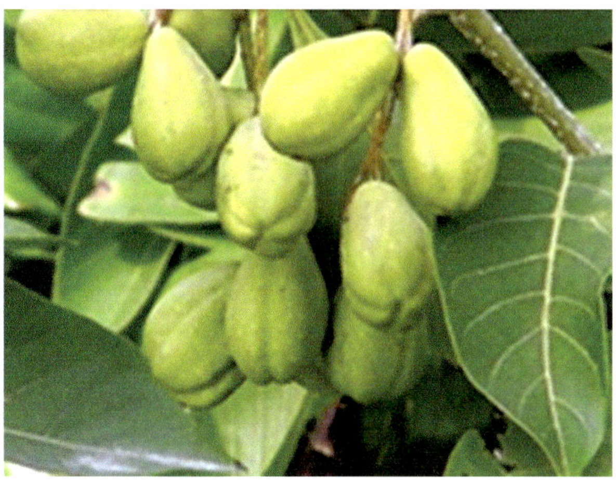

FIGURE 30.1 *Terminalia chebula* fruits.

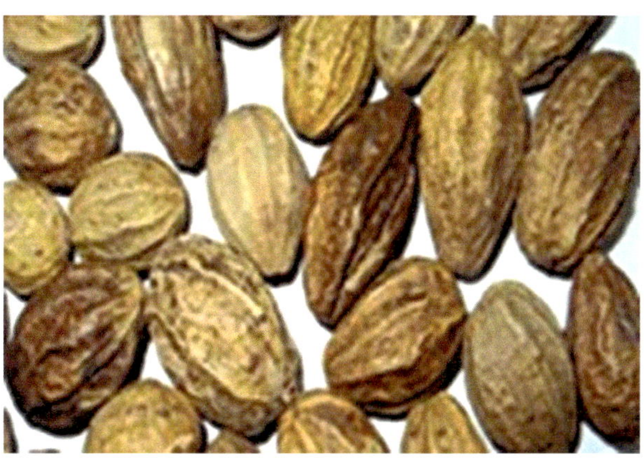

FIGURE 30.2 *Terminalia chebula* fruits (dried form).

'Vijaya' is used in almost every disease and has a gourd shape. The variety is from the Vindhya Mountain ranges in South India. The fruit of the 'Rohini' variety is round and used for wound healing; the variety is common in Jhansi and other parts of Madhya Pradesh, India. 'Abhaya' is found generally in the ancient Champadesha, currently the area of Dhaka, Bangladesh, and has fine lines on its fruit. It is mainly used for eye diseases. It is bulkier than the 'Putana' variety. The mesocarp is present in fruit and is used for shodhana karma habituation (i.e., purification purposes). It is mainly used for cleansing. 'Jeevanti' is found in the Himalayan region. Fruits of the variety are golden yellow and are used in all diseases. 'Chetaki' occurs in the Himalayas, and its fruits have three lobes. Chetaki fruits have a laxative effect and are generally used as a powder (in Sanskrit, churn). Additionally, it has two varieties of fruits in white and black appearances.[8]

However, three varieties of *T. chebula* (Haritaki) are commonly used, namely, Bala, Chambari, and Survari. The seeds of Bala are hard and are the smallest among all the varieties. The color of the fruit is deep brown to black and has homogeneous pulp. Fruits of Chambari are yellowish

DOI: 10.1201/9781003512868-32

with fewer wrinkles and furrows. It is slightly more astringent than other varieties. The fruit of Survari is about two inches long with a yellow-brown appearance and a stone.[8]

In Tibetan literature, the plant *T. chebula* is grouped into seven types, namely, Bum gyi mgrin (Kalasa Kantha), Rnam par rgyal ba (Vijaya), Gso byed (Ayuh Vardhak), Jigs med (Abhaya), Bdud-rtsi (Amrita), Skam Po (Suska), and Phel Byed (Vriddhikari).[12] 'Flora of British India' (1854) also divided the species into seven parts,[13] but only two varieties (*Terminalia chebula* var. tomentella (Kurz) C.B.Clarke, and *Terminalia chebula* var. chebula) are recognized as true varieties; the others are considered sub-varieties. The leaves and shoots are hairless or only hairy when very young in *Terminalia chebula* var. chebula, while in *Terminalia chebula* var. tomentella (Kurz) C.B.Clarke, the leaves and shoots are hairy and silvery to orange in appearance.[14] Botanically, only two more species have been reported, namely *Terminalia citrina* Roxb. (from Assam, India) and *T. pallida* (from South India and Bengal), which produce another kind of fruit, used as an adulterant and substitute for Haritaki, respectively, in different regions.[14]

The best period for the collection of *T. chebula* fruits is January to March. The first half of January is the best period to collect the fallen fruits, as these have optimum tannin content and fetch a better price. The fruits on the ground for a long period may be attacked by the mold and have a darker color.[8]

Harvesting fruits is generally done by picking them up from the ground after shaking the trees. After collection, fruits are dried in the sun for 3 weeks in an isolated area to avoid contamination. The dried fruits (myrobalans) are stored to protect them from rain, as the therapeutic compounds of the fruits decompose in the presence of water. Based on the morphological appearance, the raw myrobalan is graded under different trade names; the selection is based on its color, solidness, and health (without insect attack), and before grading generally, the second-grade fruits are separated from the first-grade and marked.[8]

ETHNOPHARMACOLOGY

Ayurvedic classics have vividly narrated the medicinal effects of the different varieties of *T. chebula*,[14] and all the classics are not unanimous about the therapeutic effects. Vijaya has the preference and is recommended for all kinds of diseases, for both the preparation of malt (Avaleha)-based products, and purificatory measures. Rohini is prescribed for wound healing and consumption. Putana has been mentioned as useful for external applications. Amrita is recommended to be used as a purgative, and Abhaya is used for eye disease. Jeevanti is used in oil therapy (Snehana), while Chetaki is for purgation. In Tibetan literature, the different parts of the plant species are used for a special therapeutic aim. The roots are used to cure the diseases of the bone, the stem is used to cure muscle-related diseases, the bark is useful for skin problems, the branches of the species are used to treat vascular disorders, leaves are used to treat visceral diseases, and fruits are used to treat the vital organs, including the heart diseases.[12,14]

The Ayurvedic and Tibetan literature on *T. chebula* (Haritaki) is divided, though both systems have a total number of seven varieties.[10–12] Ayurvedic texts, the Brihatrayee (main lexicons of Ayurveda, Charaka, Sushruta, Vagbhata Charak-Susruta-Vagbhatt), do not decipher for its varieties.[14] Only the Nighantus has stated the different varieties of the species (i.e., Amrita, Jivanti, Chetaki, Vijaya, Putana, Abhaya, and Rohini), based on the shape, color, and location of harvest.[14] Additionally, two varieties of Chetaki, namely, black and white, respectively, are mentioned in the Bhavaprakashnighantu.[11] The black variety of Chetaki [Krisnaatwekaangulamata (black chebulic myrobalan is of the size of only one fingerbreadth)] is described by Bhavamishra and may be compared with the black, small-sized fruit of *T. chebula* (immature fruit of Haritaki/Jangi Haritaki) of the present time, which is available everywhere.[14] 'Churnartha-chetaki-sasthaa' is used to make the powder form of fruits for laxative purposes, and Jangi Haritaki (Chetaki) is mainly used. The other variety (white), which has a length of up to six fingers (six-angula), is used in preparations like Vyaghri-haritakee Avaleha, Agastya-haritakee, Abhayarishta, etc.[14]

Rathinamoorthy and Thilagavathi have reported that fruits of *T. chebula* cleanse wounds and ulcers, effectively reduce swelling, fasten the healing, and prevent the accumulation of pus in skin diseases.[15] Especially, it is used to treat burn cases and fasten the wound healing. Fruits are applied for relief in conjunctivitis and used as an anticancer agent, mouth rinse, and anti-astringent.[15–17]

T. chebula is globally used for medicinal applications in countries and continents such as China, Thailand, and Africa.[18] It is used in Thai traditional medicine as an astringent, expectorant, and carminative.[19] Triphala, an Ayurvedic formulation in which *T. chebula* is an integral part, is used as a laxative to treat chronic constipation, detoxify the colon, cure food digestive problems (poor digestion and assimilation), and rejuvenate the body. Triphala stimulates appetite and is used to treat cancer and detoxify the body. Triphala is the most versatile of all herbal formulations that are prescribed to treat candida infection and as a cardiotonic.[20]

Internally, *T. chebula* fruits are used to cure several different diseases. As per Ayurveda, *T. chebula* fruits with rock salt are used to treat 'kapha' diseases, with sugar to treat 'pitta' diseases, and with ghee to treat 'vata'-related diseases are cured. *T. chebula* fruits act as a rejuvenator when ingested with various supportive ingredients (i.e., the dravyas) in different seasons. There is a specific reference to a carrier (the Anupana) as per the season (Ritu) to take orally with the fruits of *T. chebula*. For example, in the rainy season [Varsa Ritu (July–August)], it should be taken with rock salt; during September–October (Sarad Ritu), with sugar; during November–December (Hemanta Ritu), with sunthi; during January–February (Sisira Ritu), with pippali; in the spring season [Vasanta Ritu (March–April)], with honey; and in the summer season [Grisma Ritu (May–June)], with jaggery. According to Vagbhata, regular use of *T. chebula* fruit powder fried in ghee and with sufficient ghee in food promotes longevity and boosts energy.[8] Common gastrointestinal ailments such as enlargement of the liver and spleen, tumors, piles, ascites, colitis, and worms are treated well with *T. chebula* fruits.[8] The bark of *T. chebula* (Bala haritaki) fruit is swallowed after chewing, and it helps with hemorrhoids and in clearing the bowels. In obesity, the decoction of *T. chebula* fruits with honey reduces excessive body fat. The regular use of *T. chebula* fruits has a beneficial effect on the brain nerves and improves memory.[21] It is also valuable in urinary stones and dysuria.[22] *T. chebula* fruit paste has analgesic, anti-inflammatory, purifying, and healing capacity for wounds.[23,24]

CHEMICAL CONSTITUENTS

Phenolic compounds, namely chebulagic acid, ethyl gallate, gallic acid, methyl gallate, penta-O-galloyl-β-D-glucose, ellagic acid, chebulinic acid, and tetra-O-galloyl-β-D-glucose from fruits of *T. chebula*, have been isolated.[25] All phytoconstituents of *T. chebula* are hydrolyzable tannins (HTs) (assay: 20%–50%, wt./wt.)[26] and are responsible for the pharmacological properties of *T. chebula* fruits. The tannin content in *T. chebula* varies with the geological variation.[8] Tri-terpenoids, coumarin-conjugated compounds with gallic acid flavonol, and glycosides have also been isolated from *T. chebula*.[25] In various researches, it has been reported that T. chebula contains 14 components of hydrolysable tannins, and the most common compounds are gallic acid, chebulic acid, punicalagin, chebulanin, corilagin, neochebulinic, ellagic acid, chebulagic acid, 1,2,3,4,66-penta-orgalloyl-β-D-glucose, 1,6-di-o-galloyl-D-glucose, and terchebulin.[27,28] Different anthraquinone derivatives with purgative properties have been reported in *T. chebula* fruits.[29] All seven varieties of *T. chebula* are more or less used similarly but vary in specific usages and quality.[10,11,13,25] Leaves of the species have been reported to contain polyphenols such as punicalagin, punicalin, terflavin B, terflavin C, and terflavin D.[30] Different investigations have deciphered that *T. chebula* contains more phenolic compounds than any other plant.[31]

PHARMACOLOGICAL PROPERTIES OF *T. CHEBULA*

T. chebula plant has been reported for various pharmacological effects (i.e., pleiotropic effects)[32–34] such as hepatoprotective, antioxidant, renoprotective, antidiabetic, anti-anaphylactic, prokinetic, and immunomodulatory (Table 30.1).[35] Several phytochemicals of different chemical classes are associated with different biological properties (e.g., ß-sitosterol, shikimic acid, daucosterol, gallic acid, palmitic acid, triacontanoic acid, tannic acid, luteolin, ethyl ester of gallic acid, and tri-ethyl ester of chebulic acid) of *T. chebula* fruits. Moreover, numerous pleiotropic effects have been exhibited by *T. chebula*, including antidiabetic, renoprotective, antioxidant, hepatoprotective, immunomodulatory, anti-anaphylactic, and prokinetic effects. The pleiotropic effects (i.e., various pharmacological effects at a time, resulting in several therapeutic benefits) of *T. chebula* have been proved both experimentally and clinically. Besides, the plant has been significantly used to cure people having chronic intermittent fever, leprosy, heart disease, anorexia, anemia, cough, diarrhea, excessive secretion of mucus, etc.[36]

TABLE 30.1
Properties of Some Bio-Actives from *T. chebula* Fruits

Compounds	Activities
Ellagic acid	Antibacterial activity against intestinal bacteria *Escherichia coli*, *Clostridium perfringens*, antiproliferative activity.[47,48]
Chebulic acid	Antioxidant, hepatoprotective, free radical scavenging activity, cytoprotective.[49,50]
Neo chebulic acid	Antioxidant, free radical scavenging, and hepatoprotective activity.[49]
Gallic acid	Antibacterial, cytoprotective, antioxidant, antiviral activity.[50,51,52]
2,4-chebulyl-ß-D-glucopyranose	Antiproliferative activity.[47]
Chebulinic acid	Antiproliferative activity.[47]
Hydroxy-benzoic acid derivatives	Antioxidant activity.[53]
Flavonol aglycones	Antioxidant activity.[53]
Chebulagic acid	Antiarthritic, cytoprotective activity.[17,50]

As many therapies are associated with the *T. chebula* plant, its different extracts have been widely investigated for various pharmacological properties. The plant has been reported to have potent antioxidant activities due to the presence of phenolics. The aqueous extract of the fruits of *T. chebula* has antioxidant activity, as evidenced by the fact that the extract significantly decreased lipid peroxidation effects. The hepatoprotective effect of the extract, additionally evidenced by reductions in biochemical concentration, supported by histopathological observations, is a case of potent antioxidant properties of the extract.[37] *T. chebula* is highly effective against *Helicobacter pylori*, a bacterium responsible for stomach cancers, ulcers, and gastritis.[38,39] Ethanolic extract of *T. chebula* fruits has time- and concentration-dependent molluscicidal activity against the vector snail *Lymnaea acuminata*.[40]

The extract of fruits of *T. chebula* has been reported to inhibit human immunodeficiency virus-1 reverse transcriptase, and hot water extract of fruits has anti-herpes simplex virus properties.[41] Ponnusankar et al.[42] have studied the effect of 70% methanolic fruit extract of *T. chebula* on the growth of several malignant cell lines. The fraction rich in chebulagic acid from *T. chebula* fruits has potent dual inhibition against COX and 5-LOX. The chebulagic acid-rich fraction from *T. chebula* fruits has antiproliferative activity against HCT-15, MDAMB-231, COLO-205, K562, and DU-145 cell lines. Triphala is reported to inhibit cytochrome P450.

The 75% methanolic extract of *T. chebula* fruits (100 mg/kg b.w.) reduced the blood glucose level in normal and alloxan-induced diabetic rats within 4 hours of oral administration. The chloroform extract of *T. chebula* seeds has a dose-dependent reduction in the blood glucose of diabetic rats.[43] The *T. chebula*, along with other medicinal herbs, has been reported to resist many stressors in different ways. *T. chebula* reduces the serum histamine when given following anaphylactic shock and reveals the strong anti-anaphylactic activity of the species.[44]

The ethanol, chloroform, petroleum ether, and water extracts of *T. chebula* fruits have been evaluated for analgesic activity by using the tail immersion method in mice. The ethanolic extract has an analgesic response at 200, 400, and 800 mg/kg body weight per day.[45] The hydroalcoholic extract of *T. chebula* fruits has been examined in animals pretreated with 200 and 500 mg/kg body weight, exhibiting a reduction in lesion index, total affected area, and % of lesions compared with control groups in the ethanol-, aspirin-, and cold restraint stress-induced ulcer models.[46]

The hydroalcoholic extract of *T. chebula* inhibits joint swelling compared to the control in both CFA-induced and formaldehyde-induced arthritis. The use of *T. chebula* extract has been reported to reduce serum TNF-α levels and synovial expression of IL-6, IL-1β, and TNF-R1.[17]

T. chebula leaves alcoholic extract on topical administration induces faster healing of dermal wounds in vivo due to improved rates of contraction and a decreased period of epithelialization. Biochemical studies revealed an increase in collagen content in the granulation tissues of treated wounds of rats.[54] Chebulagic acid and gallic acid in different concentrations, isolated from fruit extract of *T. chebula*, have been reported to block cytotoxic and granule exocytosis.[55] The aqueous extract of the fruit of *T. chebula* (50 μg) has been reported to neutralize 1,1-diphenyl-2-picrylhydrazyl by 92.9% and protect the plasmid DNA pBR322 from radiation.[56]

The ethanolic extract of *T. chebula* fruits (500 mg/kg b.w.) has a cardioprotective effect in isoproterenol-induced myocardial damage.[57] The oral administration of the bark of *T. chebula* as an extract with different solvents has histological alterations in seminiferous tubules in the testes of treated animals.[58]

SCOPE AND OPPORTUNITIES

Fruits of *T. chebula* are used as a popular drug in different folk and traditional medicines. There is a need to collect the samples of different varieties at the same time from regions as described for every variety, analyze the active principles of each, and investigate the pharmacological properties before any conclusive remarks.

Detailed literature has revealed that *T. chebula* has significant health effects, such as hepatoprotective, cardioprotective, antimutagenic, cytoprotective, antioxidant, and adaptogenic. The ethanol, ethyl acetate, and aqueous extracts of *T. chebula* fruits do not exhibit any cellular toxicity on erythrocytes, and the acute oral toxicity in animals exceeds the recommended doses.[34,59,60] The aqueous-alcoholic extract of *T. chebula* fruits has cytochrome P-450 inhibition potential in animals[61] and does not have a genotoxic effect in both the Ames assay and VITOTOX test.[62] The lead- and aluminum-induced genotoxicity is reduced by *T. chebula* fruits,[63,64] and its HTs have antimutagenic activity against mutagens like 4-nitro-O-phenylene diamine and sodium azide.[7] These pharmacological results indicated that utilization of *T. chebula* is generally safe as a drug. *T. chebula* has a wide spectrum of medicinal and pharmacological properties due to the presence of diverse bioactive compounds, but research work on medicinal applications of the plant against multi-drug-resistant pathogens is scanty. There is a need for extensive research to explore the potential of *T. chebula* to combat drug-resistant infections. Currently, with the changed global scenario and consciousness of healthcare practices, the use of nontoxic plant products from traditional applications is in demand for a new drug development program. *T. chebula* may be a good choice for developing modern green medicines, with compound fingerprints isolated from it and validated for effectiveness against different types of pathogens, as well as overcoming the problem of drug resistance. There is a need for extensive research on its toxicity, mechanism of action, and pharmacotherapeutics to develop specifications for both raw herbs and value-added products.

REFERENCES

1. Promila P, Madan VK. 2018. Therapeutic & phytochemical profiling of *Terminalia chebula* Retz. (Harad): a review. *Journal of Medicinal Plants Studies*. 6 (2): 25–31.
2. Anonymous. 2001. *The Ayurvedic Pharmacopoeia of India*. Government of India, Ministry of Health and Family Welfare Department of Indian System of Medicine & Homoeopathy, New Delhi. pp. 47, 143.
3. Khare CP. 2007. *Indian Medicinal Plants: An Illustrated Dictionary*. Springer-Verlag, Berlin. pp. 652–653.
4. Anonymous. 2002. *The Wealth of India – A Dictionary of Indian Raw Materials and Industrial Products*. Publication and Information Directorate, CSIR, New Delhi, Vol X. pp. 522–524.
5. Prakash DV, SreeSatya N, Avanigadda S, Vangalapati M. 2012. Pharmacological review on *Terminalia chebula*. *International Journal of Pharmacy & Biomedical Research*. 3 (2): 679–683.
6. Chattopadhyay RR, Bhattacharyya SK. 2007. PHCOG REV: plant review. *Terminalia chebula*: An update. *Pharmacognosy* Reviews. 23: 145–150.
7. Bag A, Bhattacharyya SK, Chattopadhyay RR. 2013. The development of *Terminalia chebula* Retz. (Combretaceae) in clinical research. *Asian Pacific Journal of Tropical Biomedicine*. 3 (3): 244–252.

8. Singh P, Malhotra H. 2017. *Terminalia Chebula*: A review pharmacognistic and phytochemical studies. *International Journal of Recent Scientific Research*. 8 (11): 21496–21507.
9. Sandeep C, Padma MP. 2009. *Jsminum grandiflorum* Linn (chameli): Ethnobotany, phytochemistry and pharmacology: a review. *Pharmacognosy News Letters*. 2: 586–595.
10. Chunekar KC. 1999. Bhavaprakashnighantu. Chaukhamba Bharati Academy, Varanasi. pp. 3.
11. Chunekar KC, Pandey GS. 2006. *Bhavaprakash Nighantu, Haritakyadi Varga*, 1st Edition. Chaukhambha Bharti Academy. pp. 5–6. UP, India.
12. Dash BVd. 2012. The Drug *Terminalia chebula* in Ayurveda and Tibetian Literature. Available from: https://www.thlib.org/static/reprints/kailash/kailash_04_01_01.pdf, as on 21 September 2021.
13. Hooker JD. 1854. *Flora of British India (pt 2)*. Oxford, London. pp. 443–449.
14. Ratha KK, Joshi C. 2013. Haritaki (*Chebulic myrobalan*) and its varieties. *AYU*. 34 (3): 331–333.
15. Rathinamoorthy R, Thilagavathi G. 2014. *Terminalia chebula*: Review on pharmacological and biochemical studies. *International Journal of Pharm Tech Research*. 6(1): 97–116.
16. Ramani YR, Pradhan S. Antiarthritic activity of acetone extract of *Terminalia chebula*. *Webmed Central Pharmacology*. 3 (2): WMC003057.
17. Nair V, Singh S, Gupta YK. 2010. Anti-arthritic and disease modifying activity of *Terminalia chebula* Retz. in experimental models. *Journal of Pharmacy and Pharmacology*. 62 (12): 1801–1806.
18. Wetwitayaklunget P, Charoenteeraboon J, Limmatvapirat C, Phaechamud T. 2012. Antioxidant activities of some Thai and exotic fruits cultivated in Thailand. *Research Journal of Pharmaceutical Biological and Chemical Sciences*. 3 (1): 12–21.
19. Mallik J, Das P, Karon B, Das S. 2012. A review on phytochemistry and pharmacological activity of *Terminalia belerica*. *International Journal of Drug Formulation and Research*. 3 (6): 1–5.
20. Kadian R, Parle M, Yadav M. 2014. Therapeutic potential and phytopharmacology of *Terminalia bellerica*. *World Journal of Pharmacy and Pharmaceutical Sciences*. 3 (10): 804–819.
21. Afshari AR, Sadeghnia HR, Mollazadeh H. 2016. A review on potential mechanisms of *Terminalia chebula* in Alzheimer's disease. *Advances in Pharmacological Sciences*. Article ID 8964849, 14 pages. https://doi.org/10.1155/2016/8964849, as on September 22, 2021.
22. Thomas J, Joy PP, Mathew G, Skaria S, Duethi BP, Joseph TS. 2000. *Agronomic Practices for Aromatic and Medicinal Plant*. Directorate of Arecanut and Spices Development India. Calicut, Kerala, India. pp. 124–130.
23. Goossens L, Pommery N, Hénichart JP. 2007. COX-2/5-LOX dual acting anti-inflammatory drugs in cancer chemotherapy. *Current Topics in Medicinal Chemistry*. 7: 283–296.
24. Rani AA, Jeeva S, Punitha MJS. 2016. Antioxidant, anti-inflammatory, anti-proliferative and apoptotic properties of *Terminalia chebula* (fruit) towards raw 264.7 and oral KB Cell Lines. *International Journal of Applied and Pure Science and Agriculture*. 2 (5): 90–100.
25. Suchalatha S, Devi CS. 2005. Antioxidant activity of ethanolic extract of *Terminalia chebula* fruit against isoproterenol induced oxidative stress in rats. *Indian Journal of Biochemistry & Biophysics*. 42: 246–249.
26. Riaz M, Khan O, Sherkheli MA. 2017. Chemical constituents of *Terminalia chebula*. *Natural Products: An Indian Journal*. 13 (2): 112. https://www.tsijournals.com/articles/chemical-constituents-of-terminalia-chebula-13577.html, as on September 22, 2021.
27. Kumar KJ. 2006. Effect of geographical variation on contents of tannic acid, gallic acid, chebulinic acid and ethyl gallate in *Terminalia chebula*. *Natural Products*. 2 (3–4): 170–175.
28. Juang LJ, Sheu SJ, Lin TC. 2004. Determination of hydrolyzable tannins in the fruit of *Terminalia chebula* Retz. By high-performance liquid chromatography and capillary electrophoresis. *Journal of Separation Science*. 27 (9): 718–724.
29. Quanbin H, Jingzheng S, Chunfeng Q, Lina W, Hongxi X. 2006. Preparative isolation of hydrolysable tannins chebulagic acid and chebulinic acid from *Terminalia chebula* by high-speed countercurrent chromatography. *Journal of Separation Science*. 29: 1653–1657.
30. Patel M, Patel V, Patel RK. 2010. Development and validation of improved RPHPLC method for identification and estimation of ellagic and gallic acid in Triphala churna. *International Journal of ChemTech Research*. 2 (3): 1486–1493.
31. Ali M, Nandini P. 2010. Simultaneous isolation and identification of phytoconstituents from *Terminalia chebula* by preparative chromatography. *Journal of Chemical and Pharmaceutical Research*. 2 (5): 97–103
32. Na M, Bae K, Kang SS, Min BS, Yoo JK, Kamiryo Y, Senoo YI, Yokoo S, Miwa N. 2004. Cytoprotective effect on oxidative stress and inhibitory effect on cellular aging of *Terminalia chebula* fruit. *Phytotherapy* Research. 18: 737–741.
33. Rao NK, Nammi S. 2006. Antidiabetic and renoprotective effects of the chloroform extract of *Terminalia chebula* Retz. seeds in streptozotocin-induced diabetic rats. *BMC Complementary and Alternative Medicine*. 6: 17 https://doi.org/10.1186/1472-6882-6-17, as on 12 October 2021.
34. Kim JH, Koo YC, Hong CO, Yang SY, Jun W, Lee KW. 2011. Mutagenicity and oral toxicity studies of *Terminalia chebula*. *Phytotherapy Research*. 26: 39–47. https://doi.org/10.1002/ptr.3504
35. Khan MU, Rohilla A, Bhatt D, Afrin S, Rohilla S, Ansari SH. 2011. *Terminalia chebula*: A review on its pleiotropism. *Journal of Pharmacy Research*. 4 (9): 3037–3039.
36. Malekzadeh F, Ehsanifar H, Shahamat M, Levin M, Colwell RR. 2001. Anti-bacterial activity of black myrobalan (*Terminalia chebula* Retz) against *Helicobacter pylori*. *Journal of Anti-Microbial Agents*. 18:85–88.
37. Muhammad S, Khan BA, Akhtar N, Mahmood T, Rasul R, Hussain I, Khan H, Badshah A. 2012. The morphology, extractions, chemical constituents, and uses of *Terminalia chebula*: A review: *Journal of Medicinal Plants Research*. 6 (33): 4772–4775.
38. Kannan P, Ramadevi SR, Hopper W. 2009. Antibacterial activity of *Terminalia chebula* fruit extract. *African Journal of Microbiol Research*. 3 (4): 180–184.
39. Sohni YR, Bhatt RM. 1996. Activity of a crude extract formulation in experimental hepatic amoebiasis and in immune-modulation studies. *Journal of Ethnopharmacology*. 54 (2–3): 119–124.
40. Upadhyay A, Singh DK. 2011. Molluscicidal activity of *Sapindus mukorossi* and *Terminalia chebula* against the fresh-water snail *Lymnaea acuminate*. *Chemosphere*. 83 (4): 468–474.

41. Lin LT, Chen TY, Chung CY, Noyce R S, Grindley TB, McCormick C, Lin TC, Wang G H, Lin C C. Richardson C D. 2011. Hydrolyzable tannins (chebulagic acid and punicalagin) target viral glycoprotein-glycosaminoglycan interactions to inhibit herpes simplex virus 1 entry and cell-to-cell spread. *Journal of Virology*. 85 (9): 4386–4398.
42. Ponnusankar S, Pandit S, Babu R, Bandyopadhyay A, Mukherjee PK. 2011. Cytochrome P450 inhibitory potential of Triphala-A Rasayana from Ayurveda. *Journal of Ethnopharmacology*. 133 (1): 120–125.
43. Murali YK, Anand P, Tandon V, Singh R, Chandra R, Murthy P S. 2007. Long-term effects of *Terminalia chebula* Retz. On hyperglycemia and associated hyperlipidemia, tissue glycogen content and *in-vitro* release of insulin in streptozotocin induced diabetic rats. *Experimental and Clinical Endocrinology & Diabetes*. 115 (10): 641–646.
44. Shin TY, Jeong HJ, Kim DK, Kim SH, Lee JK, Kim DK, Chae BS, Kim JH, Kang HW, Lee CM, Lee KC, Park ST, Lee EJ, Lim JP, Kim KM, Leen YM. 2001. Inhibitory action of water-soluble fraction of *Terminalia chebula* on systemic and local anaphylaxis. *Journal of Ethnopharmacology*. 74 (2): 133–140.
45. Kaur S, Jaggi RK. 2010. Anti-nociceptive activity of chronic administration of different extracts of *Terminalia bellerica* Roxb. and *Terminalia chebula* Retz. Fruits. *Indian Journal of Experimental Biology*. 48 (9): 925–930.
46. Sharma P, Prakash T, Kotresha D, Ansari MA, Sahrm UR, Kumar B, Debnath J, Goli D. 2011. Antiulcerogenic activity of *Terminalia chebula* fruit in experimentally induced ulcer in rats. *Pharmaceutical Biology*. 49 (3): 262–268.
47. Saleem M, Hushum P, Harkonen K, Pihlaja. 2002. Inhibition of cancer cell growth by crude extract and phenolics of *Terminalia chebula* fruit. *Journal of Ethnopharmacology*. 81: 327–336.
48. Kim HG, Cho JH, Jeong EY, Lim JH, Lee SH, Lee HS. 2006. Growth inhibitory activity of active component from *Terminalia chebula* fruits against intestinal bacteria. *Journal of Food Protection*. 69 (9): 2205–2209.
49. Lee HS, Jung SH, Yun BS, Lee KW. 2007. Isolation of chebulic acid from *Terminalia chebula* Retz., and its antioxidant effect in isolated rat hepatocytes. *Archives of Toxicology*. 31 (3): 211–218.
50. Chang CL, Lin CS, Lai GH, Chen YH, Tuan WC, Hsu CM. 2010. Influence of *Terminalia chebula* extracts on the effect of PC12 cell growth. *Journal of Traditional Medicine*. 21 (1): 23–30.
51. Sato Y, Oketani H, Singyouchi K, Ohtsubo T, Kihara M, Shibata H, Higuti T. 1997. Extraction and purification of effective antimicrobial constituents of *Terminalia chebula* Retz. against methicillin-resistant *Staphylococcus aureus*. *Biological and Pharmaceutical Bulletin*. 20 (4): 401–404.
52. Jeong AHN, Kim CY, Lee JS, Kim TG, Kim SH, Lee CK, Lee BB, Shin CG, Huh H, Kim J. 2002. Inhibition of HIV-1 integrase by galloyl glucoses from *Terminalia chebula* and flovonol glycoside gallates from *Euphorbia pekinensis*. *Planta Medica*. 68: 457–459.
53. Chen X, Sun F, Ma L, Wang J, Qin H, Du G. 2011. In vitro evaluation on the antioxidant capacity of triethylchebulate, an aglycone from *Terminalia chebula* Retz fruit. *Indian Journal of Pharmacology*. 43 (3): 320–323.
54. Choudhary GP. 2011. Wound healing activity of ethanolic extract of *Terminalia chebula* Retz. *International Journal of Pharma and Bio Sciences*. 2(1): 48–52.
55. Manosroi A, Jantrawut P, Akihisa T, Manosroi W, Manosroi J. 2010. In vitro anti-aging activities of *Terminalia chebula* gall extract. *Pharmaceutical Biology*. 48 (4): 469–481.
56. Gandhi NM, Nair CKK. 2005. Radiation protection by *Terminalia chebula*: Some mechanistic aspects. *Molecular and Cellular Biochemistry*. 277 (1–2): 43–48.
57. Suchalatha S, Srinivasan P, Shyamala Devi CS. 2007. Effect of *Terminalia chebula* on mitochondrial alterations in experimental myocardial injury. *Chemico-Biological Interactions*. 169 (3): 145–153.
58. Gupta PC, Singh S K. 2010. Effect of different extracts of bark of *Terminalia chebula* on reproductive organs in male mice. *ICRH & 20th Annual Meeting of the Indian Society for the Study of Reproduction & Fertility*, Feb 8–10, 2010, p. 40.
59. Khan KH. 2009. The effect of regular intake of *Terminalia chebula* on oxidative stress in mice originated from *Salmonella typhimurium*. *EurAsian Journal of BioSciences*. 3: 113–121.
60. Panunto W, Jaijoy K, Lerdvuthisopon N, Lertprasertsuke N, Jiruntanat N, Soonthornchareonnon N, Sireeratawong S. 2011. Acute and chronic toxicity studies of the water extract from dried fruits of *Terminalia chebula* Rezt. in rats. *International Journal of Applied Research in Natural Products*. 3 (4): 36–43.
61. Ponnusankar S, Pandit S, Venkatesh M, Bandyopadhyay A, Mukherjee PK. 2011. Cytochrome P450 inhibition assay for standardized extract of *Terminalia chebula* Retz. *Phytotherapy Research*. 25 (1): 151–154.
62. Arora S, Brits E, Kaur S, Kaur K, Sohi RS, Kumar S, Verschaeve L. 2005. Evaluation of genotoxicity of medicinal plant extracts by the Comet and VITOTOX tests. *Journal of Environmental Pathology, Toxicology, and Oncology*. 24 (3): 193–200.
63. Rathore HS, Makwama M. 2005. Prevention of lead toxicity in *Allium cepa* root tip cells with myrobalan (fruit of *Terminalia chebula* Retz.). *Biochemical and Cellular Arch ives*. 5(2): 169–176.
64. Rathore HS, Shazia B, Sharma A, Makwana M. 2006. Prevention of aluminium chloride – induced mitodepression with myrobalan (fruit of *Terminalia chebula* Retz, Combretaceae) in *Allium cepa* model. *Ethnobotanical Leaflets*. 10: 272–279.

31 *Viburnum opulus* (Cramp Bark)

INTRODUCTION

Viburnum opulus Linn. (family: Adoxaceae) is known as crampbark, cherry-wood, European cranberry bush, water elder, rose elder, and snowball tree.[1–5] It is a popular ornamental shrub, a source of many bioactive compounds, and its common natural habitats are temperate regions of North Africa, Asia, and the European continent.[6–8] The species has been known for its medicinal and food properties for a long time.[3,9] The raw *V. opulus* fruits have an astringent-bitter-sour taste and are considered slightly toxic because of the presence of viburnine and saponins.[10,11] *Viburnum* fruits have a low pH, are rich in tannins, and have an inadequate taste, so they act as repellents, defend against predators and pathogens, and are not very attractive to frugivores.[12,13]

Typically, fruits of the family Adoxaceae are fleshy drupe-containing stones, but drupe mesocarp may dry in some cases.[14] The drupes of *V. opulus* ripen in August–September. These fruits are persistent in nature and do not shed during autumn (Figure 31.1), but remain on the plant throughout winter, often until May or June.[15]

The fruits of *V. opulus* are not generally eaten by birds after they have frozen and thawed several times but are eaten by foxes, chipmunks, deer, mice, moose, raccoons, squirrels, rabbits, skunks, grouse, songbirds, and pheasants. The dense shrub shape of the plant provides safety and nesting sites for many small animals. Pollination is by insects.

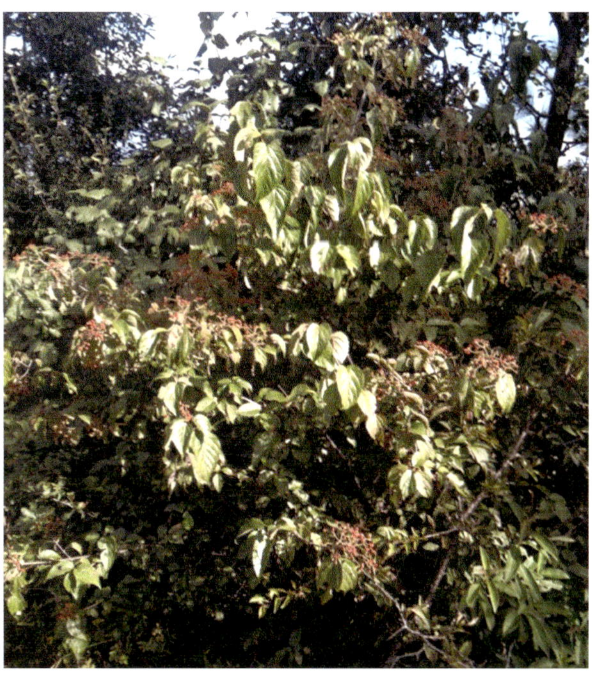

FIGURE 31.1 *V. opulus* plant (during November 2023).

A red dye is made from fruits. Stems without pith are used to make popguns.[15]

The use of the plant for health benefits is due to the presence of carotenoids, vitamin C, phenolic compounds, essential oils, iridoids, etc.[7,16–18] The pro-health properties, such as antimicrobial,[19] antidiabetic,[20] antiobesity,[21] anti-inflammatory,[22] and anticancer effects,[23] of different morphological parts of the species have been deciphered by in vivo and in vitro assays. The name 'Crampbark' is due to the ability of plant bark to treat cramps, particularly menstrual cramps.[15] The fruit extract is also used to relax muscles and blood vessels, which can relieve pain and reduce blood pressure, though there is no valid scientific evidence to support the claim.[24]

ETHNOPHARMACOLOGY

In Ukraine and Russia, the red *V. opulus* fruits are used in traditional cuisine as a component of liqueurs, marmalades, herbal teas, and jams, despite their astringent, bitter-sour taste.[16] In Scandinavia, cooked *V. opulus* fruits are popular, while in Canada, these are the substitute for cranberries.[3] In Turkey (Kayseri region), these fruits are stored to stand in plastic drums filled with tap water in a dark place at room temperature for 3–4 months to ferment and eliminate the sour, pungent flavor. The filtrate of this solution is known as 'gilaburu juice', a nonalcoholic traditional fermented beverage of Turkey, and is available in commercial outlets.[11, 25] Recently, a few value-added functional foods, such as pear juice with the addition of *V. opulus* juice or cakes incorporated with *V. opulus* fruit pomace, have been developed.[26,27] Çemtekin et al. have suggested the possibility of using concentrated *V. opulus* fruit juice in cooked minced meat in Turkey as an alternative source of antioxidants to delay oxidative changes.[28]

V. opulus fruits, flowers, and bark are widely used in folk and traditional medicines; additionally, fruits are used as cooking ingredients. *V. opulus* has some folkloric uses as an expectorant, diuretic, and for treating kidney disorders, diabetes, bile and liver disorders, epilepsy, mumps, and prostate disorders. The bioactivity of *V. opulus* fruits has been reported as antioxidant, antimicrobial, and immunostimulant.[29–31]

The dried bark of *V. opulus* (Sunaira Phul, local name) in District Muzaffarabad, Pakistan, is used as a diuretic and uterine sedative, and for treating emesis, hysteria, as a purgative, and for scurvy, infections, spasms, liver disorders, and uteritis. The decoction of the root is taken for swollen glands, entire body pain, mumps.[32] Awan et al. have described that the decoction of the plant is used to treat sore eyes, the fruits are used as food, an infusion of the plant

DOI: 10.1201/9781003512868-33

is used to treat cold and fever, in fever roots are given to babies, the decoction of branches is used to treat the fallen womb after birth, the decoction of bark is taken by overweight people facing difficulty breathing due to fatty muscles, and the inner bark is used to cure stomach cramps.[32]

PHYTOPHARMACOLOGY

The main component of *V. opulus* fruits is water (85.7%–88.3%) of the fresh weight.[5,33] The total dissolved solids content has been reported from 9.0% to 24.7%.[33–36] Sugars, one of the main groups of fruit, ranged between 4.02% and 8.80%. Sucrose content alone varied from 0.13 to 140 mg/100 g, and the ratio of glucose content to the fructose content ranged from 1.0 to 1.5.[1,5,16,33]

The *V. opulus* fruits are acidic because of the large number of different acidic molecules, with titratable acidity assay reported between 1.34% and 3.20%.[5,33,36] The organic acids vary as per geo-climatic conditions;[16] e.g., the main organic acids of *V. opulus* fruits are malic acid and citric acid in the fruits collected from Russia, while malic and tartaric acids are major ingredients in fruits from Turkey.[18] Citric acid, quinic acid, and malic acid have considerable presence in the pomace of *V. opulus* fruits.[37]

Cam et al. have reported oxalic acid and malic acid in *V. opulus* seeds.[38] Dry fruits of *V. opulus* have been reported to have lipids (9.34%–12.35% of dry weight), which include oleic acid, linoleic acid, and palmitic acid as the major ingredients.[17] In addition, unsaturated fatty acids predominate over saturated fatty acids in *V. opulus* fruits.

V. opulus fruits have their typical smell, a major cause to be disliked by consumers. The volatile ingredients identified in fruits are from different chemical classes, such as phenols, alcohols, aldehydes, terpenoids, branched fatty acids, ketones, esters, and acids.[17,39] The aroma of fruits is mainly due to 2-methylbutanoic acid, 3-methylbutanoic acid, ethyl decanoate, and linalool.[39] In fermented *V. opulus* fruit juice (gilaburu juice), butanoic acid, propanoic acid, and isovaleric acid are the major ingredients.[40,41] Sonmezdag et al. have reported a total of 47 aroma compounds in the Gilaburu juice using a highly representative aromatic extract by use of the trap and purge technique using dichloromethane and subsequently analyzed by gas chromatography-mass spectrometry.[41]

The stalks, leaves, and fruits of *V. opulus* have calcium, phosphorus, potassium, sodium, and magnesium as macro-elements, whereas copper, iron, manganese, and zinc have been reported as microelements.[5,42] Potassium regulates blood pressure and helps in maintaining cardiovascular health and muscle function through the modulation of liquid retention in the body.[43]

The pigments (carotenoids, flavonoids, and anthocyanins) in *V. opulus* fruits are mainly present in the fruit skin and, comparatively less quantity in the mesocarp. The coral color of *V. opulus* fruits is due to carotenoids, flavonoids, and anthocyanins. Carotenoids in the *V. opulus* fruits have been reported to be 10-fold higher than those of the *V. lantana* fruits. Essential oils and steroids have been reported as lipid droplets in the cuticle and cell walls of fruits. Saponins have been reported only in the fruit mesocarp of the species.[39,44]

MEDICINAL APPLICATIONS OF THE SPECIES

1. **To inhibit community-acquired infections**: Currently, there is a limited number of effective antibiotics for the prevention or treatment of *Staphylococcus aureus* and hospital-acquired infections. It is a timely need to search for alternatives, as it is still one of the leading causes of infectious diseases due to rapid changes in the morphology of the pathogen itself. The extracts from the fruits of *V. opulus* and bark have been reported as potentially effective in the prevention of staphylococcal infections. *V. opulus* extracts strongly inhibited staphylococcal sortase adhesins A activity and staphylococcal protein A expression, so these extracts have pro-health potential and are useful as dietary supplements that are beneficial to prevent staphylococcal infections. However, more research data based on animal models and clinical trials are needed before the commercial application of the species to check the *S. aureus* menace.[45]

   The anti-infective properties of different extracts of *V. opulus* are mainly due to the presence of phenolics (derivatives of hydroxycinnamic and hydroxybenzoic acids, mainly ferulic acid, chlorogenic acid, gallic acid, etc.), flavanols (procyanidin, epicatechin, catechin, etc.), flavonols (isorhamnetin glycosides, quercetin, etc.), and anthocyanins (mainly cyanidin 3-arabinosyl-glucoside, cyanidin 3-glucoside, cyanidin 3-sambubioside, cyanidin 3-rutinoside, etc.).[16,18,39,46–49] The role of macronutrients (e.g., sugars, proteins, and organic acids) is also valuable for its bioactivities. Extracts from barks are richer than the extracts from fruits by approximately seven times, three times, and more than six times in terms of the total flavonols, phenolics, and pro-anthocyanidins, respectively.[45,49]
2. **Reduce the free fatty acid load**: Different preparations from *V. opulus* fruits, including its purified juice, influence the lipid accumulation in the hepatocytes. Obesity is a nonalcoholic fatty liver disease, a state of lipid accumulation in hepatocytes resulting in inflammation and fatty liver (hepatic steatosis).[50] Excessive intake of nutrients rich with fats and fatty acids, including palmitic and oleic acids, significantly elevates the risk of hepatic steatosis induction.[51] The purified fruit juice has the strongest potential to decrease lipid accumulation in HepG2 cells, which is associated with a decrease in free fatty acid uptake. The excess free fatty acids are closely related to mitochondrial dysfunction

and a decrease in mitochondrial membrane potential. Different products of *V. opulus* are reported to increase the polarization of the mitochondrial membrane, which may be due to their antioxidant properties. As *V. opulus* phenolics control the hepatic lipo-toxicity in obese implications, and a synergistic influence of *V. opulus* phenolic compounds due to the enhanced phosphorylation and increased LKB-1 level decreases the accumulation of lipids in HepG2 cells, even during the excess of free fatty acids, *via* the downregulation of lipogenic proteins.[52]

V. opulus phenolics have been reported to enhance the signal transduction of the insulin receptor pathway and suppress insulin resistance due to hyperlipidemia. Pietrzyk et al. (2021) have concluded that the juice and pulp from *V. opulus* are rich sources of bioactive compounds with the potential to prevent and treat liver steatosis, and that the whole *V. opulus* fruit is a potential functional food ingredient.[52]

3. **Anti-adipogenic effect**: Podsędek et al. have reported that the semi-purified phenolic extract of *V. opulus* fruits has an anti-adipogenic effect in mice by reducing lipid accumulation and intracellular oxidative stress.[53] The semi-purified phenolic extract of fruits of *V. opulus* is reported to regulate the secretion level of leptin. Leptin is known to regulate pancreatic lipase activity. The semi-purified phenolic extract potentiated the inhibitory effect of orlistat (a gastrointestinal lipase inhibitor) toward lipase. Probably, it may act as a supplement or an additional component of the formulation, which may lead to the reduction of orlistat treatment dosages and their side effects. Hydroxycinnamic acids, especially chlorogenic acid, have been reported as the main ingredients of extracts.[53]

SCOPE AND OPPORTUNITIES

The current growing interest in natural food products for their unique aroma and high nutritional value is a significant issue for longevity and quality of life. *V. opulus* fruits have been reported for lipids and their derivatives (essential oils, carotenoids, saponins, and steroids), polyphenols (anthocyanins, flavonoids, and tannins), proteins, and pectin. Fruits of *V. opulus* have been reported to have higher quantities of polyphenols, carotenoids, steroids, flavonoids, and pectin than *V. lantana* drupes. *V. lantana* drupes are characterized by a higher content of essential oils, saponins, and proteins. These metabolites are different in the pericarp layers, but the highest amount is reported in the drupe skin. Detailed comparative studies on different species of the genus may lead to more clues for different biological applications in different edaphoclimatic regions.

V. opulus has rich bioactive compounds, and its diverse chemical composition is responsible for different therapeutic effects as a food ingredient and folk medicine. Currently, the evidence-based utilization of phenolics and iridoids is growing for their biological activity, including antiobesity, antimicrobial, anti-inflammatory, antioxidative, cytoprotective, antidiabetic, and anticancer properties.

Most of the research so far has been carried out on fruits of *V. opulus*, while only a few data are available on other bark, flowers, leaves, and stems. The *V. opulus* fruits have health-enhancing values due to polyphenols, flavonoids, and carotenoids. Many of the biological mechanisms are based on cell assays to explain how *V. opulus* compounds exert bioprotective action, though the molecular pathways of these effects are poorly understood.

Applications of *V. opulus* are known to decrease inflammatory responses during endometriosis, induce a diuretic effect, alleviate pain associated with uterine contractions, and reduce the formation of ureteral stones. However, the side effects associated with the use of *V. opulus* reveal the need to intensify investigations on the bioavailability of its different ingredients introduced into the body, both in the form of food and various value-added products, for careful consideration as a promising source to promote healing effects. Thus, further research, including basic and clinical validation, is the need of the hour to use *V. opulus* plant species as modern green medicine.

REFERENCES

1. Ozrenk M, Göndogdu N, Kenskin N, Kaya T. 2011. Some physical and chemical characteristics of gilaburu (*Viburnum opulus* L.) fruits in Erzincan region. *Igdir University Journal of the Institute of Science and Technology*. 1: 9–14.
2. Karaçelik AA, Küçük M, Iskefiyeli Z, Aydemir S, De Smet S, Miserez B, Sandra P. 2015. Antioxidant components of *Viburnum opulus* L. determined by on-line HPLC–UV–ABTS radical scavenging and LC–UV–ESI-MS methods. *Food Chemistry*. 175: 106–114.
3. Velioglu YS, Ekici L, Poyrazoglu ES. 2006. Phenolic composition of European cranberrybush (*Viburnum opulus* L.) berries and astringency removal of its commercial juice. *International Journal of Food Science & Technology*. 9205: 1011–1015.
4. Sagdic O, Ozturk I, Yapar N, Yetim H. 2014. Diversity and probiotic potentials of lactic acid bacteria isolated from gilaburu, a traditional Turkish fermented European cranberrybush (*Viburnum opulus* L.) fruit drink. *Food Reseach International*. 64: 537–545.
5. Akbulut M, Calsir S, Marakoglu T, Coklar H. 2008. Chemical and technological properties of European cranberrybush (*Viburnum opulus* L.) fruits. *Asian Journal of Chemistry*. 20: 1875–1885.
6. Altun ML, Çitoglu GS, Yilmaz BS, Özbek H. 2009. Antinociceptive and anti-inflammatory activities of *Viburnum opulus*. *Pharmaceutical Biology*. 47: 653–658.
7. Rop O, Reznicek V, Valsikova M, Jurikova T, Mlcek J, Kramarova D. 2010. Antioxidant properties of European cranberrybush fruit (*Viburnum opulus* var. edule). *Molecules*. 15: 4467–4477.

8. Konarska A, Domaciuk M. 2018. Differences in the fruit structure and the location and content of bioactive substances in *Viburnum opulus* and *Viburnum lantana* fruits. *Protoplasma*. 255: 25–41.
9. Cesoniene L, Daubaras R, Viskelis P. 2008. Evaluation of productivity and biochemical components in fruit of different *Viburnum* accessions. *Biologija*. 54: 93–96.
10. Wang LQ, Chen YG, Xu JJ, Liu Y, Li XM, Zhao Y. 2008. Compounds from *Viburnum* species and their biological activities. *Chemistry & Biodiversity*. 5: 1879–1899.
11. Soylak M, Elcit L, Saracoglu S, Divrikli U. 2002. Chemical analysis of fruit juice of European cranberry bush. *Asian Journal of Chemistry*. 14: 135–138.
12. Hernandez A. 2001. Are wayfaring tree *Viburnum lantana* fruits adapted for consumption by seed-disperser mammals. *Mammalia*. 65: 521–524.
13. Cazetta E, Schaefer HM, Galetti M. 2008. Does attraction to frugivores or defense against pathogens shape fruit pulp composition? *Oecologia*. 155: 277–286.
14. Donoghue MJ, Bell CD, Winkworth RC. 2003. The evolution of reproductive characters in Dipsacales. *International Journal of Plant Sciences*. 164 (S5): S453–S464.
15. Native Plants of PNW. An Encyclopedia of the Cultural and Natural History of Northwest Native Plants. https://nativeplantspnw.com/american-cranberrybush-viburnum-opulus/ as on February 23rd, 2022.
16. Perova IB, Zhogova AA, Cherkashin AV, Éller K I, Ramenskaya GV. 2014. Biologically active substances from European guelder berry fruits. *Pharmaceutical Chemistry Journal*. 48: 332–339.
17. Zarifikhosroshahi M, Tugba Z, Kafkas E, Okatan V. 2020.Variation in volatile and fatty acid contents among *Viburnum opulus* L. fruits growing different locations. *Scientia Horticulturae*. 264: 109160.
18. Polka D, Podsedek A. 2019. Phenolics composition and antioxidant capacity of guelder rose fruit, flower and bark extracts. *Food Science and Biotechnology*. 83: 37–46.
19. Turker H, Yıldırım AB. 2015.Screening for antibacterial activity of some Turkish plants against fish pathogens: a possible alternative in the treatment of bacterial infections. *Biotechnology & Biotechnological Equipment*. 29: 281–288.
20. Zakłos-Szyda M, Majewska I, Redzynia M, Koziołkiewicz M. 2015. Antidiabetic effect of polyphenolic extracts from selected edible plants as α-amylase, α-glucosidase and PTP1B inhibitors, and β pancreatic cells cytoprotective agents-A comparative study. *Current Topics in Medicinal Chemistry*. 15: 2431–2444.
21. Zakłos-Szyda M, Pietrzyk N, Szustak M, Podsedek A. 2020. *Viburnum opulus* L. juice phenolics inhibit mouse 3T3-L1 cells adipogenesis and pancreatic lipase activity. *Nutrients*. 12 (7): 2003. https://doi.org/10.3390/nu12072003
22. Zakłos-Szyda M, Nowak A, Pietrzyk N, Podsedek A. 2020. *Viburnum opulus* L. juice phenolic compounds influence osteogenic differentiation in human osteosarcoma Saos-2 cells. *International Journal of Molecular Sciences*. 21: 4909. https://doi.org/10.3390/ijms21144909
23. Ucar TA, Yildirim AB, Karakas FP. 2012. Antibacterial and antitumor activities of some wild fruits grown in Turkey. *Biotechnology & Biotechnological Equipment*. 26: 2765–2772.
24. Nicholson JA, Darby TD, Jarboe CH. 1972.Viopudial, a hypotensive and smooth muscle antispasmodic from *Viburnum opulus*. *Proceedings of the Society for Experimental Biology and Medicine*. 140: 457–461.
25. Baschali A, Tsakalidou E, Kyriacou A, Karavasiloglou N, Matalas AL. 2017. Traditional low-alcoholic and non-alcoholic fermented beverages consumed in European countries: a neglected food group. *Nutrition Research Reviews*. 30: 1–24.
26. Lachowicz S, Oszmianski J. 2018.The influence of addition of cranberrybush juice to pear juice on chemical composition and antioxidant properties. *Journal of Food Science and Technology*. 55: 3399–3407.
27. Al O, Ulger H, Eetekin T, Nisari M, Susar H, Ceylan D, Karatoprak GS. 2017. The effect of gilaburu (*Viburnum opulus*) juice on Ehrlich ascites tumor (EAT) cell culture. *Proceedings*. 1: 1051.
28. Çemtekin B, Kilinc E, Karabacak L, Dagtekin T, Aa evaluation of guelder rose (*Viburnum opulus* L.) and hawthorn (*Crataegus monogyna*) concentrates as alternative antioxidant sources to BHT and nitrite in poultry meat model system. *Scientific Papers: Series D, Animal Science*. LXII: 217–227.
29. Akgül G, Yılmaz N, Celep A, Celep F, Çakılcıoğlu U. 2016. Ethnobotanical purposes of plants sold by herbalists and folk bazaars in the center of Cappadocica (Nevşehir, Turkey). *Indian Journal of Traditional Knowledge*. 15 (1): 103–108.
30. Korkmaz M, Karakuş S. 2015.Traditional uses of medicinal plants of Üzumlu district, Erzincan, Turkey. *Pakistan Journal of Botany*. 47 (1): 125–134.
31. Koşar M, Orakçı EE, Karatoprak GS. 2011. Antioxidant properties and phenolic composition of *Viburnum opulus* from Turkey. *Planta Medica*. 77: 39. https://doi.org/10.1055/s-0031-1282688
32. Awan ZI, Rehman HU, Awan AA, Minhas FA, Khan MN. 2013. Ethnobotanical importance of some highly medicinal plants of District Muzaffarabad, Pakistan with special reference to the species of the Genus *Viburnum*. *IOSR Journal of Pharmacy and Biological Sciences*. 6 (2): 53–66.
33. Cesoniene L, Daubaras R, Vencloviene J, Viškelis P. 2010. Biochemical and agro-biological diversity of *Viburnum opulus* genotypes. *Central European Journal of Biology*, 5: 864–871.
34. Ersoy N, Ercisli S, Gundogdu M. 2017. Evaluation of European cranberry bush (*Viburnum opulus* L.) genotypes for agro-morphological, biochemical and bioactive characteristics in Turkey. *Folia Horticulturae*. 29: 181–188.
35. Ozkan G, Ercisli S, Ibrahim H, Gulce S. 2020. Diversity on fruits of wild grown European cranberry bush from coruh valley in Turkey. *Erwerbs-Obstbau*. 62: 275–279.
36. Moskalets TZ, Moskalets V, Vovkohon AH, Knyazyuk OV. 2019. Fruits of new selection forms and varieties of snowball tree for manufacture of products of therapeutic and prophylactic purpose. *Regulatory Mechanisms in Biosystems*. 10: 432–437.
37. Dienaite L, Pukalskiene M, Pereira CV, Matias AA, Venskutonis PR. 2020. Valorization of European cranberry bush (*Viburnum opulus* L.) berry pomace extracts isolated with pressurized ethanol and water by assessing their phytochemical composition, antioxidant, and antiproliferative activities. *Foods*. 9: 1413.

38. Cam M, Hisil Y, Kuscu A. 2007. Organic acid, phenolic content and antioxidant capacity of fruit flesh and seed of *Viburnum opulus*. *Chemistry of Natural Compounds*. 43: 379–380.
39. Kraujalyte V, Leitner E, Rimantas P. 2012. Chemical and sensory characterisation of aroma of *Viburnum opulus* fruits by solid phase microextraction-gas chromatography-Olfactometry. *Food Chemistry*. 132: 717–723.
40. Yilmaztekin M, Sislioglu K. 2015. Changes in volatile compounds and some physicochemical properties of European cranberrybush (*Viburnum opulus* L.) during ripening through traditional fermentation. *Journal of Food Science*. 80: C687–C694.
41. Sonmezdag AS, Sevindik O, Kelebek H, Selli S. 2017. Aroma compounds of non-alcoholic fermented beverage: Gilaburu juice. *EuroBiotech Journal*. 1: 226–229.
42. Taskin O, Asik BB, Izli N. 2019. Mineral content of leaves, stalks and fruits of European cranberrybush plant (*Viburnum opulus* L.). *KSU Tarım Do ga Derg*. 22: 178–182.
43. Udensi UK, Tchounwou PB. 2017. Potassium homeostasis, oxidative stress, and human disease. *International Journal of Clinical and Experimental Pathology*. 4: 111–122.
44. Yilmaz N, Yayli N, Misir G, Karaoglu S, Yayli N. 2008. Chemical composition and antimicrobial activities of the essential oils of *Viburnum opulus*, *Viburnum lantana* and *Viburnum orientala*. *Asian Journal of Chemisty*. 20: 3324–3330.
45. Wojcik-Bojek U, Rywaniak J, Bernat P, Podsedek A, Kajszczak D, Sadowska B. 2021. An *in-vitro* study of the effect of *Viburnum opulus* extracts on key processes in the development of staphylococcal infections. *Molecules*. 26: 1758. https://doi.org/10.3390/molecules26061758
46. Kajszczak D, Zaklos-Szyda M, Podsedek A. 2020. *Viburnum opulus* L.-A review of phytochemistry and biological effects. *Nutrients*. 12: 3398.
47. Kraujalyte V, Venskutonis PR, Pukalskas A, Cesoniene L, Daubaras R. 2013. Antioxidant properties and polyphenolic compositions of fruits from different European cranberrybush (*Viburnum opulus* L.) genotypes. *Food Chemistry*. 141: 3695–3702.
48. Ozrenk M, Gundogdu N, Keskin N, Kaya T. 2011. Some physical and chemical characteristics of gilaburu (*Viburnum opulus* L.) fruits in Erzincan region. *Igdir University Journal of the Institute of Science and Technology*. 1: 9–14.
49. Polka D, Podsedek A, Koziolkiewicz M. 2019. Comparison of chemical composition and antioxidant capacity of fruit, flower and bark of *Viburnum opulus*. *Plant Foods for Human Nutrition*. 74: 436–442.
50. Festi D, Colecchia A, Sacco T, Bondi M, Roda E, Marchesini G. 2004. Hepatic steatosis in obese patients: clinical aspects and prognostic significance. *Obesity Reviews*. 5 (1): 27–42. https://doi.org/10.1111/j.1467-789X.2004.00126.x
51. Kien CL, Bunn JY, Stevens R, Bain J, Ikayeva O, Crain K, Koves TR, Muoio DM. 2014. Dietary intake of palmitate and oleate has broad impact on systemic and tissue lipid profiles in humans. *American Journal of Clinical Nutrition*. 99 (3): 436–445. https://doi.org/10.3945/ajcn.113.070557
52. Pietrzyk N, Zakłos-Szyda M, Koziołkiewicz M, Podsędek A. 2021. *Viburnum opulus* L. fruit phenolic compounds protect against FFA-induced steatosis of HepG2 cells via AMPK pathway. *Journal of Functional Foods*. 80: 104437. https://doi.org/10.1016/j.jff.2021.104437
53. Podsędek K, Zakłos-Szyda M, Polka D, Sosnowska D. 2020. Effects of *Viburnum opulus* fruit extracts on adipogenesis of 3T3-L1 cells and lipase activity. *Journal of Functional Foods*. 73: 104111. https://doi.org/10.1016/j.jff.2021.104437

32 *Zanthoxylum armatum* (Timur)

INTRODUCTION

Zanthoxylum armatum DC. (fam.: Rutaceae, synonyms of *Z. armatumare*, *Z. planispinum*) is an aromatic, deciduous, spiny evergreen shrub of height up to 6 m (also known as winged prickly ash or Timur, Figure 32.1).[1] The fruit is reddish and around 5 mm in diameter.[1] The flower of *Z. armatum* is green to yellowish, and the seeds are bitter and shiny. In India, fruits, seeds, and their bark are used to cure dyspepsia, fever, and cholera.[2] Fruits and seeds are useful for dental troubles and are utilized in many kinds of dental pastes, while their powder has antiseptic properties.[2] The species is mainly found in the Himalayas' warmer valleys from 1,000 to 2,100 MSL, ranging from Jammu Kashmir to Assam, Meghalaya, Mizoram, and Manipur (Figure 32.2).[3,4]

In India, mainly in Uttarakhand, collection of the species for medicine, and food is cottage employment, and its trade on the barter system still prevails.[5] The Bhotiyas of the Pithoragarh district of the Kumaon region use Timur fruits, while those from the Chamoli district of the Garhwal region have developed their collection practices. The sticks made from the branches of the species are used by the pilgrims visiting the shrines of Badrinath, Gangotri, Yamunotri, and Kedarnath. This practice still exists between these two communities, but since the last decade, herbal-based pharmaceutical companies have started purchasing *Z. armatum* fruits in bulk from this region, resulting in competitive commercial activity and negotiations.[5] Although there is scattered information on the use of *Z. armatum*,[6,7] the current commercialization trend, the impact of trade on traditional harvesting mechanisms, and its ownership have not been adequately documented, resulting in a gap in the conservation of the species in the Himalayan region.

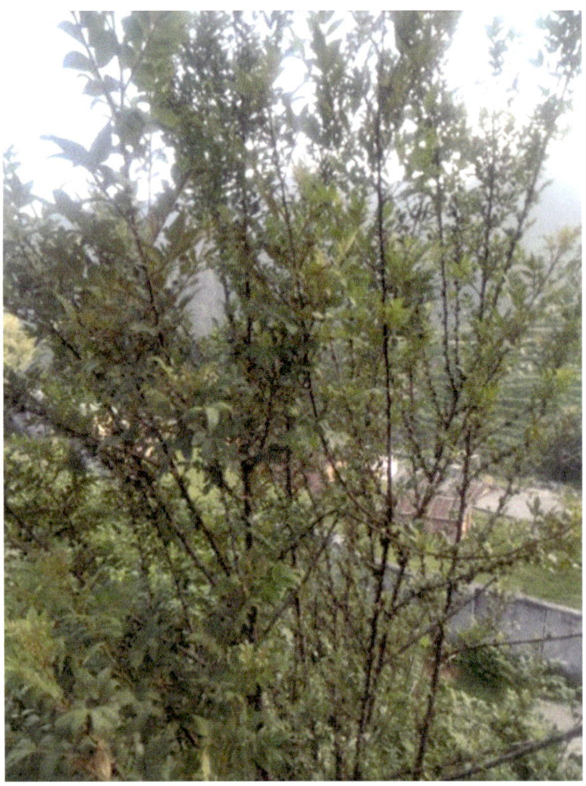

FIGURE 32.1 *Z. armatum* in forest.

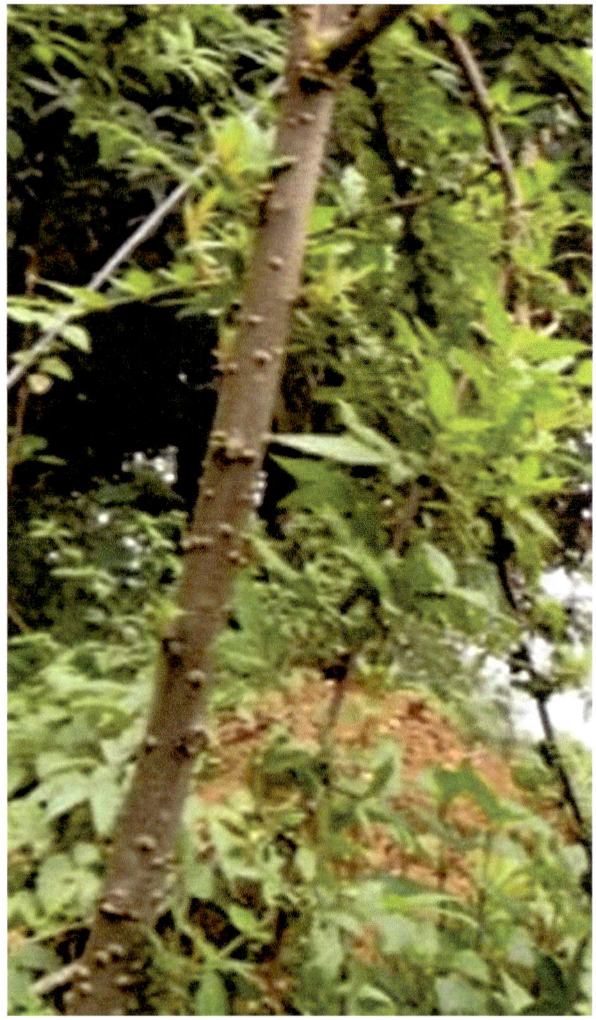

FIGURE 32.2 Close view of *Z. armatum* stem.

ETHNOPHARMACOLOGY

Since ancient times, the plant *Z. armatum* has been used as a medicine by different folks to cure various diseases (Table 32.1),[8] such as gum bleeding, toothache, and problems related to the tooth, asthma, fever, dyspepsia, tonics, etc.[9,10] Fruits of the species are used to repel insects and to

DOI: 10.1201/9781003512868-34

TABLE 32.1
Folk Applications of *Z. armatum* in Different Countries

Country	Used Parts	Application
India	Aerial parts	Insecticidal[2]
	Seeds and bark	Cholera, dyspepsia, and fever[2]
Japan	Seeds	Depression and GIT problems[11]
Nepal	Fruits	i. Decoction is used to cure abdominal pain.[12] ii. Pickles are used to treat colds and coughs, tonsillitis, high altitude sickness, limb numbness, and vertigo/dizziness. Decoction of powdered fruits is used to treat diarrhea, dysentery, and stomachache.[12]
	Berries	Antirheumatic, antispasmodic, carminative, and skin diseases.[12]
	Barks	Asthma, cholera, and diabetes[12]
Malaysia, Thailand	Branches and stems	Stomach tonic and to treat snake bites[13]
China	Aerial parts	An infusion is applied to expel worms or bugs infecting the ear. Its lotion is used to treat scabies.[14]
Pakistan	Fruits	i. Used as spice and condiment.[11,12] ii. Powdered dried fruit mixed with dried leaves of *Mentha longifolia*, seeds of *Trachyspermum ammi*, and black salt is taken with water to treat indigestion and cholera.[11,12] iii. Twigs are used as toothbrushes during gum problems and toothache.[11,12]

purify the water. Its wood is rich in tannins, resulting in its use as a strong stick for walking.[8]

Z. armatum fruits are used by the Bhotiyas community of Uttarakhand, India, for medicine and value-added products and subsequent trade.[15] Fruits, barks, and leaves of *Z. armatum* are used as a spice in the Indian system of medicine.[16] Bhotiya, a transhumant pastoral community in the Uttarakhand Himalaya, India, collects the *Z. armatum* plant for food, medicine, and barter trade.[5] In Uttarakhand, social groups in different geographical regions have adopted different strategies for the acquisition of *Z. armatum*. The Bhotiya community uses fruits in the form of medicine, spices, and condiments. It is used in curing various common ailments such as fever, toothache, cough, and the common cold. The dry or fresh fruit of the species is pressed over the affected tooth to treat toothache and reduce the severity of realized pain due to pungency. The fruit soup is used to cure stomach problems.[1]

Fruits of *Z. armatum* are used to brew liquor. Both fruits and seeds are a source of an aromatic tonic to treat dyspepsia and fever.[1] The bark of *Z. armatum* is used for the treatment of cholera.[2] In China, the infusion of *Z. armatum* in vinegar is used to expel bugs or worms infecting the ear.[17] The plant is used to treat scabies as a lotion applied to the skin.[18] It has a stimulating effect on the circulatory and lymphatic systems and acts as a stimulating liniment for rheumatism and fibrositis.[19] Since ancient times, *Z. armatum* has been a plant of more interest due to its historical claims as well as anticancer properties. Several other species of the genus, including the *Z. armatum*, have cytotoxicity against various human cancer and tumor cell lines.[20]

The greater utilization of the plant *Z. armatum* by the Bhotiya tribal community is due to its availability near their winter settlements in Uttarakhand, rather than in those of other communities.[1] *Z. armatum* is used in the preparation of certain traditional dishes, and it is a flavoring item and spice that is very popular. 'Hag', a traditional soup made from dried fruits, is consumed during winter by the entire family to keep them warm. The sauce, locally known as 'Dunkcha', is also a popular food item among the Bhotiya community. Young shoots of the plant are used as toothbrushes, and the powder is made from dried fruits for cleaning teeth. Timur soup is a common medicine among Bhotiyas to treat stomachaches. The brewed liquor from *Z. armatum* is palatable, and most members of the Bhotiya community consider the plant to have magical properties and religious significance. The use of Timur in alcohol, as a spice, as a leech repellent, etc., is a more common application of the species (Table 32.2).

Over the years, an indigenous business pattern related to *Z. armatum* trade in the region has evolved into a social mechanism for exchange and distribution to villages and people in surrounding areas, although it had not found previously. In return, cereals, millets, fruits, and pulses that do not grow in their native villages are collected, along with other items such as woolen garments. This type of reciprocity also exists with people who have moved from the mountains and now living in far-off cities and towns. With the rise of pharmaceutical companies, *Z. armatum* has become a profitable non-timber forest product, and its fruit is used to make various types of toothpaste, which has increased market demand (Table 32.3).

PHYTOPHARMACOLOGY

The biological activities of plants are dependent on the composition of their secondary metabolites (i.e., phytochemicals). These compounds are non-nutritive and synthesized by plants in response to external biotic and abiotic factors. Different chemical classes of phytochemicals have been identified in *Z. armatum* species, such as alkaloids, coumarins, flavonoids, terpenes, and phenolic acids,

TABLE 32.2
Uses of *Z. armatum* among the Bhotiyas[1]

S. No.	Usages	Regularity of Use (n=86) %			
		Frequently	Sometimes	Very Rarely	Out of Use
1	Alcohol preparation	Nil	Nil	3.48	96.51
2	Cure for cough and cold	32.55	34.88	32.55	Nil
3	Cure for fever	36.04	36.04	27.90	Nil
4	Cure for *bai-gola*	100	Nil	Nil	Nil
5	*Dunkcha*	31.39	33.72	34.88	Nil
6	Leech repellent	11.62	32.55	10.46	45.34
7	Spice	Nil	20.93	11.62	67.44
8	*Timur hag* (soup)	44.18	32.55	23.25	Nil
9	Toothbrush	9.30	Nil	67.44	23.25
10	Toothache cure	Nil	44.18	24.41	31.39
11	Vermicide	81.39	11.62	6.97	Nil

TABLE 32.3
Traditional uses of *Z. armatum* Vis-à-Vis Modern Applications[1]

Plant Part Used	Traditional Uses	Modern Uses
Fruits	1. Alcoholic beverages	1. Dabur Red Gel Toothpaste
	2. Cure for cough and cold	2. Dabur Toothpaste
	3. Cure for toothache	3. Dabur Lal Dant Manjan
	4. Cure for fever	4. Insect repellent
	5. Dunkcha	5. MDH Dant Manjan
	6. Leech repellent	6. Vermicide
	7. Spices	
	8. Vermicide	
	9. Cure a locally understood ailment called 'bai-gola'	
Stem	Sticks i. Toothbrush	
	ii. Walking sticks	

the most reported among all the classes.[1] Carbonyl compounds, linalool, α-phellandrene, linalyl acetate, sesquiterpenes, hydrocarbons, fragarine, dictamine, skimmianine, xanthoplanine, and magnoflorine are the main ingredients of the *Z. armatum* species.[21,22] Many more fragrances in food and beverages, e.g., citronella, fennel, geranium, lavender, and rosemary, are known to be added with *Z. armatum* essential oil.[23,24] Plant *Z. armatum* also contains β-sitosterol, tambulatin, linalool, aramatamide, tamblin, asarinin, fragesin, and lignans. The bark of the plant contains berberine, a yellow crystalline compound.[25] Due to the unique chemical composition of phytochemicals, plant *Z. armatum* is expected to be a more focused plant species in future investigations for modern green medicines.[25]

The *Z. armatum* plant is mainly used to treat cramps in the legs, gum bleeding, toothache, rheumatism, skin disease, varicose ulcers, varicose veins, fever, low blood pressure, fibrositis, inflammation, circulation disorders, lymphatic system disorders, etc.[26] Fruits and seeds are usually used as a chow mein condiment and spice in momos, thukpa, biscuits, sweetened cakes, etc. The fruit part of the plant is used as an insect repellent and to purify the water.[27] Its fruits are used as a flavoring agent due to the aromatic fragrance present in them.[26]

Folk applications of *Z. armatum* have good results in diabetic management. Biological investigations confirm the antidiabetic activity of oral medication, which significantly reduces blood glucose levels, low-density lipids, and *very-low-density lipoprotein*.[28]

The depressant activity of plant *Z. armatum* has been checked out by bioassay-guided fraction, which reveals its potency as an antidepressant. Biochemical and molecular studies have revealed the seed part of the species as a potent antidepressant moiety.[29] The ethanolic extract of *Z. armatum* has hepatoprotective properties. It increases the levels of hepatic enzymes against CCl_4-damaged liver, more particularly decreasing the marker enzyme leakage.[30]

Z. armatum has an antispasmodic effect,[31] and its hexane extract has been reported to have a good antispasmodic effect.[32,33] Crude extract of *Z. armatum* has been identified for enhancing the improvement in gastrointestinal and cardiovascular health by the concentration effect of potassium and calcium.[34] A detailed study of the memory-enhancing herb on *Z. armatum* was conducted using its hydroalcoholic extract, which reveals it as a good memory-enhancing plant species.[35] The stem bark extract in animal studies has revealed the inhibition of cyclo-oxygenase[36] and an analgesic effect.[37,38] The alcoholic extracts of *Z. armatum* fruits have free radical scavenging activities.[39] These activities may affect microorganisms such as *Bacillus subtilis*, *Alternaria brassicicola*, etc.[40,41]

The *Z. armatum* plant has been reported to have larvicidal properties against the *Culex pipiens*, *Aedes aegypti*, and *Anopheles stephensi*.[42] Fruits of the *Z. armatum* have been reported for piscicide activity. Alcoholic extract of *Z. armatum* is rich in minerals (e.g., magnesium, potassium, sodium, etc.) and has been reported harmful to air-breathing catfish, and different investigations have revealed its effect on piscicide activities.[43] Research on the essential oil of *Z. armatum* has confirmed its repellent activity.[44] The insecticidal activity of *Z. armatum* is associated with the acetylcholinesterase (AChE) activity of its volatile oil. Potent fumigant toxicity of the species has been observed, but no direct correlation between AChE inhibition and fly toxicity could be established.[45]

SCOPE AND OPPORTUNITIES

The information gathered from various articles, annual reports, books, journals, proceedings, and web-based materials reveals that *Z. armatum* has a potent trade value with a high manifold application in allopathy, Ayurveda, general pharmacy, and other industries. The market rates of *Z. armatum* have been reported as INR (Indian National Rupee) 12–15 per kg in villages and local markets before 2000 AD. The local market price was Rs. 45 per kg in hilly Uttarakhand, India, whereas it was INR 150–200 per kg in the plains at the same time in the year 2000 AD. As a result, average household incomes in the Dharchula and Munsiyari blocks of District Pithoragarh (Uttarakhand) were around INR 700 in a season. About 4 hours of work in collection earned over INR 50 per head per day, an amount more than the minimum wage rate in the state policy then. Mostly, children, women, and elderly people who were otherwise unproductive collect the herb, and *Z. armatum* was recorded for the significant cash flows in the Malla and Talla Dumor villages and earned together around INR 82,620.[1] The *Z. armatum* species is extensively used in the different formulations of the Indian system of medicine. A few tricks of the collection mechanisms adopted by the local people are harmful to the existence of the *Z. armatum* population, and it looks for immediate efforts for its conservation. Because of its current demands, the plantation of the species is a viable source of income for poor villagers. *Z. armatum* can be grown on unproductive, marginal land and in forested land as an understory shrub.

With its diverse applications and current trade demands, the plant species can be utilized to develop different commodities of daily use, and more extensive investigations on the species for individual ingredients can lead to novel innovations in green medicines.

REFERENCES

1. Kala CP, Farooquee NA, Dhar U. 2005. Traditional uses and conservation of Timur (*Zanthoxylum armatum* DC.) through social institution in Uttaranchal Himalaya, India. *Conservation & Society*. 3 (1): 224–230.
2. Thokchom PS, Okram MS. 2011. Phytochemical and pharmacological profile of *Zanthoxylum armatum* DC: An overview. *Indian Journal of Natural Products and Resources*. 2 (3): 275–285.
3. Gupta S, Bhaskar S, Andola HC. 2011. Altitudinal variation in essential oil in leaves of *Zanthoxylum alatum* Roxb. A high value aromatic tree from Uttarakhand. *Journal of Medicinal Plants Research*. 5 (3): 348–351.
4. Vana PD. 2008. *Agro-Technique Study Carried Out by Regional Station, National Bureau of Plant genetic Resources, Dist Niglat*, Nainital, Uttarakhand, B- RRL, CSIR, Itanagar, Arunachal Pradesh. Teri Press. India, New Delhi. pp. 231–234.
5. Farooquee NA. 1994. Transhumance in the Central Himalaya: a study of its impact on environment. Ph.D. thesis, HNB Garhwal University, Srinagar, Garhwal, India.
6. Kala CR. 2004. Revitalizing traditional herbal therapy by exploring medicinal plants: a case study of Uttaranchal State in India. In: *Indigenous Knowledges: Transforming the Academy*. Farmer BL, Maretzki A, Semali L. (Eds.) Pennsylvania State University, Pennsylvania. pp. 15–21.
7. Den Hertog, WH, Wiersum KF. 2000. Timur (*Zanthoxylum armatum*) production in Nepal: dynamics in non-timber forest resource management. *Mountain Research and Development*. 20: 1.
8. Bhattacharjee A, Biplab Kumar D, Das B, Dkhar D, Kachari D. 2019. *Zanthoxylum armatum*: a systemic review of its ethnomedicinal properties, phytochemistry, pharmacology and toxicology. *Advances in Pharmacology and Clinical Trials*. 4 (3): 000162.
9. Barkatullah IM, Hussain F. 2009. Ethnobotanical studies of plants of Charkotli Hills, Batkhela District, Malakand, Pakistan. *Frontiers of Biology in China*. 4: 539–548.
10. Abbasi AM, Khan MA, Ahmed M, Zafar M. 2010. Herbal medicines used to cure various ailments by the inhibitants of Abbottabad district, Northwest Frontier Province, Pakistan. *Indian Journal of Traditional Knowledge*. 9: 175–183.
11. Negi JS, Bisht VK, Bhandari AK, Singh P, Sundriyal RC. 2011. Chemical constituents and biological activities of the genus *Zanthoxylum*: a review. *African Journal of Pure and Applied Chemistry*. 5 (12): 412–416.
12. Barkatullah M, Muhammad N, Rehman I, Rehman MU, Khan A. 2013. Chemical composition and biological screening of essential oils of *Zanthoxylum armatum* DC leaves. *Journal of Clinical Toxicology*. 3 (5): 1–6.
13. Tiwary M, Naik SN, Tewary DK, Mittal PK, Yadav S. 2007. Chemical composition and larvicidal activities of the essential oil of *Zanthoxylum armatum* DC (Rutaceae) against three mosquito vectors. *Journal of Vector Borne Diseases*. 44 (3): 198–204.
14. Singh G, Kapoor IPS, Singh P, Carola SH, Lampasona MP, Catalan CA. 2013. Chemistry and antioxidant properties of essential oil and oleoresins extracted from the seeds of tomer (*Zanthoxylum armatum* DC). *International Journal of Food Properties*. 16 (2): 288–300.

15. Ramidi R, Ali M, Negueruela AV, Pérez-Alonso MJ. 1998. Chemical composition of the seed oil of *Zanthoxylum alatum* Roxb. *Journal of Essential Oil Research*. 10 (2): 127–130.
16. Barua CC, Yasmin N, Elancheran R. 2018. A review on effective utilization, phytochemical compounds, pharmacological intervention of a popularly used plant for developing a new drug: *Zanthoxylum armatum* with reference to its anticancer activity. *MOJ Bioequivalence & Bioavailability*. 5(3): 156–167. https://doi.org/10.15406/mojbb.2018.05.00097
17. Watson E. 2013. *The Principal Articles of Chinese Commerce*, 2nd Edition. Statistical Department of the Inspectorate General of Customs, Shanghai. pp. 491.
18. Roi Jacques SJ. 1955. *Traite des plantes medicinales chinoises*. Lechevalier, Paris. pp. 198.
19. Brijwal L, Aseesh P, Tamta S. 2013. An overview on phytomedicinal approaches of *Zanthoxylum armatum* DC: an important magical medicinal plant. *Journal of Medicinal Plants Research*. 7 (8): 366–370.
20. Özkan M, Mutiso PB, Nahar L, Liu P, Brown S, Wang W, Sarker SD. 2013. *Zanthoxylum usambarense* (Engl.) Kokwaro (Rutaceae) extracts inhibit the growth of the breast cancer cell lines MDA-MB-231 and MCF-7, but not the brain tumour cell line U251 in vitro. *Phytotherapy Research*. 27 (5): 787–790.
21. Kapoor LD. 1990. *Handbook of Ayurvedic Medicinal Plants*. CRC Press, Boca Raton, FL. pp. 339–340.
22. Curtis CF, Lives JD, Baolib LU, Renz A. 1998. Natural and synthetic repellents. In: *Appropriate Technology in Vector Control*. Curtis CF (Ed.) CRC Press, Boca Raton, FL. pp. 75–92.
23. Brown M, Hebert AA. 1997. Insect repellents: an overview. *Journal of the American Academy of Dermatology*. 36: 243–249.
24. Ranawat LS, Bhatt J, Patel J. 2010. Hepatoprotective activity of ethanolic extracts of bark of *Zanthoxylum armatum* DC. in CCl_4 induced hepatic damage in rats. *Journal of Ethnopharmacology*. 127: 777–780.
25. Siddhanadham AS, Yejella R, Prava R. 2017. Isolation, characterization, biological evaluation of two new lignans from methanolic extract of bark of *Zanthoxylum armatum*. *International Journal of Pharmacognosy and Phytochemistry*. 9 (3): 395–399.
26. Zoolfa N, Singh S, Kumar D, Tandon SS. 2017. Characterization and evaluation of bioactive polyphenolic constituent form *Zanthoxyllum armatum*. A traditionally used plant. *Biomedicine and Pharmacotherapy*. 89: 366–375.
27. EPPO Global Database. 2021. *Zanthoxylum armatum* (ZANAP) EPPO.
28. Karki H, Upadhayay K, Pal H. 2014. Antidiabetic potential of *Zanthoxylum armatum* bark extract on streptozotocin-induced diabetic rats. *International Journal of Green Pharmacy*. 8 (2): 77–83.
29. Barua CC, Haloi P, Saikia B. 2018. *Zanthoxyllum alatum* abrogates lipopolysaccharides-induced depression-like behaviours in mice by modulating neuroinflammation and monoamine neurotransmitters in the hippocampus. *Pharmaceutical Biology*. 56 (1): 245–252.
30. Verma N, Khosa, RL. 2010. Hepatoprotective activity of leaves of *Z. armatum* DC in CCl_4-induced hepatotoxicity in rats. *Indian Journal of Biochemistry and Biophysics*. 47 (2): 124–127.
31. Saikia B, Barua CC, Haloi P. 2017. Anticholinergic, antihistaminic, and antiserotonergic activity of n-hexane extract of *Zanthoxylum alatum* seeds on isolated tissue preparations: an ex vivo study. *Indian Journal of Pharmacology*. 49 (1): 42–48.
32. Hemming JM, Guarraci FA, Firth TA. 2010. Actions of histamine on muscle and ganglia of the guinea pig gallbladder. *American Journal of Physiology Gastrointestinal and Liver Physiology*. 279 (3): 622–630.
33. Matsumoto T, Horiuchi M, Kamata K. 2009. Effects of *Bidens pilosa* L. var. radiata SCHERFF treated with enzyme on histamine-induced contraction of guinea pig ileum and on histamine release from mast cells. *Journal of Smooth Muscle Research*. 45 (2–3): 75–86.
34. Gilani SN, Khan A, Gilani AH. 2010. Pharmacological basis for the medicinal use of *Zanthoxylum armatum* in gut, airways, and cardiovascular disorders. *Phytotherapy Reserach*. 24 (4): 553–558.
35. Saikia B, Barua CC, Sarma J. 2018. *Zanthoxyllum alatum* ameliorates scopolamine-induced amnesia in rats: behavioral, biochemical, and molecular evidence. *Indian Journal of Pharmacology*. 50 (1): 30–38.
36. Sati SC, Sati MD, Raturi R, Badoni PP. 2011. A new flavonoidal glycoside from stem bark of *Zanthoxylum armatum*. *IJPI'S Journal of Pharmacognosy and Herbal Formulations*. 1 (2): 29–32.
37. Kaur V, Kumar T, Bora SK. 2011. Pharmacological evaluation of *Zanthoxylum armatum* root extract on analgesic and anti-inflammatory activity. *Journal of Pharmacy Research*. 4 (8): 25–61.
38. Guo T, Denq YX, Xie H, Yao CY, Cai CC, Pan SL, Wanq YL. 2010. Antinociceptive and anti-inflammatory activities of ethyl acetate fraction from *Zanthoxylum armatum* in mice. *Phytotherapy*. 82 (3): 347–351.
39. Parajuli RR, Tiwari RD, Chaudhary RP, Gupta VN. 2005. Fungitoxicity of the essential oils of some aromatic plants of managing against *Alternaria brassicicola*. *Scientific World*. 3 (3): 39–43.
40. Batool F, Sabir SM, Rocha JBT, Shah AH, Saify ZS, Ahmed SD. 2010. Evaluation of antioxidant and free radical scavenging activities of fruit extract from *Zanthoxylum alatum*: a commonly used spice from Pakistan. *Pakistan Journal of Botany*. 42 (6): 4299–4311.
41. Upadhyaya K, Ashok PK. 2010. Concentration dependent antioxidant activity of *Zanthoxylum armatum*. *Journal of Pharmacy Research*. 3 (7): 1581–1582.
42. Yun Z, Ying-Hui P, Dong-Qin Z, Fei-Fei C, Qio-Hui Q, Yi H. 2010. Insecticidal activity of essential oil from *Zanthoxylum armatum* fructification against two mosquito species. *Guihaia*. 30 (2): 274–279.
43. Ramanujam SN, Ratha BK. 2008. Effect of alcohol extract of a natural piscicide-Fruits of *Zanthoxylum armatum* DC. on Mg2+- and Na+, K+ATPase activity in various tissues of a freshwater air-breathing fish, *Heteropneustes fossilis*. *Aquaculture*. 283 (4): 77–82.
44. Dube S, Kumar A, Tripathi SC. 1961. Antifungal and insect repellent activity of essential oil of *Zanthoxylum armatum* linn. *Current Science*. 30: 223–224.
45. Nirmala P, Pramod KJ, Pankaj PR, Sangeeta R. 2018. *Zanthoxylum armatum* DC: current knowledge, gaps, and opportunities in Nepal. *Journal of Ethnopharcology*. 32 (4): 84–96.

33 *Ziziphus mauritiana* (Ber)

INTRODUCTION

Z. mauritiana Lam. (synonym: *Z. jujuba*, fam.: Rhamnaceae) is a flowering tree, widely grown for its edible fruit and found on roadsides, in the wild, and in bushes throughout the Indian subcontinent.[1] Its fruits are of variable shape and size. At the unripe stage, fruits are a bit juicy and have a pleasant aroma. The skin of fruits is glossy, smooth, and thin but tight. Fruits are edible and used in other forms such as candied, dried, juiced (Ber butter), and pickled. *Z. mauritiana* is a plant of the tropical and subtropical regions, and originally it is native to India. Currently, it is widely naturalized in the tropical regions of Africa, China, Afghanistan, Malaysia, Australia, and some Pacific regions.[2]

In India, *Z. mauritiana* is distributed in warm-temperate, tropical, and subtropical regions of the Himalayas, Bihar, Madhya Pradesh, Rajasthan, Uttar Pradesh, Meghalaya, Sikkim, Maharashtra, Arunachal Pradesh, and Thar Desert regions of the Indian subcontinent. Species *Z. mauritiana* is globally distributed in the Paleotropics.[3] Its fruits are a rich source of dietary nutrients utilized in Ayurvedic medicine to treat various body ailments.[4] *Z. mauritiana* (Hindi name: Ber, Eng.: Indian jujube)[5] is the most nutritious fruit in the world and has gained much horticultural attention in India.[6] In semi-arid regions of the world, species *Z. mauritiana* is considered an underutilized fruit crop and is successfully cultivated in the marginal ecosystem of the subtropics and tropics.[7] The fruits of *Z. mauritiana* enhance the livelihood of the rural people and reduce land degradation in the region. Sustained production of fruits of the species can improve household incomes irrespective of drought, as the tree is tolerant to salinity and drought and can even grow on poorly degraded land.[8] A study revealed that peach trees exhibited severe drought stress signs after 100 days, whereas *Z. mauritiana* plants in the same area showed no signs of drought stress, indicating that the species avoids drought stress by using the deep soil water reserves.[9] The study concluded that the tree is suitable for drought-prone areas where crop production is limited. The *Z. mauritiana* plant is hoped to be used for eradicating extreme hunger and poverty in drought-prone tropical and subtropical areas. Currently, there is an international focus on ending hunger, improving nutrition, achieving food security, and promoting sustainable agriculture practices globally. Fruits of *Z. mauritiana* can compensate local farmers for food scarcity due to poor crop harvests and provide a potential source of income in local markets.[9]

The *Ziziphus* genus is comprised of approximately 170 species and is commonly used to treat various diseases. The ripe fruits of the species are mostly consumed raw globally, and the leaves are cooked and eaten in Indonesia.[10]

ETHNOMEDICAL APPLICATIONS

The plant *Z. mauritiana* has been described in the Ramayana and has been used as food for centuries in the subcontinent. In India, the plant species is sacred to the Lord Siva and is respected as 'the tree which removes sorrow', maybe because of its calming properties.[11] Chalise et al. described the centuries-old medicinal properties of *Z. mauritiana* fruits for various purposes, especially in Korean and Chinese traditional medicine,[12] which has a successful history of folk applications for many ailments and diseases in China for over 4,000 years.[13] Ethnobotanical data reveals that leaves of the *Z. mauritiana* plant are used to treat typhoid, diarrhea, liver troubles, wounds, asthma, and fever. It is used as an astringent in different folklore.[14]

Z. mauritiana fruits are used in folk medicine for treating wounds, anodynes, and abscesses. It is used as a styptic, for purifying blood, and as a tonic.[15] The root paste of *Z. mauritiana* is traditionally used to treat worms.[16] According to Ayurveda, *Z. mauritiana* root is commonly used as a cooling and bitter tonic, relieving headaches, coughs, and biliousness. The bark is astringent, cures boils, and is a common remedy for diarrhea and dysentery.[17] The roots are bitter and used to treat chronic fever, old wounds, cephalalgia, ulcers, and headaches. The leaves are antipyretic, bitter, anthelmintic, and cooling, and are useful in asthma, typhoid fever, and stomatitis.[18] The fruits are sweet, mucilaginous, aphrodisiac, appetizing, and nutritious. The seeds are applied to treat leucorrhea, astringent purposes, and eye disorders. Its tonic is helpful for the good health of the brain and heart.[19] The seeds are acrid and help to relieve asthma, thirst, burning sensation, vomiting, cough, and diarrhea, and are also helpful in physical weakness, pain, rheumatic symptomology, and insomnia.[20]

A few medicinal applications of *Z. mauritiana* in India are similar to those of *Z. mucronata* in Africa for treating dysentery, vomiting, diarrhea, rheumatism, nausea, ulcers, mental retardation, fever, and wounds.[21] Roots, leaves, seeds, and bark are the common parts used as medicine, and in some instances, flowers are also part of traditional therapy. Ingredients such as alkaloids (amphibines, mauritines, hysodricanin, frangufoline, aralionin, and scutianin) have been reported in *Z. mauritiana*.[22] Generally, fresh fruits of *Z. mauritiana* are consumed and are dehydrated for future use, which are very nutritious.[23] The ripe fruits, after drying, are ground to make powder[24] to be used for preparing jam, baking, and making a traditional loaf in sub-Saharan Africa.[25] A famine food with flour is prepared after pounding the *Z. mauritiana* fruits. In Southeast Asia, ripened fruits are eaten with salt. Mature, unripe green fruits are used in India to prepare jelly, pickles, and chutney.[26] A very popular cold

DOI: 10.1201/9781003512868-35

drink is prepared from ripened fruits after crushing them with water. The powder of the ripened fruits after sun drying is prepared for out-of-season consumption. The sweet, fleshy *Z. mauritiana* fruits are used in India to prepare a nutritious drink called 'jujube tea', which is enriched with vitamins A, B1, and C, natural sugar, and is commonly used to treat various health ailments ranging from anemia to sore throat.[11] In Indonesia, cooked young leaves are eaten as a relish.[26] In Venezuela, a jujube liqueur is sold under the name 'Crema de Ponsigue'.[27] Seed kernels of *Z. mauritiana* are also eaten during drought and famine. In Sudan, the pulp of the fruit is fermented, dried, and soaked in water to produce a refreshing drink that is rich in vitamin C.[28] The surplus fruits of the species in drought-prone areas of Zimbabwe are sun-dried and made into porridge, while an intoxicating spirit, 'kachasu', is distilled from the pulp of fermented fruits.[29]

A liquor, 'crema de ponsigue', is prepared from the fruits of *Z. mauritiana* in South America.[30] The dried fruits are fermented for 6–7 days after pounding and distilled; the distillate is known as 'kachasu', an intoxicating spirit, and its sale generates income as well as in 'nhimbe', a cooperative work in Zimbabwe for community development programs. A 25 L bucket of *Z. mauritiana* produces 5 L of the 'kachasu'. Kachasu is also used during funerals and in traditional rainmaking ceremonies in Zimbabwe.[31] A traditional non-alcoholic refreshing drink, a brew from *Z. mauritiana* fruits known as 'Gununzvi' in Zimbabwe, is used by villagers during fieldwork or between meals.[31]

In Ethiopia, fruits are used to stupefy fish, while in Burma, the fruits are used in silk dyeing. The root bark and stem bark of the species are used in tanning. The bark is pounded and mashed in water to generate reddish, grey, and brown dyes, which are sold to earn a living.[30] The Indian *Z. mauritiana* plant is used to rear the *Kerria lacca*, a lac insect, which sucks the juice from the leaves and covers them with an orange-red resinous substance known as lac. Additionally, the leaves are also gathered to feed silkworms to generate a highly prized tussar silk.[32]

PHYTOPHARMACOLOGY

Z. mauritiana is a fruiting tree that has folk implications against many diseases and ailments. Plant *Z. mauritiana* is used to treat liver troubles, typhoid, fever, diarrhea, asthma, and wounds, and as an astringent in ethnomedicine.[10] Leaves contain alkaloids, reducing sugar, steroids, glycosides, and tannins.[33] Chromatographic analysis of the plant extract followed by isolation, purification, and structure elucidation reveals the presence of β-sitosterol, α-amyrin, lupeol, stigmasterol, γ-fagarine, and β-amyrin.[34] Palmitic acid, methyl stearate, and α-linolenic acid are the major constituents of leaves of the species.[35] Pharmacological studies on leaf extract revealed promising antimicrobial, analgesic, sedative,[36] antidiarrheal,[34] antitumor, antidiabetic, cardiovascular, immunostimulant,[37] hepatoprotective,[38] anti-inflammatory,[39] and phagocytic[40] activities. Hossain et al. and Ashraf et al. have reported that chloroform-soluble extracts of leaves have thrombolytic and anticancer properties.[34,35] It has been reported that the fruits,[41] seeds,[2] roots,[42] and bark of the species possess promising antioxidant and cytotoxic properties.[43]

The leaves of the species are reported to prevent leucopenia significantly and noise-induced enhancement of neutrophil function compared with diazepam.[44] Seeds of the species have been reported for their antidiabetic and anticancer potentials. The ethanolic extracts of seeds of the species are reported to induce the death of cancer cells and significantly reduce tumor volume, as well as tumor cell count, after 13 days of treatment with a dose ranging from 100 to 800 mg/kg b.w.[2] The same extract has been reported for hypoglycemic properties on the administration of a dose of 800 mg/kg, b.w., along with the weight loss and reduced mortality of alloxan-induced diabetic animals.[45]

Mahesh and Satish have reported that the fruit of the species is medicine for indigestion, stomach problems, biliousness, astringency, laxatives, nausea, blood purification, throat troubles, and vomiting.[46] Mishra et al. reported the anticarcinogenic potential of the seed extract and mentioned that it reduces viable tumor cell count and tumor volume. Medical studies using the *Z. mauritiana* fruits and its extracts have deciphered that they inhibit the growth of tumor cells, lower blood pressure, reverse liver disease, and treat anemias.[2] The fruit extracts of *Z. mauritiana* have skincare properties and are used to diminish skin moisture and wrinkles and treat sunburn skin pain.[18] The fruits mixed with chili peppers and salt are eaten to treat biliousness and indigestion. The seeds are taken with buttermilk to stop vomiting, abdominal pains, and nausea during pregnancy. In traditional Chinese medicine, the crushed seeds of *Z. mauritiana* are used to treat insomnia and anxiety. The freshly prepared seed powder is mixed with oil and rubbed on rheumatic areas.[18]

The leaves of the species are applied as poultices to cure fever, asthma, and liver troubles.[18] The bark decoction is prescribed to cure dysentery and diarrhea. According to Dahiru et al., bark paste is applied to cure ulcers, sores, and wound dressings. The pounded roots are added to drinking water and given to humans for indigestion and to poultry suffering from diarrhea. Juice of the root bark is claimed to reduce rheumatism, epilepsy, and gout.[47] In northern parts of Nigeria, the dried root is used to treat diarrhea, one of the principal causes of infant death, though a strong dose of the root or bark may be toxic, resulting in poisoning of the patients.[18]

An infusion of flowers is used as an eye lotion.[6] The aqueous and methanolic extracts of the bark of the species have antimicrobial properties against *Pseudomonas aeruginosa*, *Streptococcus faecalis*, *Staphylococcus aureus*, *Enterobacter faecalis, Escherichia coli*, *Klebsiella pneumoniae*, *Proteus mirabilis*, and *Enterobacter faecium*.[48] The bark extracts of *Z. mauritiana* plants have potent antibacterial activity against pathogens causing urinary tract infections. The bark extracts of the species are used to treat vaginal infections.[48] The flowers of the species are internally used to cure jaundice and externally to treat skin ulcers and eye disease.[11]

SCOPE FOR INNOVATION

Value-added products, using modern technology like modified atmosphere packaging, may have increased benefits through international trade for household business of the species *Z. mauritiana*. Modern packaging techniques help maintain quality and prolong the shelf-life period during storage and subsequent marketing. Modified atmosphere packaging is a replacement of air in the pack with a desired gaseous combination. The fruit of the *Z. mauritiana* species can be processed into traditional non-alcoholic and alcoholic beverages that can be marketed like any other beverage. Traditional foods are currently in vogue due to their health-friendly contents compared to food products rich in fat; hence, there is a high market opportunity for the *Z. mauritiana* traditional food products.

Z. mauritiana, a fruiting crop of arid and semi-arid regions of the world, can be successfully cultivated in the marginal ecosystem of the subtropics and tropics for poverty alleviation and food security. The species tolerates extremely dry, very high temperatures, waterlogging, and saline soils. The tree is utilized for making furniture, fodder for animals, medicinal uses, and flowers for nectar. The tree reduces land degradation as it survives harsh environments where other tree species can hardly survive. *Z. mauritiana* can serve as an alternative source of livelihood through the trade of its value-added products.

REFERENCES

1. Ghani A. 2003. *Medicinal plants of Bangladesh: Chemical Constituents and Uses*. Asiatic Society of Bangladesh, Dhaka. pp. 434.
2. Mishra T, Kullar N, Bhatia A. 2011. Anticancer potential of aqueous ethanol seed extract of *Ziziphus maurtiana* against cancer cell lines and Ehrlich *Ascites Carcinoma. Evidence Based Complementary and Alternative Medicines*. Article ID 765029. 2011: 1–11.
3. Awasthi OP, More TA. 2009. Genetic diversity and status of *Ziziphus* in India. *Acta Horticulturae*. 840: 33–40.
4. Bisla SS, Daulta BS. 1988. Variability and heritability of some growth characters in ber (*Zizyphus mauritiana* Lamk). *Indian Journal of Horticulture*. 45: 29–33.
5. Kaaria S. 1998. *Ziziphus mauritiana*: a valuable tree for arid and semi-arid lands. https://winrock.org/ziziphus-mauritiana-a-valuable-tree-for-arid-and-semi-arid-lands/#:~:text=This%20species%20which%20is%20also%20known%20as%20ber%2C,and%20produce%20fruits%20in%20arid%20or%20semi-arid%20regionsas on 3rd June 2025.
6. Morton JF. 1987. *Indian Jujube. Fruits of Warm Climates*. Florida Fair Books, Miami.
7. Pareek S, Kitinoja L, Kaushik RA, Paliwal R. 2009. Postharvest physiology and storage of Ber. *Steward Postharvest Review*. 5 (5): 1–10.
8. Pareek OP. 2001. *Fruits for the Future 2: Ber. Ziziphus mauritiana Lam.- Field Manual for Extension Workers*. Published online, Cambridge University Press. ISBN 854-327-525.
9. Arndt SK, Clifford SC, Wanek W, Jones HG, Popp M. 2001. Physiological and morphological adaptations of the fruit tree *Ziziphus rotundifolia* in response to progressive drought stress. *Tree Physiology*. 21: 705–715.
10. Goyal M, Nagori BP, Sasmal D. 2012. Review on ethnomedicinal uses, pharmacological activity and phytochemical constituents *of Ziziphus mauritiana* (Z. jujuba Lam.). *Spatula DD*. 2(2): 107–116.
11. Meena S, Meena HP, Meena RS. 2014. Diversified uses of Ber (*Ziziphus* spp*). Popular Kheti*. 2 (1): 154–159.
12. Chalise JP, Acharya K, Gurung N, Bhusal R, Gurung R, Skalko-Basnet N. 2010. Antioxidant activity and polyphenol content in edible wild fruits form Nepal. *International Journal of Food Sciences and Nutrition*, 61 (4): 425–432.
13. Pareek S. 2013. Nutritional composition of jujube fruit. *Journal of Food and Agriculture*. 25 (6): 463–470.
14. Goyal M, Sasmal D, Nagori BP. 2012. Review on ethnomedicinal uses, pharmacological activity and phytochemical constituents of *Ziziphus mauritiana* (Z. jujuba Lam.)-. Spatula D D Tamamlayıcı Tıp ve İlaç Geliştirme Alanında Hakemli Dergi. 2: 107–116.
15. Marwat SK, Khanetal MA. 2009. Fruit plant species mentioned in the Holy Quran and Ahadith and their ethnomedicinal importance. *American-Eurasian Journal of Agricultural Environmental Sciences*. 5 (2): 284–295.
16. Taylor RSL, Manandhar NP, Hudson JB, Towers GHN. 1996. Antiviral activities of Nepalese medicinal plants. *Journal of Ethnopharmacology*. 52 (3): 157–163.
17. Kirtikar KR, Basu BD. 1994. *Indian Medicinal Plants*, 2nd Edition. Bishen Sigh, Mahendrapal Singh, Dehradun. Vol. II. pp. 1–34.
18. Mishra T, Paice AG, Bhatia A. 2011. Use of seeds of Malay apple (*Ziziphus mauritiana*) and related species in health and disease. *Nuts and Seeds in Health and Disease Prevention*. 87: 733–739.
19. Kim KS. 2002. Effects of the *Zizyphus jujuba* seed extract on the lipid components in hyperlipidemic rats. *Journal of Food Science and Nutrition*. 7: 72–77.
20. Khare CP. 1995. *Ziziphus mauritiana. Encyclopedia of Indian Medicinal Plants*. Springer, New York. pp. 493 and 498.
21. Ara H, Abul Hassan MD, Khanam M. 2008. Taxonomic study of the genus *Ziziphus* Mill. (Rhamnaceae) of Bangladesh. *Bangladesh Journal of Plant Taxonomy*. 15 (1): 47–61.
22. Jossang A, Zahir A, Diakite D. 1996. Mauritine J, A cyclopeptide alkaloid from *Zizyphus mauritiana*. *Phytochemistry*. 42 (2): 565–567.
23. Memon AA, Memon N, Bhanger MI, Luthria DL. 2012. Phenolic acids composition of fruit extracts of Ber (*Z. mauritiana* L). *Pakistan Journal of Analytical & Environmental Chemistry*, 13 (2): 123–128.
24. Saran PL, Godara AK, Dalal RP. 2007. Biodiversity among Indian Jujube (*Z. mauritiana* L) Genotypes for powdery mildew and other traits. *Notulae Botanicae Horti Agrobotanici Cluj-Napoca*. 35 (2): 1–15.
25. Williams TO. 1998. Multiple uses of common pool resources in semi-arid West Africa: A survey of existing practices and options for sustainable resource management. *Natural Resource Perspectives*. https://media.odi.org/documents/2885.pdf, as of 18th June 2025.
26. Gupta MK, Bhandari AK, Ramesh KS. 2012. Pharmacognostical evaluations of the leaves of *Ziziphus mauritiana*. *Journal of Pharmaceutical and Research*. 3 (3): 818–812.

27. Azam-Ali S, Bonkkoungou E, Bowe C, deKock C, Godara A, Williams JT. 2006. *Fruits for the Future 2: Ber and Other Jujube*, 2nd Edition. International Centre for Under Utilised Crops, Southampton.
28. Baumer M. 1983. *Notes on Trees and Shrubs in Arid and Semi-Arid Regions*. FAO, EMASAR Phase.
29. Nyanga LK, Nout MJR, Tendekayi H, Gadaga TH, Boekhout T, Zwietering MH. 2008. Traditional processing of masau fruits (*Ziziphus mauritiana*) in Zimbabwe. *Food Microbiology*. 47 (1): 95–107.
30. Gadaga TH, Mutukumira AN, Narvhus JA, Feresu SB. 1999. A review of traditional fermented foods and beverages of Zimbabwe. *International Journal of Food Microbiology*. 53: 1–11.
31. Chazovachii B, Mutangi GT, Chitongo L, Mushuku A. 2012. Dry land livelihood strategies: Merlot (masawu) fruit utilisation in Dande area, Zimbabwe. *Journal of Sustainable Development in Africa*. 14 (3): 98–110.
32. Maruza IM, Musemwa L, Mapurazi S, Matsika P, Munyati VT, Ndhleve S. 2017. Future prospects of *Ziziphus mauritiana* in alleviating household food insecurity and illnesses in arid and semi-arid areas: a review. *World Development Perspectives*. 5: 1–6.
33. Parmar P, Bhatt S, Dhyani S, Jain A. 2012. Phytochemical studies of the secondary metabolites of *Ziziphus mauritiana* Lam. Leaves. *International Journal of Current Pharmaceutical Research*. 4: 153–155.
34. Hossain MJ, Sikder MAA, Kaisar MA, Haque MR, Chowdhury AA, Rashid MA. 2015. Phytochemical and biological investigations of methanol extract of leaves of *Ziziphus mauritiana* Lam. *Boletín Latinoamericano y del Caribe de Plantas Medicinales y Aromáticas*. 14: 179–189.
35. Ashraf A, Sarfraz RA, Anwar F, Shahid SA, Alkharfy KM. 2015. Chemical composition and biological activities of leaves of *Ziziphus mauritiana* L. native to Pakistan. *Pakistan Journal of Botany*. 47: 367–376.
36. Karon B, Ibrahim M., Mahmood A, Huq AKMM, Chowdhury MMU, Hossain A, Rashid MA 2011. Preliminary antimicrobial, cytotoxic and chemical investigations of Averrhoa bilimbi Linn. and Zizyphus mauritiana Lam. *Bangladesh Journal of Pharmacology*. 14: 127–131.
37. Sharma GN, Gaur A. 2013. *Ziziphus mauritiana* Lam.; An overview. *Indo American Journal of Pharmaceutical Sciences*. 3: 4560–4566.
38. Dahiru D, Obidoa O. 2007. Pretreatment of albino rats with aqueous leaf extract of *Ziziphus mauritiana* protects against alcohol-induced liver damage. *Tropical Journal of Pharmaceutical Research*. 6: 705–710.
39. Kumar RM, Gayatri N, Sivasudha T, Ruckmani K. 2017. Profiling of bioactive components present in *Ziziphus mauritiana* Lam for *in-vitro* antioxidant and *in- vivo* anti-inflammatory activities. *International Research Journal of Pharmacy*. 8: 19–24.
40. Wadekar RR, Patil KS. 2008. Effect of *Ziziphus mauritiana* leaf extracts on phagocytosis by human neutrophils. *Journal of Pharmacy Research*. 1: 79–83.
41. Esteki T, Urooj A. 2012. Antioxidant components and activity in the peel of *Ziziphus jujuba* Mill. *Journal of Pharmacy Research*. 5: 2705–2709.
42. Afzal S, Batool M, Ch BA, Ahmad A, Uzair M, Afzal K. 2017. Immunomodulatory, cytotoxicity, and antioxidant activities of roots of *Ziziphus mauritiana*. *Pharmacognosy Magazine*. 13: 262–265.
43. Rahman S. 2012. Antioxidant, analgesic, cytotoxic and antidiarrheal activities of ethanolic *Zizyphus mauritiana* bark extract. *Oriental Pharmacy and Experimental Medicine*. 12: 67–73.
44. Vakharia B, Adhvaryu M., Reddy N. 2014. Evaluation of adaptogenic potential of *Curcuma longa* and *Zizyphus mauritiana* against acute noise stress induced changes in guinea pigs. *The Journal of Alternative and Complementary Medicine*. 20 (5): A37–A37.
45. Bhatia A, Mishra T. 2010. Hypoglycemic activity of *Ziziphus mauritiana* aqueous ethanol seed extract in alloxan-induced diabetic mice. *Pharmaceutical Biology*. 48 (6): 604–610.
46. Mahesh B, Satish S. 2008. Antimicrobial activity of some important medicinal plant against plant and human pathogens. *World Journal of Agricultural Sciences*. 4: 839–843.
47. Dahiru D, Sini JM, John-Africa L. 2006. Anti-diarrhoeal activity of *Z. mauritiana* root extract in rodents. *African Journal of Biotechnology*. 5 (10): 941–945.
48. Dubey R, Dubey K, Scridhar C, Jayaveera KN. 2011. Human vaginal pathogen inhibition studies on aqueous, methanolic and saponins extracts of stem barks of *Ziziphus mauritiana*. *International Journal of Pharmaceutical Sciences and Research*. 2 (3): 659–663.

Section III

Conclusion

34 Safety and Regulatory Aspects

INTRODUCTION

Currently, there are rapid changes in socio-economic and environmental conditions, resulting in rapid biodiversity loss globally, and reduced possibilities for food alternatives. Researchers have enlisted several foods that were consumed during wars, famines, prolonged natural disasters, or pandemics, especially from Asia, on wild edible plant resources.[1] Wild edible plants grow without human help, by simply using the available natural resources, and are undervalued due to a lack of knowledge about their therapeutic ingredients and nutritional properties. There is a need to focus on their socio-economic relevance and their worthiness in the agri-food industry. Consumption of 100 and 200 g of some of the wild edible plants covers up to 50% of the endorsed daily intake of fiber and proteins, along with minerals.[2]

The Food and Agriculture Organization estimated in 2016 that about 100 million people consumed wild edible plants in Europe.[2] The importance of these species is highlighted by different studies conducted in the Mediterranean region, which has a high diversity of wild edible plants, especially in Spain, Italy, Portugal, and Greece. These plant species are rich in macronutrients (i.e., fat, fiber, protein, alcohol, and carbohydrates). Nowadays, traditional diets have been replaced partially by society due to changed lifestyles, and diets rich in sugars and refined fats have large caloric results, resulting in increased incidences of metabolic syndromes, e.g., coronary heart disease, obesity, strokes, and type II diabetes.[2] *Bryonia dioica* Jacq. is a plant with 440 kcal per 100 g (dry weight), the highest energy value ever calculated.[2]

Sugars are the main source of energy for plants and play a role in metabolism, controlling multiple biological processes, including embryogenesis. Sugars are categorized as monosaccharides, disaccharides, and polysaccharides and remain the source of energy for cells to stay alive.[2] Organic acids in plants are weak acids and can be categorized in four ways based on (i) the nature of the carbon chain (aromatic, aliphatic, etc.); (ii) saturated or unsaturated properties; (iii) substituted or unsubstituted parameters; and (iv) number of functional groups. All these acids have an essential role in the physiology of plants, such as the Krebs cycle, balancing the redox potential of cells, pH regulation, organoleptic properties (such as aroma, taste, and color of both vegetables and fruits), etc.[2] Mainly three organic acids (malic, oxalic, and shikimic) are found in wild edible plants,[2] and oxalic acid is common for the Asteraceae family.[2]

The nutritional quality of the Mediterranean diet (MD) is appraised as one of the best in the world. The unique combination of vitamins and minerals is its main potential.[2,3] Minerals contribute 6.1% to body weight (typically 65 kg) and rank fourth in body composition,[2] underscoring their health significance, particularly for nutrients like zinc, iron, and iodine. Deficiency of iron affects about 18% of the world's infants under 5 years of age, along with expecting mothers.[2,4] Zinc deficiency is about 17%, and iodine affects about 28% of the world's population.[2,4] The soil is the main source of minerals and passes them to plants and to humans through the food chain. The daily intake of each element has been listed by the Food & Drug Administration (FDA).[5]

Floristic inventories on the use of wild edible plants have been reported in the Americas, Africa, Asia, and Europe,[5,6] with 1103 taxa have been reported from Italy as alimurgic species,[6] describing the significance of knowledge on edible vascular plants in Italy, mainly focused on the cultural enhancement. Plants cultivated in rural kitchen gardens have been examined, but in fewer numbers in Europe, though they have been high in tropical areas.[7,8] Results from these inventories have revealed that local knowledge is valuable to utilizing plants along with land protection strategies. The information obtained from these inventories is useful in marginal areas of agriculture to increase the availability of crops tolerant to extreme climatic factors, e.g., low rainfall, salinity, and high temperatures, and develop strategies for the impacts of climate change and altered conditions of agriculture.[9] Similar studies on wild edible fruiting plants may play a key role in the 'Sustainable Development Agenda-2030. Wild edible fruiting plants are a potential source of health-friendly ingredients, and biochemical research on these species, including documentation of folk applications, procedures, and their phytochemical profiles, is the need of the hour. Additionally, investigations to improve sensory quality and nutritional composition with other foods and to find innovative methods to develop value-added products are still open vistas.

PREFERRED CHOICE: A LOOK AT HERBAL RESOURCES

Physical, mental, and cognitive health have been reported manyfold better with frequent consumption of vegetables and fruits.[10] Though wild fruiting edible plants alone do not fully explain the health-promoting effects of their consumption, researchers have searched for and reported health-promoting compounds (i.e., a combination of phytochemicals, vitamins, trace elements, etc.) from these species and have developed specifications for a few by this time.[10] Polyphenols have been reported as the main ingredients in these compounds, generated in plants in response to abiotic stress.[11] There are over 8,000 polyphenols,

DOI: 10.1201/9781003512868-37

which share common properties.[11] The structure of polyphenols varies extensively, but the presence of more than one OH^- (hydroxyl) group attached directly to one or more aromatic rings is the main characteristic of the chemical class. Polyphenols are measured as 'total polyphenol content', a marker of the bioactivity of the herbal product.[11,12] Researchers have experimentally tested these ingredients for other health-promoting properties, and in vitro studies have realized a gap between the high dosage of these phytochemicals and the low bioavailability of most of these in actual human metabolism.[13] Further, in foods, herbal polyphenols exert a synergistic effect with different chemical classes of herbal origin in the human body, resulting in increased anti-inflammatory effects and antioxidant capacity. These compounds, as an herbal mixture, interact with the gut microbiome and target signaling pathways. Researchers have reported over 5,000 dietary phytochemicals in fruits, vegetables, whole grains, and nuts, with many more are still not known. Their consumption as green edible plants promotes health and longevity.[14]

Further detailed biomolecular research on these molecules has depicted their mechanisms of action in promoting health, though the quantity of these ingredients varies because of environmental and genetic variation, stage of utilization, and the plant part used. The Mediterranean-style boiled vegetable mixture, the MD, is rich in different classes of phytochemicals, ranging from traces to milligrams, and enhances the availability of at least a little of each health-promoting ingredient, though they may be unhealthy in higher quantities.[15] The Mediterranean-style boiled wild edible vegetable food has mainly 10 unique ingredients (namely, lutein, caffeic acid, flavonoids, polysaccharides, melatonin, carotenoids, phenolic acids, polyphenols, and silicon along with silicates), which are supposed to prevent Alzheimer's disease.[12] Similar studies on MD to prevent atherosclerosis, arthritis, diabetes, different cancers, etc., and protect different body organs and body systems (e.g., the nervous system, cardiovascular system, liver, kidneys, etc.) have been tested and concluded to consume green edible plants, whether cultivated or wild.[12] Though the herbals used in MD often contain 52 chemical ingredients as health-promoting ingredients and ions, it is necessary to examine new parts of otherwise edible plants that do not have any non-nutrient or toxic ingredients.[12,15]

INNOVATIVE SPIRIT, RISK, AND REMEDY

Currently, many people are interested in domesticating wild edible fruiting plants in their domestic gardens, though the inexpert pickers can easily confuse the morphological characteristics of the young plant of edible species with those of toxic ones. Cornara et al. (2018) have reported cases of hospitalization, and a few of these with a fatal end, due to accidental ingestion of wild plants.[16] In the Mediterranean region, the faith and spirit to use MD on a special occasion, plant species are collected either from the forests or semi-domesticated sources and are used for culinary purposes, e.g., *Spinacia oleracea* L. (spinach), *Borago officinalis* L. (borage), etc. The young leaves of spinach and borage have many similarities with poisonous plants, and it is difficult to ascertain their identity. Borage, an annual herb, is traditionally used for medicinal and culinary purposes, and its seed oil has a commercial value. Borage leaves have a cucumber-like taste and are used in salads and as vegetables. Young leaves of borage have many similarities with *Mandragora autumnalis* Bertol. (mandrake), and it is difficult to distinguish between the leaves of *S. oleracea* and *Digitalis purpurea* L. (foxglove), both of which are highly poisonous.[16] There have been 50 cases of accidental poisoning by mandrake, and six cases of foxglove in Italy from 1995 to 2007.[16] Further, two different cases of mandrake poisoning and hospitalization were reported alone in Italy in 2017 due to confusion/misidentification/adulteration with spinach in a commercial frozen vegetable.[16] Furthermore, poisoning due to Datura (*Datura stramonium* L.) leaves, although they are an edible wild vegetable[17] and a popular Ayurvedic medicinal herb,[18] due to overdose also deciphers the need for proper dose determination for its food and medicinal utility.

The incidence of phyto-intoxication can be checked by a multidisciplinary approach and using a product specification for wild edible plants, such as the % of foreign material and % poisonous plant product, along with standard protocols for collection and reliable identification, which may be useful for different stakeholders. Additionally, molecular markers for the species, using techniques like TLC, HPTLC, HPLC, GC, UV-Vis., FTIR, etc. along with DNA fingerprints, confirm the possibility of differentiating among species due to high interspecific genetic variability. The chromatographic and spectral fingerprints of each plant species are useful in the identification of poisonous and edible plants.

REGULATORY PROVISIONS AND THE GLOBAL SCENARIO

Currently, the regulatory status of wild edible fruiting plants is included along with herbal products/drugs, in different forms across different countries. They are allowed to be traded as herbal products, and their pre-marketing requirements are as per herbals. However, there is no global harmonization system. Furthermore, the trade of these products is categorized based on consumer acceptance of herbal products, such as beauty care, healthcare, and food supplementation, globally. There is a focus of concerned industries on the herbal sector for economic reasons, and the legalized trade of wild edible fruiting plant products in their countries indicates growth opportunities as an herbal product. There are challenges also, as developing a globally acceptable product is an issue due to differences in regulatory requirements.[19]

In India, herbal drugs are regulated under the Drug and Cosmetic Act (D and C) with regulatory provisions for Ayurveda, Siddha, and Unani medicines, and the Ministry of AYUSH is the regulatory authority. Official formularies and pharmacopeia are available to define quality standards and lay down rules for good manufacturing practice in the manufacture of herbal products. In Malaysia, herbals and related products are regulated, and prior registration with the Malaysia Registrar of Business is a must for those intending to enter the market. Similarly, in the Philippines, it requires prior application based solely on traditional uses, with at least five or more decades of documented application in medical and ethnobotanical literature. In Nigeria, herbal medicines and related products are regulated by the National Agency for Food and Drug Administration and Control (NAFDAC). In Saudi Arabia, herbal products are allowed if they have at least 50 years of continuous traditional use, and their dose and the process of manufacturing should be the same as in traditional practices.[19]

In Australia, the Therapeutic Goods Administration Act regulates herbal products under the category of complementary medicine. Ayurvedic medicine, traditional Chinese medicine, and Australian indigenous medicines are all covered under this category. The United States of America enforces the US FDA (United States Food and Drug Administration Act) regulations for herbals, and herbs are classified as drugs, foods, or dietary supplements based on their claims or end use. Herbal products do not require premarket approval, and it's the responsibility of the marketing organization to ensure the safety and quality compliance of their products. However, all claims should comply with the FDA regulatory guidelines. In Canada, 'Health Canada' regulates herbals, such as Ayurvedic products, which are categorized as natural health products, and all the concerns need to have a prior registration with Health Canada. In the European Union, the European Medicines Agency has laid down the procedure to register herbal medicinal products.[19]

SOCIO-RELIGIOUS ASPECTS

The wild edible fruiting plants, a crucial section of the human diet since the prehistorical period have been a hopeful focus on miracles for fighting different body ailments. The diversity and associated traditional knowledge of the flowering plants can be deciphered in the Ramayana, a holy epic of Hindu, which describes that Lord Hanuman also became confused to identify the proper plant species from Himalayan flora, as there were similarities among many of them. Under these circumstances, a wistful and brief decision was taken by the lord to overcome the problem, and he presented a foolproof match of the specification laid down by the Royal herbal Man, Sushen Vaidya.[20,21]

This historical incident narrates the importance of detailed agricultural studies and documentation of each plant species to foster bioconservation strategies, sustainable production and utilization, along with biochemical knowledge to evaluate the health benefits and physiological effects, for which there is currently a need to develop a vision and strategy.

Further, Islamic scholars also encouraged the use and exploration of herbals, as the quote of the Prophet Mohammed [Peace Be Upon Him (PBUH)] says, '*There is no disease that Allah has created, except that Allah also has created its cure*'.[22] The impact of different ancient cultures on the utilization of natural products is documented in Islamic scriptures, and the divine teachings of Islam combine natural and practical healing with the incorporation of inherited science and technology.[22]

There is a description of 206 biblical medicinal plants, of which 95 have been recognized,[23] implying that the rest are still in nature and emphasizing the need to decipher all for the good of humans; probably most of them may be edible flowering species. As once spoken by King Solomon, 'That which has been what will be, that which is done is what will be done, and there is nothing new under the sun'.[23]

Buddhist herbal healing practices and therapies employ many methods to diagnose disease and imbalances using herbs collected from nature. It offers patients a carefully designed personalized treatment strategy to promote balance with the environment and develop the ability to prevent the reoccurrence of disease.[24] Traditional Sikh medicine, mostly of herbal origin, is undergoing rapid changes in the diaspora situation[25] to manage better treatment of minor ailments and chronic diseases.[25]

Anthropological developments reveal that at the beginning of Jainism, some Buddhist and Hindu monks were originally Brahmanas, and their caste could not be dissolved after ordination, which affected their healing practices; however, little is known about this among the Jains. As Jain tradition did not allow treatment to the body, it was basically aimed at relieving and healing the body through suffering, the eradication of karma, and even bodily discomfort,[26] but in general, there is always a social practice to provide the best medical treatment to infants, kids, and expecting mothers in every religion.

Further, the chemical composition of a plant species is affected by biotic and abiotic factors, resulting in variation in therapeutic properties, as *Viburnum opulus* L. (Family: Adoxaceae) is among the near-endemic valuable folk medicinal Himalayan shrubs[27] and is available in Europe, Russia, and some parts of North Africa. In folk medicine, the species is used to treat body ailments such as diabetes, liver and prostate disorders, rheumatic aches, obesity, kidney problems, coughs, colds, etc.[27] Currently, evidence-based utilization of herbals is on the rise, but most of the research so far has been carried out on its fruits, while only a few data are available on bark, flowers, leaves, and steam. Research results have revealed that organic acids in fruits vary as per geo-climatic conditions.[28] The main organic acids of *V. opulus* fruits are malic acid and citric acid in fruits collected from Russia, while malic and tartaric acids are major ingredients from Turkey.[29] To overcome such barriers, the use of a geographical indicator tag is currently in practice.

CONCLUSION

The concept of wild edible fruiting plants reflects traditional practices that are gaining attention as a business opportunity due to globalization and technological advancement. However, many youths and entrepreneurs interested in cultivating these plants lack sufficient training, increasing the risk of confusion with poisonous plant species and resulting in cases of intoxication. There is a need to develop a policy to effectively utilize various wild edible fruiting plants from around the world while also emphasizing the importance of conserving underutilized species. Research into these plants may lead to the discovery of new molecules or combinations of molecules that could help alleviate human suffering, particularly in overcoming metabolic syndromes. Discussions around the dietary practices of different regions, such as the Himalayan diet and Chinese diet, could provide valuable insight for stakeholders and lead to the development of industrial products with the necessary nutritional composition. Finally, it is crucial to gather toxicological information for each species to ensure their acceptance as food materials on a global scale by both consumers and regulators.

REFERENCES

1. Mandal SK, Saha S, Saha S. 2023. The importance of wild edible plant and macro-fungi diversity to attain food security for the tribes of eastern India-a quantitative study. *Frontiers in Sustainable Food Systems*. 7: 1198187. https://doi.org/10.3389/fsufs.2023.1198187
2. Clemente-Villalba J, Burlo F, Hernandez F, Carbonell-Barrachina AA. 2023. Valorization of wild edible plants as food ingredients and their economic value. *Foods*. 12: 1012. https://doi.org/10.3390/foods12051012
3. Mesias M, Seiquer I, Delgado-Andrade C. 2020. The mediterranean diet and mineral composition. In: *The Mediterranean Diet*, 2nd Edition. Preedy VR, Watson RR (Eds.) Academic Press, Amsterdam, The Netherlands. pp. 151–163.
4. Shankar AH. 2020. Mineral deficiencies. In: *Hunter's Tropical Medicine and Emerging Infectious Diseases*, 10th Edition. Ryan ET, Hill DR, Solomon T, Aronson NE, Endy TP (Eds.) Elsevier, London, UK. pp. 1048–1054.
5. Motti R. 2022. Wild edible plants: a challenge for future diet and health. *Plants*. 11: 344. https://doi.org/10.3390/plants11030344
6. Paura B, Di Marzio P, Salerno G, Brugiapaglia E, Bufano A. 2021. Design a database of Italian vascular alimurgic flora (AlimurgITA): preliminary results. *Plants*. 10: 743.
7. Ivanova T, Bosseva Y, Chervenkov M, Dimitrova D. 2021. Enough to feed ourselves! – Food plants in Bulgarian rural home gardens. *Plants*. 10: 2520.
8. Vitasovic-Kosic I, Kaligaric M, Juracak J. 2021. Divergence of ethnobotanical knowledge of Slovenians on the Eege of the Mediterranean as a result of historical, geographical and cultural drivers. *Plants*. 10: 2087.
9. Costa-Becheleni FR, Troyo-Dieguez E, Nieto-Garibay A, Bustamante-Salazar LA, Garcia-Galindo HS, Murillo-Amador B. 2021. Hydro-environmental criteria for introducing an Eeible halophyte from a rainy region to an arid zone: a study case of *Suaeda* spp. as a new crop in NW Mexico. *Plants*. 10: 1996.
10. Gehlich KH, Beller J, Lange-Asschenfeldt B, Kocher W, Meinke MC, Lademann J. 2020. Consumption of fruits and vegetables: improved physical health, mental health, physical functioning and cognitive health in older adults from 11 European countries. *Aging & Mental Health*. 24 (4): 634–641. https://doi.org/10.1080/13607863.2019.1571011
11. Samec D, Karalija E, Sola I, Vujcic Bok VV, Salopek-Sondi B. 2021. The role of polyphenols in abiotic stress response: the influence of molecular structure. *Plants*. 10 (1): 118. https://doi.org/10.3390/plants10010118
12. Ahlberg MK. 2021. A profound explanation of why eating green (wild) edible plants promote health and longevity. *Food Frontiers*. 2: 240–267. https://doi.org/10.1002/fft2.106
13. Zhang L, Virgous C, Si H. 2019. Synergistic anti-inflammatory effects and mechanisms of combined phytochemicals. *The Journal of Nutritional Biochemistry*. 69: 19–30. https://doi.org/10.1016/j.jnutbio.2019.03.009
14. Nunes MA, Rodrigues F, Vinha AF, Alves RC, Beatriz PP, Oliveira MBPP. 2018. Nutrigenomics and polyphenols. In *Polyphenols: Properties, Recovery, and Applications*. Galanakis CM (Ed.) Woodhead Publishing. pp. 103–132. https://doi.org/10.1016/B978-0-12-813572-3.00004-X
15. Thakur M, Singh K, Khedkar R. 2020. Phytochemicals: extraction process, safety assessment, toxicological evaluations, and regulatory issues. In *Functional and Preservative Properties of Phytochemicals*. B. Prakash (Ed.) Academic Press. pp. 341–361. https://doi.org/10.1016/B978-0-12-818593-3.00011-7
16. Cornara L, Smeriglio A, Frigerio J, Labra M, Di Gristina E, Denaro M, Mora E, Trombetta D. 2018. The problem of misidentification between edible and poisonous wild plants: reports from the Mediterranean area. *Food and Chemical Toxicology*. 119: 112–121. https://doi.org/10.1016/j.fct.2018.04.066
17. Chang SS, Wu ML, Deng JF, Lee CC, Chin TF, Liao SJ. 1999. Poisoning by datura leaves used as edible wild vegetables. *Veterinary and Human Toxicology*. 41 (4): 242–245. PMID: 10434380.
18. Soni P, Siddiqui AA, Dwivedi J, Soni V. 2012. Pharmacological properties of *Datura stramonium* L. as a potential medicinal tree: an overview. *Asian Pacific Journal of Tropical Biomedicine*. 2 (12):1002–1008. https://doi.org/10.1016/S2221-1691(13)60014-3
19. Sharma S. 2015. Current status of herbal product: regulatory overview. *Journal of Pharmacy and Bioallied Sciences*. 7: 293–296.
20. Lahkar S, Kalita P, Chakraborty A. 2015. An overview on properties, therapeutic efficacy of the Indian magical herb- "SANJEEVANI". *American Journal of Pharmacy and Health Research*. 3 (2): 1–10.
21. Tejaswi JKD, Rajan RG. 2018. A review on Indian magical herb, Sanjeevani. *World Journal of Advance Healthcare Research*. 2 (5): 118–122.
22. El-Seedi HR, Khalifa SAM, Yosri N, Khatib A, Chen L, Saeed A, Efferth T, Verpoorte R. 2019. Plants mentioned in the Islamic scriptures (Holy Quran and Ahadith): traditional uses and medicinal importance in contemporary times. *Journal of Ethnopharmacology*. 243:112007. https://doi.org/10.1016/j.jep.2019.112007

23. Dafni A, Bock B. 2019. Medicinal plants of the Bible-Revisited. *Journal of Ethnobiology and Ethnomedicine*. 15: 57. https://doi.org/10.1186/s13002-019-0338-8
24. Roberti di Sarsina P, Ottaviani L, Mella J. 2011. Tibetan medicine: a unique heritage of person-centered medicine. *EPMA Journal*. 2 (4): 385–389. https://doi.org/10.1007/s13167-011-0130-x.
25. Sandhu DS, Heinrich M. 2005. The use of health foods, spices, and other botanicals in the Sikh community in London. *Phytotherapy Research*. 19 (7): 633–642. https://doi.org/10.1002/ptr.1714
26. Stuart MJ. 2014. Mendicants and medicine: ayurveda in Jain monastic texts. *History of Science in South Asia*. 2: 63–100.
27. Pant S, Samant. 2006. Diversity, distribution, uses and conservation status of plant species of the Mornaula Reserve Forests, West Himalaya, India, *The International Journal of Biodiversity Science and Management*. 2: 97–104. https://doi.org/10.1080/17451590609618102
28. Perova IB, Zhogova AA, Cherkashin AV, Eller KI, Ramenskaya GV. 2014. Biologically active substances from European guelder berry fruits. *Pharmaceutical Chemistry Journal*. 48: 332–339.
29. Polka D, Podsedek A. 2019. Phenolics composition and antioxidant capacity of guelder rose fruit, flower, and bark extracts. *Food Science and Biotechnology*. 83: 37–46.

35 Wild Edible Plants
Research Avenues

INTRODUCTION

Wild edible fruiting species were used in the olden days to cure various body ailments such as acidity, asthma, anemia, bronchitis, colds, diarrhea, jaundice, diabetes, dysentery, etc.[1] The different parts of these species, including fruits, are rich in vitamins, carbohydrates, minerals, fats, fiber, potassium, iron, calcium, phosphorus, zinc, magnesium, sodium, copper, manganese, etc.,[1] and have health and medical benefits. There are several plant species that are confined to the kitchen gardens over time and have not been domesticated fully but are a good source of therapeutic nutrition.[2]

Humans depend on plants for food and fresh air to breathe throughout their lives. There are different chemical classes and thousands of natural compounds in plants, and polyphenols are one of the biggest chemical classes, which have more than 8,000 known compounds to date. These compounds are defined as 'naturally occurring substances that are used to maintain or restore good health'. These compounds have biological activities, such as anti-parasitic, antibiotic, repelling predators, promoting cellular health, and reducing environmental stress, etc.[3] These plants are repositories of nutrition, food security, and livelihoods for the vulnerable population living near the forests. There is a need to bridge the current molecular knowledge with traditional practices for better utilization in nutritionally balanced diets, dietary diversity, health, food, medicine, fodder, and fuel. As natural sources of food and botanical resources are shrinking globally with increasing population, wild edible fruiting plant species are emerging as new sources of our food and natural medicine. The wild edibles integrate with food policies as defensive strategies to increase food security in human nutrition programs,[4] which needs more focused scientific research and policy exploration beyond the phytopharmacology for utilization of these species, and their more bio-application for the next century may be categorized as follows.

CLUES TO ERADICATE FATAL DISEASES

Currently, there has been growing interest in the therapeutic use of folk and traditional herbs to minimize or cure metabolic syndromes, e.g., all parts of the *Azadirachta indica* A. Juss. (Hindi: Neem) tree are used in folk and traditional medicines (Unani, Ayurveda, Homeopathy, Chinese, African, etc.) to control smallpox, leprosy, fever, malaria, diarrhea, cholera, intestinal helminthiasis, and respiratory disorders and to treat many infectious, metabolic, and cancerous diseases. In folk medicine, Nigerians consume its leaves in unspecified quantities without considering its toxicological effects in treating malaria.[5] In India, in the olden days, relatives of departed patients suffering from chickenpox slept in the *A. indica* leaves to get their medicinal value. Biomolecular studies have revealed and supported all the folk and traditional applications of *A. indica* plants in healthcare practices,[5] and various health products based on *A. indica* are available in the market globally as over-the-counter products.

Additionally, the development of the smallpox vaccine, based on an ancient practice of variolation, has saved millions of lives globally. In the olden days, variolation was widely practiced in Asia and some parts of Africa, in which the smallpox sore material was transferred to the healthy individual, resulting in a milder infection. Lady Mary Wortley Montagu (1721) successfully inoculated her child against smallpox, and the incident has raised much-needed attention on extensive molecular testing that resulted in an effective vaccine and has eradicated smallpox globally.[6] Another traditional Ayurvedic practice of exposing babies with jaundice (hyperbilirubinemia) to sunlight is also accepted by modern medical science as a form of phototherapy, as bilirubin converts into a water-soluble derivative (unconjugated form) in the presence of sunlight.[7]

PHYTO-INGREDIENTS TO BALANCE DIFFERENT MICROBIOTA FOR OVERALL HEALTH

The beneficial phyto-ingredients and their metabolites instigate protective effects on peripheral organs and are more readily accessible than the brain. These compounds alter the composition of the circulatory system. The gut-microbiota-brain axis plays a protective role via afferent spinal and efferent vagal nerves, an intriguing property to communicate to the brain about the ingested materials. Moreover, the gut microbiome mediates stress, produces neuromodulating molecules, and releases them into the systemic circulatory system. The dietary compounds instigate the renovation of the peripheral organs, resulting in neurological enhancement, though the final impact is dependent on the nature of resident microorganisms in the specific organ.[3] Similarly, dietary interventions targeting improvements in cardiometabolic, renal, respiratory health, etc., may be investigated for various neurodegenerative and other bodily ailments using new and more potent bioactive compounds from wild edible fruiting plants.

DOI: 10.1201/9781003512868-38

PHYTO-INGREDIENTS TO CROSS THE BLOOD–BRAIN BARRIER

Different plant species are used as hallucinogens in different cultures globally, and the genus *Ipomoea* is one of these. Different species of *Ipomoea* are practiced calming down the central nervous system (CNS), and a few of them from the pre-Columbian period attain a state of mind during religious ceremonies and magical healing practices. Additionally, in the Catholic religion, *Ipomoea* seeds are respected as a gift from God and are known as 'Seeds of the Virgin', 'Virgin's Cloak', and 'Holy Mary Herb'. During the Candomblé (i.e., dance in honor of the gods), the 'father of saint' uses seeds and leaves of *Ipomoea purpurea* in traditional preparations offered to adepts of the religion to help them attain a state of mind suitable for divination.[8] Several pharmacological studies have revealed and confirmed these folk and traditional claims on *Ipomoea* seeds. Lysergol, an ingredient from *I. purpurea* seeds, has serotonin receptor properties and has a potential role in the treatment of anxiety, depression, and other psychiatric disorders.[8] Based on the concentration of lysergol used for the health benefits, its impact on target cells, tissues, or organs is different.[3] Lysergol affects the CNS via several mechanisms, after crossing the blood–brain barrier, influencing the brain parenchyma, and finally imparting benefit to brain health.[3] The biomolecular mechanism is characterized by the lipid composition and release of signaling proteins as a result of lysergol. The possible stereoselectivity of natural ingredients in brain cells reveals that a few more molecules may also interact with endothelial transporters, which regulate the entry of circulating phyto-molecules, and that a few of them may have specific tropisms toward defined brain regions.[3] This concept needs investigation of the molecular process of entry of natural products and metabolites into the brain parenchyma, identification of their tropism for targets, and their neuroprotective effects, along with randomized clinical trials to reveal results for the best recommendations.

EXPANDING KNOWLEDGE THROUGH RECENT TECHNOLOGIES AND ARTIFICIAL INTELLIGENCE

The folk and traditional knowledge of the world around us is a torch to discover new value-added food and natural well-being medicine. The rapid and remarkable technological innovations may provide a deeper understanding of the tangible benefits of utilizing wild edible fruiting plants. Artificial intelligence (AI) is an emerging significant revolution that is transforming the study and folk practice of healing systems. AI, advanced algorithms, and machine learning capabilities facilitate researchers to explore extensive folk knowledge, identifying once elusive patterns and trends, and mapping evidence. A validated base enables us to develop appropriate regulatory mechanisms and policies for quality control and monitoring the folk healing products and practices. Functional magnetic resonance imaging enabled us to study brain activity and measure the relaxation responses of individuals. It is increasingly in practice to reduce stress and enhance mental health and overall well-being.[3]

Currently, with the increased interest in wild edibles and the protection and conservation of biodiversity, the associated folk knowledge on wild edible fruiting plants is to be preserved for the benefit of future generations.[9] Therefore, better resource management with participatory practice for sustainable conservation along the positive attributes can be utilized for bioprospecting and modern green medicines, an additional source of income for the marginal population.

NUTRITIONAL SECURITY TO VULNERABLE GROUPS

Wild edible fruiting plant species are a source of cheaper and inexpensive foodstuffs, and it is worthwhile to incorporate edible wild plant resources into marginal and vulnerable populations. The richness of these products in nutrients and phytochemicals is crucial in tackling the issue of nutritional security among rural populations and combating the pathogenesis of many challenging diseases.[10] Genetic engineering and hybridization among these wild-fruiting species may lead to higher productivity, potentially meeting food and nutritional requirements, and playing a vital role in combating malnutrition as a substitute for common, expensive, and rare plant-based foods. Systematic studies of wild edible fruiting plant species for their consumption and socio-economic benefit to the native population through value addition can help in situ conservation of rainwater. The scientific validation of the health benefits of wild edible fruiting species will spread an additional source of nutritional security among the rural population.[10]

USE OF ENDOPHYTES

Endophytes are microbial entities that reside inside plant tissue with a symbiotic relationship and have the potential to synthesize novel bioactive compounds.[11] Currently, endophytes have gained considerable recognition from the pharmaceutical industries as a source of a variety of compounds that have antifungal, anti-inflammatory, antibacterial, and antiviral properties and may be a source of new therapeutic ingredients for treating cancer, diabetes, and neurological disorders.[11] There are various methods for isolation and culture of endophytes. The isolated endophytes are screened for their therapeutic ingredients and are characterized by chromatographic and spectral techniques such as high-performance liquid chromatography, mass spectrometry, nuclear magnetic resonance (NMR) imaging, etc., and can be synthesized and tested for bioactivity in animal models.[11] Pharmaceutical industries have identified many bioactive compounds from endophytes and are currently investigating them for their potential therapeutic applications. Despite these activities, there is still much to be revealed about the potential of endophytes, a treasure house of novel bioactive compounds.[12] Endophytes have the potential to revolutionize the pharmaceutical industry with additional modern green medicines, and research to identify novel compounds and develop methods for their extraction, purification, and characterization, along with safety data, is the prime concern. Extensive research is needed to acknowledge the potential impacts of endophyte-based treatment on human and animal health, as well as the environmental impact on combating drug-resistant pathogens in the future. Sharma et al. have reported a range of endophytes that have been isolated from roots, leaves, and stems of the *Berberis aristata* plant and tested against a range of different pathogens. These endophytes have been reported effective against all the tested pathogens, and a few have exhibited up to 90% inhibition of bacterial growth.[13]

USE OF GREEN CORROSION INHIBITOR

Plants and their extracts are rich in phytochemicals, including hetero compounds. Hetero compounds are large-size molecules containing heteroatoms (N, P, O, and S), which are potential candidates for developing passivity over the metallic surface; such compounds are known as green inhibitors. Heteroatomic molecules either have multiple bonds in conjugation or have aromatic rings, in which the heteroatom is an active center in conjugation. Most of these natural compounds contain functional groups such as primary amino ($-NH_2$), ketonic (=C=O), and aldehydic (–CHO), and are known to be viable corrosion inhibitors. These compounds are adsorbed on the metal surface through thermodynamically spontaneous adsorption processes, forming a defensive/protective thin layer that protects the metal surface from environmental exposure.[14]

As most synthetic corrosion inhibitors are toxic to the environment and ecology and are expensive, green inhibitors are the best alternatives due to their easy availability, sustainability, non-toxicity properties, cheapness, and friendliness to the environment. Additionally, a few green inhibitors have comparable results to synthetic and anodic inhibitors[15] and are obtained from all the plant parts, i.e., fruits, leaves, flowers, bark, roots, and seeds.[14]

SUITABLE CONTAINER TO STORE BEVERAGES

The ^{1}H-NMR technique has revealed changes in aliphatics, carbohydrates, and phenolics of the wine during storage and deciphered that 12 molecules were modified in an oak barrel during the maturation phase. The maturation period of wine is between the end of the maceration and the bottling stages, and it can be stored in different containers, such as concrete tanks, stainless steel tanks, oak (*Q. leucotrichophora*) barrels, etc.[16] Nowadays storage in oak barrels is very popular because it enhances the quality and aromas of wines. Wine aging in an oak barrel develops a balance between the ingredients and available oxygen and affects aromas, tannins, colors, enzymes, and proteins. During this phase, wine interacts with its available enzymes in the staves and compounds extracted from oak barrels in the presence of available oxygen, resulting in many chemical changes. Further, with time, catechin, amino acids, acetoin, and epicatechin decrease, while ethyl lactate, acetic acid, and sugars increase.[16] The NMR-based technology to determine the molecular modification is useful in the maturation phase of wine. Similar studies on barrels of other wild fruiting species may be conducted.

NUTRIENTS RECYCLE AND REDUCE THE IMPACT OF GLOBAL WARMING

Litter decomposition determines the potential return of nutrients and organic matter to the soil. An example may be cited from the different litter components of *Coriaria nepalensis* Wall., which have been recorded for 57%–100% mass loss for 1 year, revealing that nutrients and organic matter resulting from decomposing litter improve the soil conditions. Low soil availability of N and P seems to be the major constraint in the reclamation of degraded regions.[17] Additionally, the ability of *C. nepalensis* to form a symbiotic association with nitrogen-fixing microorganisms makes it suitable for the management of fragile lands and conservation of plant biodiversity. Simultaneously, climate change may have a negative or positive impact on litter decomposition or change in its composition as well as environmental variables. Optimum conditions for quick or healthy decomposition are favored, but conditions such as prolonged drought may reduce litter modification because of unfavorable conditions.[17] In the long run, climate change may influence the growth of flora and the recycle rate of their litter.

NANO-COMBINATIONS FOR PATHOGENESIS

Viruses are the cause of frequent respiratory infections. A co-capsulated nano-emulsion consisting of quercetin and curcumin for nasal administration has been reported as a promising medicine to treat viral respiratory infection with 99% inhibition.[18] The experiment deciphers the need for different possible combinations of the potent biologically active ingredients for synergistic therapy against viral respiratory infections.

NANO-COMBINATION TO TARGET TUMORS

Currently, the use of herbal-origin nanomedicines is in demand due to their health-friendly properties.[19] Jiaoyang et al. have reported that a composite nanomedicine consisting of a combination of quercetin and doxorubicin used for chemotherapy and photothermal therapy at the same time completely suppressed tumor growth. Treatment of a tumor has long been a challenge due to drug resistance and side effects of chemotherapy. The study has concluded with the development of a simple and high drug-loading composite nanoparticle with excellent tumor-targeting properties in the acidic environment, which reduces the toxicity of doxorubicin to healthy cells and inhibits the function of P-glycoprotein, resulting in an effective blocking drug efflux.[19]

Wild fruits hold better nutritional value and protective properties than their cultivated counterparts. There has been great focus in recent years to upgrade such variants for their value-added utilization in nutraceutical and pharmaceutical applications, and large-scale attempts at isolation and identification of bioactive compounds responsible for therapeutic properties have been made. Literature surveys from various sources revealed that phytochemical and pharmacological studies on selected wild fruit species have been limited to the isolation and characterization of compounds from different parts of the plants.

CONCLUSION

The plants we grow today have evolved from wild edible species through thousands of years of human intervention, involving the selection of favorable traits. Currently, the strategy for domesticating wild plants is different from the past, as available land for these species is fragile due to a shortage of fertile land. However, using fragile land can improve the livelihoods of vulnerable social groups, as it is easily available in remote and marginal areas. Wild fruiting edible plants are an important part of the human diet, and scientific research focused on plant diversity, traditional knowledge, and domestication of wild edible plants will promote their conservation and sustainable food production. Clinical investigations are needed to determine appropriate doses and understand the safety and efficacy of value-added products from these species before commercialization. Plant-based foods rich in antioxidants have a positive impact on health, and wild-fruiting edible plants can be an additional source of these beneficial items in the future.

REFERENCES

1. Urs D, Narayanappa M, Sophiya P, Krishnaram H, Pramod SN, Dharmappa KK. 2022. Medicinal and nutritional aspects of wild edible fruits from Western Ghat of India. *International Journal of Green Pharmacy*. 16 (4): 334–354.
2. Cruz-Garcia GS. 2017. Management and motivations to manage wild food plants. A case study in a mestizo village in the amazon deforestation frontier. *Frontiers in Ecology and the Environment*. 5: 127. https://doi.org/10.3389/fevo.2017.00127
3. de Rus Jacquet A, Laye S, Calon F. 2023. How nutrients and natural products act on the brain: beyond pharmacology. *Cell Reports Medicine*. 4 (10): 101243. https://doi.org/10.1016/j.xcrm.2023.101243
4. Johns T, Powell B, Maundu P, Eyzaguirre PB. 2013. Agricultural biodiversity as a link between traditional food systems and contemporary development, social integrity and ecological health. *Journal of the Science of Food and Agriculture*. 93: 3433–3442.
5. Vidhya Rekha U, Anita M, Bhuminathan S, Sadhana K. 2022. Known data on the therapeutic use of *Azadiracta indica* (neem) for type 2 diabetes mellitus. *Bioinformation*. 18 (2): 82–87. https://doi.org/10.6026/97320630018082
6. WHO. Traditional medicine has a long history of contributing to conventional medicine and continues to hold promise. https://www.who.int/news-room/feature-stories/detail/traditional-medicine-has-a-long-history-of-contributing-to-conventional-medicine-and-continues-to-hold-promise, as on 6th June 2024.
7. Horn D, Ehret D, Suresh G, Soll R. 2019. Sunlight for the prevention and treatment of hyperbilirubinemia in term and late preterm neonates. *Cochrane Database System Reviews*. 2019 (3): CD013277. https://doi.org/10.1002/14651858.CD013277
8. Meira M, Silva EP, David JM, David JP. 2012. Review of the genus *Ipomoea*: traditional uses, chemistry and biological activities. *Revista Brasileira De Farmacognosia-Brazilian Journal of Pharmacognosy*. 22: 682–713.
9. Asfaw Z. 2009. The future of wild food plants in southern Ethiopia: ecosystem conservation coupled with enhancement of the roles of key social groups. *Acta Horticulturae (ISHS)*. 806: 701–708.
10. Tripathi YC, Kumar R, Verma P K. 2020. Nutritional and quality evaluation of selected wild edible plants as a source of functional food – Project Completion Report, Forest Research Institute, Dehradun, India. https://www.researchgate.net/publication/359924537, as on 7th June 2024.
11. Sharma S, Chaitanya MVNL, Sharma S, Kumar S, Rustagi S, Singh S, Shreaz S, Rai AK, Negi R, Yadav AN. 2024. The medicinal plant *Berberis aristata* and its endophytes for pharmacological applications: current research and future challenges. *Journal of Applied Biology and Biotechnology*. X (XX): 1–10. https://doi.org/10.7324/JABB.2024.167591
12. Pimentel MR, Molina G, Dionísio AP, Marostica Junior MR, Pastore GM. 2011. The use of endophytes to obtain bioactive compounds and their application in biotransformation process. *Biotechnology Research International*. 2011: 576286.
13. Sharma S, Gupta S, Dhar MK, Kaul S. 2018. Diversity and bioactive potential of culturable fungal endophytes of medicinal shrub *Berberis aristata* DC.: a first report. *Mycobiology*. 46: 370–381.
14. Oli HB, Thapa Magar J, Khadka N, Subedee A, Bhattarai DP, Pant B. 2022. *Coriaria nepalensis* stem alkaloid as a green inhibitor for mild steel corrosion in 1 M H_2SO_4 Solution. *Electrochem*. 3: 713–727. https://doi.org/10.3390/electrochem3040047
15. Asipita SA, Ismail M, Majid MZA, Majid ZA, Abdullah C, Mirza J. 2014. Green *Bambusa arundinacea* leaves extract as a sustainable corrosion inhibitor in steel reinforced concrete. *Journal of Cleaner Production*. 67: 139–146.
16. Le Mao I, Da Costa G, Leleu G, Richard T. 2024. Monitoring red wine maturation in oak barrels using ^{1}H NMR-based metabolomics. *OENO One*. 58 (2). https://doi.org/10.20870/oeno-one.2024.58.2.7465

17. Awasthi P, Bargali K, Bargali SS and Khatri K. 2022. Nutrient return through decomposing *Coriaria nepalensis* litter in degraded hills of Kumaun Himalaya, India. *Frontiers in Forests and Global Change*. 5: 1008939. https://doi.org/10.3389/ffgc.2022.1008939
18. Vaiss DP, Rodrigues JL, Yurgel VC, do Carmo Guedes F, da Matta L L M, Barros PAB, Vaz GR, Dos Santos R N, Matte BF, Kupski L, Garda-Buffon J, Bidone J, Muccillo-Baisch AL, Sonvico F, Dora CL. 2024. Curcumin and quercetin co-encapsulated in nano-emulsions for nasal administration: a promising therapeutic and prophylactic treatment for viral respiratory infections. *European Journal of Pharmaceutical Sciences*. 197: 106766. https://doi.org/10.1016/j.ejps.2024.106766
19. Pan J, Ge Q, Wang B, Chen J, Hu H, Qiu L, Wang J, Wang C, Xu H. 2024. One-pot preparation of quercetin-doxorubicin dual-drug co-loaded nano-system for multimodal treatment of tumors. *Journal of Drug Delivery Science and Technology*. 97: 105742. https://doi.org/10.1016/j.jddst.2024.105742

Index

Note: **Bold** page numbers refer to tables and *italic* page numbers refer to figures.

For Product Safety Concerns and Information please contact our EU representative GPSR@taylorandfrancis.com Taylor & Francis Verlag GmbH, Kaufingerstraße 24, 80331 München, Germany